BAR INTERNATIONAL SERIES 3186 | 2024

Roman Feet and Shoes

The cultural significance of feet, footwear, and their representations in the north-western provinces

Elizabeth Shaw

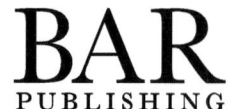

Published in 2024 by
BAR Publishing, Oxford

BAR International Series 3186

Roman Feet and Shoes

ISBN 978 1 4073 6154 3 paperback
ISBN 978 1 4073 6153 6 e-format

DOI https://doi.org/10.30861/9781407361543

A catalogue record for this book is available from the British Library

© Elizabeth Shaw 2024

COVER IMAGE *Two sandal-shaped glass flasks from a Roman burial in Cologne (Photo: Carole Raddato).*

The Author's moral rights under the 1988 UK Copyright, Designs and Patents Act, are hereby expressly asserted.

All rights reserved. No part of this work may be copied, reproduced, stored, sold, distributed, scanned, saved in any form of digital format or transmitted in any form digitally, without the written permission of the Publisher.

Links to third party websites are provided by BAR Publishing in good faith and for information only. BAR Publishing disclaims any responsibility for the materials contained in any third party website referenced in this work.

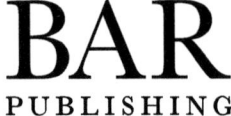

BAR titles are available from:

BAR Publishing
122 Banbury Rd, Oxford, OX2 7BP, UK
info@barpublishing.com
www.barpublishing.com

Of Related Interest

Latin Lexicon of Textiles
Clothes, adornments, materials and techniques of Ancient Rome
Elena Miramontes Seijas

BAR International Series **3051** | 2021

Dress and Identity
Edited by Mary Harlow

BAR International Series **2356** | 2012

Belonging and Belongings
Portable artefacts and identity in the civitas of the Iceni
Natasha Harlow

BAR British Series **664** | 2021

London's Roman Tools
Craft, agriculture and experience in an ancient city
Owen Humphreys

BAR British Series **663** | 2021

Dress and Cultural Identity in the Rhine-Moselle Region of the Roman Empire
Ursula Rothe

BAR International Series **2038** | 2009

Ear-Rings in Roman Britain
Lindsay Allason-Jones

BAR British Series **201** | 1989

Personal Ornamentation as an Indicator of Cultural Diversity in the Roman North
Timothy Webb

BAR British Series **547** | 2011

Ritual Significance of Personal Ornament in Roman Britain
Sonia Puttock

BAR British Series **327** | 2002

Sacred and Civic Stone Monuments of the Northwest Roman Provinces
S. L. McGowen

BAR International Series **2109** | 2010

The End of Paganism in the North-Western Provinces of the Roman Empire
The example of the Mithras cult
Eberhard Sauer

BAR British Series **634** | 1996

For more information, or to purchase these titles, please visit **www.barpublishing.com**

Acknowledgements

This book would not have been possible without the help and support provided by many people. My thanks go firstly to my supervisors, James Gerrard and Ian Haynes, who guided my footsteps from the very beginning, helping me form the ideas which have been explored throughout the study, and providing continuous advice and encouragement.

I have been overwhelmed by the generosity of the Roman archaeology community in sharing their (often unpublished) work with me. My gratitude goes to Lindsay Allason-Jones, Joshua Basey, Quita Mould, Alex Croom, Hella Eckardt, Alice Lyons, Adam Parker, Berni Seddon, Elizabeth Greene, and Frances McIntosh. Others who have provided help and encouragement include Carol van Driel-Murray, Tony Willmott, Mark Jackson, Andrew Birley and Barbara Birley.

I am beholden to the curators of various museums across Europe for providing me with data on unpublished artefacts, and for answering my queries. My particular thanks go to Andrew Parkin of the Great North Museum: Hancock; Eduard Pollhammer of Museum Carnuntinum, Austria; Sylvie Rorive of the Forum Antique, Bavay, France; Alan Fuller of the Chippenham Museum; Alison Pollard of the Ashmolean Museum, Oxford; Susan Fox of the Roman Baths Museum, Bath; and Pernille Richards of Maidstone Museum.

The following have generously given me permission to use their images in this work: Michel Feugère, Rien Bongers, Mathias Higelin for Archéologie Alsace, Rein Bongers, Roberto Castrana, Chiara Bianchi, Pete Savin, Tim Padley, Carole Raddato of 'Following Hadrian', and the Vindolanda Trust. All best efforts were made to obtain permission to reproduce any third-party images included in this book, but in some cases the copyright holder was not contactable. If any issues arise with the use of any images within this book, please contact the publisher who will help in resolving this.

Finally, I would like to thank my family and friends who supported me through this project, in particular my husband, Iain, who discussed every chapter with me, took literally thousands of photographs for me, and kept me supplied with tea.

Contents

List of Figures xi
List of Tables xvi
Abstract xvii

1. Introduction 1
    1.1 Theoretical Pathways 1
        1.1.1 Object biography 1
        1.1.2 Contextual Archaeology 2
    1.2 Steps taken in this research 2
    1.3 Recurring strands of significance 3
    1.4 Terms and limitations 3
    1.5 The significance of feet in other cultures 4
    1.6 Conclusions 4

2. Ancient and modern attitudes to Roman feet and footwear 7
    2.1 Background to Roman footwear 7
        2.1.1 Classifying Roman footwear 8
        2.1.2 Roman footwear fashion 10
    2.2 What the ancient Romans wrote 10
    2.3 An art-based approach 11
    2.4 Antiquarian footwear finds 12
    2.5 Some influential Roman calceologists 14
    2.6 Recent Roman shoe research 14
    2.7 Research into hobnailing 15
    2.8 Spiritual shoes 15
    2.9 Other foot-related research 15
    2.10 Conclusions 16

3. The point of Roman hobnailing 17
    3.1 Background to Roman hobnailing 17
    3.2 The significance of Roman hobnailing for archaeologists 18
        3.2.1 Hobnailing as evidence of the wearers 18
    3.3 The significance of hobnailing for people in the Roman Empire 19
        3.3.1 Hobnailing and domination 19
        3.3.2 Nailing and fashion 19
        3.3.3 The cosmological side of hobnailing 20
    3.4 Hobnailing and group identity 21
    3.5 Hobnailing in iconography 22
    3.6 Conclusions 22

4. The social significance of deposited Roman footwear 23
    4.1 The deposition of Roman footwear in graves 23
        4.1.1 Why deposit shoes in graves? 25
    4.2 The deposition of Roman footwear in wells 28
        4.2.1 Distinguishing deposits 30
        4.2.2 Evidence for the ritual deposition of Roman shoes in wells 31
        4.2.3 Roman beliefs and water 32
        4.2.4 Footwear and rituals surrounding the biography of Roman wells 33
        4.2.5 The ritual importance of left and right 33
    4.3 Why were shoes thought to be appropriate ritual deposits? 35
    4.4 Conclusions 35

5. The ubiquity of Roman foot- and shoe-shaped artefacts 37

- 5.1 Foot-shaped amulets 37
- 5.2 Jugs with handles ending in feet 39
- 5.3 Knife or razor handles in the shape of feet 45
- 5.4 Furniture feet 48
- 5.5 Flasks in the form of feet 51
- 5.6 Conclusions 55

6. Roman footlamps: a case study 59
- 6.1 Methodology 61
- 6.2 Background data 61
- 6.3 Fashion and footwear style 64
- 6.4 Hobnailing on Roman footlamps 67
- 6.5 Patterns in ornamentation 68
- 6.6 Footlamp distribution and socio-economic status 70
- 6.7 The role of the army in footlamp distribution 71
- 6.8 Footlamps and religion 72
- 6.9 Footlamps and Christianity 72
- 6.10 Footlamps and Graeco-Roman deities 73
- 6.11 Magic footlamps? 74
- 6.12 Funerary footlamps 75
- 6.13 Conclusions 77

7. Roman sandal fibulae: a case study 79
- 7.1 Data sources for shoe brooches 79
- 7.2 Typologies 81
- 7.3 Numbers 82
- 7.4 Chronological Distribution 84
- 7.5 Spatial Distribution 84
- 7.6 Distribution by site type and find setting 84
- 7.7 How sandal fibulae were worn 87
- 7.8 Left or right 88
- 7.9 Ornamentation 89
  - 7.9.1 Hobnailing on sandal fibulae 91
- 7.10 The apotropaic qualities of shoe brooches 92
- 7.11 Sandal fibulae in funerary settings 93
  - 7.11.1 The data for funerary fibula finds 93
- 7.12 Shoe brooches and religion 94
  - 7.12.1 Why were shoe brooches appropriate religious offerings? 96
- 7.13 Conclusions 96

8. The social significance of Roman footprints 97
- 8.1 Footprints carved in stone 97
- 8.2 Stamp matrices and seals in planta pedis 101
- 8.3 Official *planta pedis* stamps in CBM 104
- 8.4 Human footprints in Roman CBM 107
- 8.5 Conclusions 113

9. Assessing the significance of Roman statue foot-fragments from Britain 115
- 9.1 Chronological and spatial distribution 116
- 9.2 Material considerations 117
- 9.3 For whom the foot fragments stand 117
- 9.4 Distribution by site type and find setting 118
- 9.5 Patterns of deposition 119
- 9.6 Conclusions 122

10. Discussion and Conclusions 135
- 10.1 Chronological distribution 135
- 10.2 Geographical distribution 136
- 10.3 Distribution of site types and find settings 138
- 10.4 The ritual significance of Roman representations of feet and footwear 138

    10.4.1 Foot-shaped artefacts found in sanctuaries 138
    10.4.2 Offerings in watery places 139
    10.4.3 Funerary feet and footwear 140
10.5 *Pars pro toto* 140
    10.5.1 The feet of the gods 140
10.6 Apotropaic feet 141
    10.6.1 The sinister side 141
10.7 The importance of hobnailing 141
10.8 How far evidence from ancient texts applied to the north-western provinces 142
10.9 The limitations of this research 143
10.10 Conclusions 143

Bibliography 145
    Ancient Sources 145
    Modern Sources 148

List of Figures

Figure 2.1: 'Fishnet' shoe, Vindolanda Trust 7

Figure 2.2: A child's carbatina, Vindolanda Trust 8

Figure 2.3: Mainz calceus 8

Figure 2.4: 'Lepidina's' sandal, Vindolanda Trust 9

Figure 2.5: Man's wide sandal sole, Vindolanda Trust 9

Figure 2.6: 'Hero' boot on the Farnese Lar 10

Figure 2.7: Crepida on a statue of Aesculapius 10

Figure 2.8: Toga calcei 12

Figure 3.1: Sculponea from Vindolanda 17

Figure 3.2: X-ray of hobnails 18

Figure 3.3: Hobnails depicted on the Arch of Constantine 19

Figure 3.4: Shoe with ornate nailing pattern, Vindolanda Trust 20

Figure 3.5: Shoe with lozenge nailing pattern, Vindolanda Trust 20

Figure 3.6: Baby's nailed shoe, Vindolanda Trust 22

Figure 3.7: Flask or lamp with hobnailed inscription 'follow me' in Greek 22

Figure 4.1: a) Bonneuil-en-France shoe A; b) Bonneuil-en-France shoe E 25

Figure 4.2: Graph to show the chronological distribution of footwear in 1,756 Roman graves 25

Figure 4.3: Chart to show Roman funerary sites with footwear by region 26

Figure 4.4: Purple and gold shoe from Southfleet 26

Figure 4.5: Chart to show the sex and approximate age of 139 people buried with shoes in Lankhills
Late Roman cemetery 27

Figure 4.6: Chart to show the proportion of 1,311 Roman wells containing evidence of shoes 28

Figure 4.7: Chart to show the proportions of 321 Roman wells containing shoes according to site type 29

Figure 4.8: Chart to show the number of Roman wells with shoes by county/region 29

Figure 4.9: Chart to show the chronological distribution of 323 Roman wells containing footwear
according to date of construction and decommission 30

Figure 4.10: Chart to show the number of recognised ritual markers per site from 42 Roman wells with footwear 32

Figure 4.11: Chart to show the proportions of chirality in Roman shoes found in 42 wells with ritual associations 34

Figure 5.1: a) Egyptian sandal amulet, MAN Madrid. b) Iron Age foot-shaped amulets 37

Figure 5.2: a) Tongeren foot amulet. b) Gold boot charm. c) Jet foot amulet 38

Figure 5.3: Left foot amulet 39

Figure 5.4: 'Sandal' rings from near Bunnik-Vechten 39

Figure 5.5: 'Sandal' rings from Vindonissa and RGM, Cologne 39

Figure 5.6: a) Hobnailed ring from Pommerœul. b) Hobnailed sandal ring: Berganza. c) Shoe-sole ring
with Christian symbols 39

Figure 5.7: Chart to show the relative numbers of Roman copper-alloy jugs with handles terminating in
human heads or feet 40

Figure 5.8: Chart to show the date of 82 Roman jugs with handles ending in feet 40

Figure 5.9: a) Western type jug from Gallo-Romeins Museum, Tongeren b) Eastern type jug from Weißenburg 41

Figure 5.10: Chart to show the site type of 82 Roman jugs with handles ending in feet 41

Figure 5.11: Map to show the geographical distribution of the different types of Roman foot-jug 42

Figure 5.12: Chart to show the chirality of 82 Roman jugs with handles ending in feet 42

Figure 5.13: Chart to show the find settings of 82 Roman jugs with handles ending in feet 43

Figure 5.14: Map to show the geographical distribution of Roman knife/razor handles in the form of feet 45

Figure 5.15: Knife/razor handles from: Ostia; Schwirzheim; Cologne; Alba Fucens, Chartres, and Espejo 46

Figure 5.16: Roman knife/razor handles showing socks with sandals 46

Figure 5.17: Chart to show the site type of 37 foot-shaped Roman knife/razor handles 47

Figure 5.18: Chart to show the proportions of ornamentation type in 258 Roman knife/razor handles with representative designs in the PAS database 48

Figure 5.19: Chart to show the chirality of 54 sets of Roman furniture 'feet' 49

Figure 5.20: Map to show the distribution of Roman furniture 'feet' 49

Figure 5.21: Roman folding stools with human feet 50

Figure 5.22: a) Sestertius RIC II Trajan 666: b) Panzer statue of Hadrian from the theatre at Hierapytna, Crete 51

Figure 5.23: Chart to show the site type of 54 sets of Roman furniture 'feet' 52

Figure 5.24: Chart to show the find setting of 54 sets of Roman furniture 'feet' 52

Figure 5.25: Chart to show the modern find country of 23 Roman oil flasks in the shape of feet 53

Figure 5.26: Chart to show the date range of 23 Roman oil flasks in the shape of feet 53

Figure 5.27: Chart to show the site type of 23 Roman flasks in the shape of feet 53

Figure 5.28: Chart to show the find setting of 23 Roman flasks in the shape of feet 54

Figure 5.29: Two sandal-shaped glass flasks from a Roman burial in Cologne 54

Figure 5.30: Balsamarium from a grave in Hoeselt 54

Figure 5.31: Roman perfume bottle from Knidos showing hobnailing 55

Figure 5.32: The Hardwick Boot (Author's drawing) 55

Figure 5.33: Map to show the distribution of 217 selected Roman foot-shaped artefacts 56

Figure 5.34: Chart to show the date range of 217 sets of selected Roman foot-shaped artefacts 56

Figure 5.35: Chart to show the chirality of 217 sets of selected Roman foot-shaped artefacts 57

Figure 5.36: Chart to show the site type of 217 sets of selected Roman foot-shaped items 57

Figure 5.37: Chart to show the find setting of 217 sets of selected Roman foot-shaped artefacts 57

Figure 6.1: Map to show the known geographical distribution of 178 footlamps across the Roman Empire 59

Figure 6.2: Map to show the known geographical distribution of Roman footlamps across the north-western provinces 60

Figure 6.3: Footlamp in a 'crepida' with a bird on the lid from Pompeii 60

Figure 6.4: Footlamp from Licetus 1652: 770 60

Figure 6.5: Ancient Greek foot-shaped guttus 61

Figure 6.6: Ancient Greek Foot-shaped perfume bottle 62

Figure 6.7: 2nd century BCE votive footlamp 62

Figure 6.8: Chart to show the date of manufacture for 245 Roman footlamps 62

Figure 6.9: Chart to show the length in millimetres, and the materials, of 170 Roman footlamps 63

List of Figures

Figure 6.10: Lamp from a Roman-Egyptian tomb: Muzeum Archeologiczne, Krakow 63

Figure 6.11: Life-size footlamp in private ownership 63

Figure 6.12: Chart to show the site type of 245 Roman foot-shaped lamps 63

Figure 6.13: Chart to show the find settings for 245 Roman footlamps 64

Figure 6.14: Chart to show the proportions of chirality in 245 Roman footlamps 65

Figure 6.15: Left-footed lamp 65

Figure 6.16: Two-footed lamp 65

Figure 6.17: Pair of footlamps from Lillebonne, France 65

Figure 6.18: Pair of footlamps, Loeb collection, Munich 65

Figure 6.19: a) Footlamp in a solea. Xanten LVR-Römermuseum 33775; b) solea from the Comacchio shipwreck; c) Low caliga 16 from Mainz; d) Southwark footlamp in strappy sandal 66

Figure 6.20: Footlamp (or flask) in the Louvre 66

Figure 6.21: 'Ramshaw' boot and reconstruction, Saalburg 67

Figure 6.22: Example of a crepida on a footlamp 67

Figure 6.23: Footlamp wearing a 'caliga' 67

Figure 6.24: Mainz caliga 9 67

Figure 6.25: Hobnailing on a footlamp from Cologne 68

Figure 6.26: Hobnailing on a shoe from Carlisle 68

Figure 6.27: Hobnailing on a footlamp from Cologne 68

Figure 6.28: Hobnailing on a caliga 68

Figure 6.29: Hobnailing on the footlamp from Southwark 68

Figure 6.30: Hobnailing on a shoe from Valkenburg 68

Figure 6.31: Hobnailing as a potter's mark on a footlamp from Cologne 68

Figure 6.32: Footlamp with a cross depicted in hobnailing 68

Figure 6.33: Fairly plain footlamp, Saalburg 69

Figure 6.34: Double footlamp with crescent moon handle 69

Figure 6.35: Eagle footlamp found in Augst 69

Figure 6.36: Bally Schuhmuseum eagle footlamp 70

Figure 6.37: Footlamp with Gryphon, Allard Pierson Museum 70

Figure 6.38: Footlamp with head 70

Figure 6.39: Footlamp with Satyr's head from Cologne 70

Figure 6.40: Map showing the spread of Roman footlamps along the Limes 72

Figure 6.41: Footlamp with Diana statuette 73

Figure 6.42: Double footlamp with soleae and Uraeus 74

Figure 6.43: Right-footed lamp with solea and Uraeus 74

Figure 6.44: Bacchic figures on the Holborough sarcophagus 74

Figure 6.45: Ornate copper alloy footlamp 74

Figure 6.46: Double footlamp with Medusa masks 75

Figure 6.47: Right-footed lamp with Medusa mask and crescent 75

Figure 6.48: Possible Medusa mask, Museo Lázaro Galdiano, Madrid. (Photo: author's own) 76

Roman Feet and Shoes

Figure 6.49: Footlamp in a funerary assemblage, Koenigshoeffen, Strasbourg 76
Figure 6.50: Detail of footlamp from rue de Koenigshoeffen, Strasbourg 77
Figure 7.1: Heat map showing the geographical distribution of 363 Roman shoe brooches 79
Figure 7.2: Chart to show the known length in millimetres of 344 Roman shoe brooches... 80
Figure 7.3: Typology of Roman shoe brooches 82
Figure 7.4: Chart to show the proportions of type in 447 Roman sandal fibulae 82
Figure 7.5: Distribution map of 324 Roman shoe brooches of a known type with a known find location 83
Figure 7.6: Chart to show comparative numbers of different Roman brooches from the PAS database......................... 83
Figure 7.7: Chart to show the date range of 447 Roman sandal fibulae 84
Figure 7.8: Map to show the geographical distribution of Romano-British shoe brooches 85
Figure 7.9: Two Roman sandal fibulae in the National Roman Legion Museum, Caerleon 85
Figure 7.10: Chart to show the site type of 447 Roman sandal fibulae 86
Figure 7.11: Chart to show the find setting of 447 Roman sandal fibulae... 87
Figure 7.12: The tweeted sandal fibula 88
Figure 7.13: Type 4 shoe brooch from Alcester.. 88
Figure 7.14: PAS LEIC-84F493 original and flipped identifiable as left sole 89
Figure 7.15: Chart to show the proportions of chirality in each site type for 447 Roman sandal fibulae 89
Figure 7.16: Shoe brooch from London showing twisted rim design... 90
Figure 7.17: Chart to show the enamel colour of 421 Roman sandal fibulae 90
Figure 7.18: Chart to show the colour proportions for 247 Type 1 Roman sandal fibulae.. 91
Figure 7.19: Different techniques for depicting hobnails 91
Figure 7.20: Un-enamelled shoe brooch with hobnailing design 92
Figure 7.21: Shoe brooch with hobnailing around the rim 92
Figure 7.22: Shoe brooch from Sanxay compared with a real hobnailing pattern from Vindonissa................................ 92
Figure 8.1: Replica plaque with vestigia, Italica, Spain 97
Figure 8.2: Vestigia plaques from Italica 99
Figure 8.3: Plaque from the Italica theatre threshold dedicated by Marcia Voluptas to Isis... 101
Figure 8.4: Ceramic planta pedis stamp matrix from Holdeurn 102
Figure 8.5: Potter's stamp in the shape of a complete foot... 102
Figure 8.6: Chart to show the types of inscription on 165 Roman planta pedis stamps... 103
Figure 8.7: Stamp matrix from Venice, Italy, inscribed P CORNELI ACERAEL... 103
Figure 8.8: Stamp matrix inscribed VIVAS: Staatliche Museen zu Berlin, Inv. No. Misc. 3716................................... 103
Figure 8.9: Stamp matrix inscribed OLYMPIA VIVAS 103
Figure 8.10: Stamp matrix inscribed ΎΓΙΑ ΖΟΗ 104
Figure 8.11: Stamp matrix inscribed SPES IN DEO 104
Figure 8.12: Stamp matrix inscribed εισ θεοσ.. 104
Figure 8.13: Stamp matrix with a Christogram, National Archaeological Museum, Madrid.. 104
Figure 8.14: Stamp matrix featuring a cross... 104
Figure 8.15: Stamp matrix with an ivy leaf at the toe... 104
Figure 8.16: VTERE FELIX stamps: Pollenzo (after Ricci 1898); in the Louvre (after Ridder 1913: no. 4052).......... 105

List of Figures

Figure 8.17: Chart to show the frequency of inscriptions on 153 pieces of Roman foot-stamped CBM 105

Figure 8.18: Chart to show the ornamentation on 153 pieces of Roman foot-stamped CBM 106

Figure 8.19: Hadrian treading a conquered non-Roman underfoot 106

Figure 8.20: Different ornamentation on foot-stamped CBM: Hobnailing, toes and leaves 106

Figure 8.21: Chart to show the site type of 124 pieces of Roman CBM with footprints 108

Figure 8.22: Chart to show the find setting of 124 pieces of Roman CBM with human footprints 108

Figure 8.23: Dating evidence: wide soles from Corseul 109

Figure 8.24: X-shaped hobnailing pattern on CBM from Vindobona 109

Figure 8.25: S-shaped hobnailing pattern on CBM 109

Figure 8.26: Asymmetrical S-shaped hobnailing pattern on CBM from Heerlen 110

Figure 8.27: Triple nailing pattern from Aachen 110

Figure 8.28: Chart to show the clarity of footprints in 124 pieces of Roman CBM 110

Figure 8.29: Chart to show the chirality of footprints in 124 pieces of Roman CBM 111

Figure 8.30: Roman tile from Carnuntum with multiple footprints 112

Figure 8.31: Roof tile with footprints from Pietrabbondante 112

Figure 8.32: A tegula from Caerleon with Legio II Augusta stamp 112

Figure 8.33: CBM from Dover with Classis Britannica stamp 113

Figure 8.34: Footprint on CBM from Berg en Dal tilery with VEX EX GER stamp 113

Figure 9.1: Chart to show the proportions of different sculpture types in 75 sets of foot-fragments 115

Figure 9.2: Chart to show the dating of 75 sets of feet separated from Roman sculpture 116

Figure 9.3: The 'Ouse' style (Author's drawing) and detail of York funerary monument 117

Figure 9.4: Heat map to show the spread of foot-fragments from Roman sculpture 117

Figure 9.5: Chart to show whose feet are represented on 75 sets of Roman sculpture fragments 118

Figure 9.6: Chart to show the site type of 75 sets of feet separated from Roman sculpture 118

Figure 9.7: Chart to show the find setting of 75 sets of Roman sculpture foot-fragments 119

Figure 9.8: Chart to show the patterns of deposition for 75 sets of Roman sculpture foot-fragments 119

Figure 9.9: Segontium: Cellar in the sacellum: section at south-east end 121

Figure 9.10: The Milsington leg, National Museum of Scotland 122

Figure 10.1: Chart to show the artefact type of 1,492 Roman foot-shaped objects 135

Figure 10.2: Chart to show the date-range of 1,492 Roman foot-shaped artefacts 136

Figure 10.3: Chart to show the known date-range of 1,249 Roman foot-shaped artefacts 136

Figure 10.4: Distribution map of 1,145 Roman foot-shaped artefacts with a known find location 137

Figure 10.5: Distribution map of Roman foot-shaped artefacts from the north-western provinces 137

Figure 10.6: Chart to show the site type of 1,492 Roman foot-shaped artefacts 138

Figure 10.7: Chart to show the find setting of all 1,492 Roman foot-shaped artefacts 139

Figure 10.8: Chart to show the known find setting of 682 Roman foot-shaped artefacts 139

Figure 10.9: Chart to show the overall chirality for 1,492 Roman foot-shaped artefacts 141

Figure 10.10: Chart to show details of chirality for 1,492 Roman foot-shaped artefacts 142

List of Tables

Table 2.1: Numbers of surviving steps on Roman temples 11

Table 4.1: The percentage of Roman graves containing footwear for each time period 24

Table 8.1: The proportions of CBM with human footprints on 14 selected sites 107

Table 9.1: The body fragment statistics from CSIR GB series 1 124

Table 9.2: Cases where there is not enough information to interpret why the feet were preserved 125

Table 9.3: Foot-fragments repurposed as building stone in the Roman era..................................... 127

Table 9.4: Roman sculpted feet repurposed after the Roman era 129

Table 9.5: Preserved statue feet from Roman villas... 130

Table 9.6: Foot-fragments associated with Roman religious activity... 131

Table 9.7: Roman sculpted feet preserved by ritual/religious deposition.. 133

Abstract

Roman artefacts depicting human feet are found across the empire, but what did they mean to people living in the north-western provinces? To answer this question, a corpus of 1,492 foot-shaped artefacts across 12 different categories was assembled using data from museums, archaeological reports and other publications. Their geographical and chronological distribution, whether they depicted left or right feet (chirality), style of footwear, and the type of setting they were found in were noted. A mixture of theoretical approaches including object biography and contextual archaeology were applied during the data analysis.

The opening chapters discuss main theoretical and methodological approaches used and why these were appropriate for this work, give background information about Roman footwear and what we can learn from Roman shoe fashion, examine and critique relevant literature including recurrent themes surrounding feet and footwear in Roman authors. Trends and symbolism in Roman hobnailing patterns, often depicted on foot- and shoe shaped artefacts, are then considered. This chapter examines the links between hobnailing and group identity, attempting to assess how far the adoption of Roman footwear technologies represented an adoption of Roman culture and beliefs. Roman ritual use of shoes as evidenced by data for actual footwear from 18,465 burials and 1,311 wells is examined. This initial section lays the foundations for case studies of the 12 categories of artefact, including jugs with feet on their handles, knife or razor handles, oil flasks, footlamps, sandal fibulae, carved footprints and statue fragments.

The research identifies recurring strands of significance. In the Roman world, the foot could stand pars pro toto, representing a person as a whole. Shoe-shaped artefacts may symbolise deities, and thus express a particular religious affiliation. The ritual use of foot-shaped objects, including funerary and other votive use, may be a consequence of this. The footprint acted as a sort of signature, especially for those normally invisible in Roman studies such as women and slaves. Foot-shaped metal stamps were used to mark goods, as makers or owners.

Roman footwear played a metaphorical role. Shoes protect the feet from dirt, cold and injury, and are associated with crushing an enemy underfoot, which could be a supernatural enemy. Shoe-shaped artefacts may have been apotropaic, defending against the evil eye and, in particular, protecting travellers on a journey, which could be the journey of life, or to the Underworld.

Thus, we see that Roman feet and footwear do not just have a single meaning. Roman foot-shaped artefacts are polysemic, running from novelty items, through markers of fashion and status, to symbols of beings, both divine and human, appropriate votive offerings and grave goods, and apotropaic charms, frequently at the same time.

Introduction

The foot is not a very ornamental body part, associated as it is with dirt, sweat and odour, so it might seem an odd choice for decorative objects. However, many Roman artefacts were produced in the shape of feet wearing shoes. This work investigates why this apparently unprepossessing body-part was chosen as the iconography for some ornaments, what we might learn from Roman footwear and shoe-shaped artefacts about the people who owned and used them, and the ideological significance of feet in the Roman world, particularly in the north-western provinces.

As part of this process further, related questions need to be considered. The ideological significance of feet and footwear in the Roman world must be established. The ancient evidence in texts and art for how feet and footwear were regarded has to be taken into account, and the extent to which this Rome-centric, adult, male, elite evidence applied to the north-western provinces of the Roman Empire considered. It is also necessary to examine what we might learn from Roman foot- and shoe-shaped artefacts about the identity and beliefs of the people who owned them.

While there are many studies, for example, of Roman lamps and brooches, specific studies of foot- or shoe-shaped artefacts are very rare, as Eckardt points out (2013: 229). This book aims to rectify this matter by studying such objects in depth. It builds on, and extends, previous research by synthesising, and adding to, earlier findings, filling a substantial gap in our knowledge.

1.1 Theoretical Pathways

From a pragmatic stand-point, this work regards research approaches as a toolkit, applying them where appropriate. Its attitude to archaeological theories is similar: theoretical 'bricolage', rather than purism. Preucel (2006: 257) concludes that 'there can be no single, self-contained theory of material culture' and Hodder (2005: 68) suggests that a general unified theory of material culture should be regarded with some scepticism. The test for this theoretical bricolage approach is whether it works consistently in relation to the research objectives; that is, it enables a better understanding of things that are too complex for any single philosophy or social theory (Olsen 2010: 14). To cover all the archaeological theories that informed this study would require several volumes, so this section discusses those which are most relevant to the social significance of Roman foot-shaped artefacts and which helped to shape the methodology used.[1]

1.1.1 Object biography

Hoskins (2006: 77) affirms that 'asking questions about the agency of objects has led to the development of a more biographical approach', pointing out that Gell's work suggests a more active model of an object's biography, in which the object may not only assume a number of different identities, but may also 'interact' with those who look at it, use it, and try to possess it (Hoskins 2006: 76). The theory has influenced many scholars dealing with the life history of archaeological objects and sites (for example: Holtorf 1998; Gosden and Marshall 1999; Fontijn 2002; Meskell 2004; Joy 2009; van Haasteren and Groot 2013). The object biography approach has been useful for this study, particularly in researching the significance of footwear deposited in Roman wells, but also for interpreting the symbolism of some foot-shaped artefacts, since it provides a method to reveal the relationships between people and objects (Joy 2009: 540).

The idea of object biographies is generally attributed to the work of anthropologists Appadurai and Kopytoff (Harris and Cipolla 2017: 80). However, Tassinari (1973: 132) developed somewhat earlier the idea of a '*curriculum vitae*' for artefacts, by which she means the steps for reconstructing the life of an object: finding its place of origin, its date of manufacture, and establishing its movements around the Roman Empire. Kopytoff himself (1986: 66) cites the work of Rivers's 1910 paper, 'The genealogical method of anthropological inquiry', as an influence.

Appadurai (1986: 5) posits that the meanings of objects are inscribed in their forms, uses, and trajectories and that is these trajectories that illuminate their social and human context. Kopytoff (1986: 66) discusses the idea that the biographies of objects could be treated like those of people, pointing out that 'Biographies of things can make salient what might otherwise remain obscure' (Kopytoff 1986: 67), and suggesting the questions to ask of an object in order to establish its biography: its dates; where it is from and where it was found; what are the cultural markers for the stages in a thing's 'life'; what happens to it when it reaches the end of its usefulness (Kopytoff 1986: 66–67).

Hoskins (2006: 78) identifies two dominant forms of object biography: those which begin with ethnographic research, attempting to give a narrative of how certain objects are perceived by the people to whom they are linked, and those which begin with historical or archaeological research, and try to 'interrogate objects themselves by placing them in a historical context'. This second form is particularly useful for archaeologists interested in the dynamic nature of

---

[1] Further approaches, such as fragmentation theory, are discussed in the germane chapters.

artefacts (Harris and Cipolla 2017: 80), whose meanings and functions can change in different contexts (Holtorf 1998: 23).

1.1.2 Contextual Archaeology

The contextual analysis of symbolic meanings is a theoretical approach first discussed by Hodder (1987). While there is widespread recognition that the significance, or meaning, of artefacts changes over time and space, the way in which this understanding is applied to artefact studies can be uneven. Thomas (1991: 18–19) points out that the meaning given to artefacts is not intrinsic, but is attributed through practice and changes according to context. Tilley (2001: 260) states that an object's meaning comes from situated, contextualized social action which is in continuous dialectical relationship with procreative rule-based structures thus forming a medium for and an outcome of action. In other words, an artefact is given significance when it is used by a group for a particular purpose. Eckardt (2002: 26) opines that the social significance of material culture is not monolithic; it could have changed with time and according to social context. Since the symbolic and social meaning of Roman artefacts is 'not inherent and immutable, but rather determined by past actions and contexts' (Eckardt 2002: 27), a 'contextual archaeology' approach seems appropriate for studying the significance of Roman representations of feet.

When explaining the 'contextual archaeology' approach, Hodder (1987: 1) defines three types of contextual meaning: function (how the object functions in its social and physical environment), structure (its place within a code or set), and content (historical, situated within the changing ideas and associations of the object itself). The first stage of his analytical procedure is to identify the network of patterned similarities and differences in relation to the object being examined and the questions being asked. This is done by taking the four variable dimensions available to archaeologists: the temporal, spatial, depositional and typological (Hodder 1987: 6). Hodder (1987: 6) goes on to define meaningful pattern as showing statistically significant similarities and differences. He defines context as the whole of the relevant environment and all those associations relevant to its meaning (Hodder 1992: 13). The relationship between an object and its context is both complex and dialectic, as the context gives meaning to and gains meaning from the object (Hodder 1992: 13). Contextual archaeology has proved a useful approach for this study.

1.2 Steps taken in this research

Understanding foot-shaped artefacts as part of a social code, and their historically specific significance, calls for a detailed examination of the cultural context of their usage (Eckardt 2002: 28). In order to explore the meanings of artefacts in depth, Eckardt (2014: 2) explains the necessity of first selecting artefacts that may be of social or cultural significance, then compiling a corpus, mapping their distribution, and examining their contexts. In her 1973 study of Roman jugs with a handle ending in feet, Tassinari (128–130) outlines an artefact study method that produces an 'identity card', which includes, as far as possible, the date and place of discovery, context, dimensions, state of preservation, a detailed description, photographs and drawings. This, coupled with the theoretical approaches discussed above, provided a model for database entries.

This study assembled a corpus of 1,492 Roman representations of feet and footwear across 12 categories of artefacts, gathering a range of different types of data, for example, find locations, geographical and chronological deposition, and the types of site where the artefacts were found. Evidence for the deposition of actual footwear in 18,465 Roman graves and 1,311 Roman wells was also examined to explore their meanings, and the significance of Roman hobnailing patterns and how this was extended to depictions of hobnailing considered.

The data were collected from published sources and museum collections. Details of the published foot-shaped artefacts were obtained through a systematic literature review, which included artefact studies, museum catalogues, site reports and specialist Roman articles. Data for some artefacts were obtained through social media, for example, details of a foot-shaped lamp from Corsham originated on X (formerly Twitter) (Roman Britain News 2020), and were followed up with Chippenham Museum. Those for the foot-shaped lamp found at Rue de Koenigshoffen, Strasbourg, in 2019, were published on Facebook (Archéologie Alsace 2019) and researched further online (Crouvezier 2019). These data from modern media should help to counterbalance antiquarian reports. Unpublished foot-shaped artefacts were identified by contacting museums with Roman collections and through internet searches.

Although every effort has been made to ensure that this research is as thorough as possible, no survey of this kind of material can ever hope to be, or remain, complete. However, the combination of a systematic literature survey, where references were carefully followed up, and an examination of unpublished examples should ensure that the samples are as representative as possible (Eckardt 2002: 29). Details of each corpus were entered into a Microsoft Access database, since this permits the inclusion of illustrations, and allows the material to be sorted according to a variety of criteria such as findspot, map coordinates (where available), material, size, chirality, date, and type. The greatest benefit of this method was that it facilitated the observation of chronological, spatial, and depositional distribution patterns. It also enabled the use of some quantitative data, which were entered into Microsoft Excel spreadsheets, so that graphs and charts could be produced to illustrate the data analysis. Distribution maps were created using QGIS software.

The most crucial field in the database for this study, the context, was difficult to name. Various terms were experimented with. 'Social distribution' is inexact, because it assumes that we are seeing different blocks of society at different locations, when, in reality, people moved between them, and they changed over time. 'Context' is an ambiguous term in Roman archaeology, signifying both the common usage meaning, and the specific circumstances (the more precisely definable, discrete, observable 'event') in which an artefact was found. Contextual information also has two levels: the type of site where an artefact was found, which it was decided to call 'site type'; and the nature of the context, which was eventually labelled 'find setting' in order to obviate the terminological problems.

There are inherent problems in classifying both 'site types' and 'find settings', since the categories are very broad and tend to lump sites together. Millett's suggestion (2001: 64) that forts should be considered as small towns does not help the situation. This problem is also evident in dividing up site types for archaeological numismatics (Reece 1995: 182; Lockyear 2000: 399). The implications for military assemblages are made clear by Allason-Jones's work (1988) comparing small finds assemblages from Hadrian's Wall forts with those from turrets, which elicited that these differ markedly from each other. It may, however, be necessary to generalise categories of site to create sufficiently large numbers of artefacts (Eckardt 2005:144) in order to gain a representative sample.

There is a danger that the categories are used for convenience, or historically derived (Eckardt 2002: 29), although it is possible to modify these so as to incorporate material culture patterns and possible regional or status differences (Eckardt 2002: 30). Some sites call for more than one label, for example, Uley could be defined as 'rural' and 'religious'. Other sites, such as Corbridge Roman town, changed status over time, but maintained a military presence. Eckardt (2002: 30) suggests that a pragmatic approach should be adopted. The category labels used for this study, therefore, vary a little, depending on the types of site and find setting encountered: the case study of shoe brooches also includes a 'small town' category for the sake of better accuracy; for obvious reasons, the category 'tile works' was added to the study of footprints in Roman ceramic building materials; the category labels for footprints carved in stone relate to the type of building in which they were found, since there is little variety of general find setting. However, most of the case studies adopt the following categories:

Site types

- Military: legionary fortresses, forts, marching camps or mile castles;
- Urban: cities, *coloniae*, large towns, civitas capitals and small towns;
- Villa/rural: this category is biased towards villas, which have received more attention than rural settlements;
- Other: anything not covered by the above, and;
- Unknown: due to the lack of adequate recording and reporting, this tends to be the largest category.

Find settings

- Domestic: from an area or building of habitation;
- Funerary: burials, whether cremation or inhumation, and cemeteries;
- Industrial: for example tile works, potteries, ports;
- Religious: temples, sanctuaries, shrines and lararia;
- Water: wells, rivers, and bogs;
- Other, and;
- Unknown.

This contextual approach helps to facilitate a focus on patterns of usage and deposition, and thus to interpret the social significance of Roman representations of feet and footwear.

1.3 Recurring strands of significance

During the analysis of this study's corpus it became apparent that a number of strands, or themes, of social significance are common across the different categories of artefact. Feet, to the Romans, could signify a whole individual, whether human or divine, and could function as a signature, or as a symbol of power, authority, and status. Roman representations of feet and footwear could symbolize certain deities, and played a role in Roman ritual activities, particularly in burial rites. They may also have been regarded as having apotropaic properties to ward off the evil eye (Forrer 1942: 43-78; Riha 1979: 42; van Driel-Murray 1999a: 131; Galavaris 2006: 44; Eckardt 2013: 231). Chirality, whether feet were left or right, was significant to communities living within the Roman Empire, and the role it played relating to good or bad luck will be investigated. Roman hobnailing was another important part of the significances of feet and footwear, since the patterns of the nails bore symbols which could be religious or apotropaic. Roman hobnailing was also associated with ideas of authority, power and domination. How these themes relate to the different categories of objects studied is discussed in detail in the relevant chapters. This work argues that, far from being merely whimsical or fashionable, foot- and shoe-shaped artefacts could be polysemous, although they did not necessarily mean the same thing at the same time to everyone.

One should, of course, be aware that feet were not the only significant body part in Roman ideology. Heads could represent a whole person (Ferris 2003: 14) and were regarded as powerful (Eckardt 2014: 168). Hands could symbolise a being (Croxford 2003: 92) and had apotropaic properties (Eckardt 2014: 161). The human phallus is also a known apotropaic symbol (Collins 2020: 274).

1.4 Terms and limitations

'Roman' is a very slippery term, being used for a fairly long period of time and over a wide and changing geographical area in which not everyone was always considered Roman. 'Roman' in this study means within the bounds of the Roman Empire for a timeline that runs from the early first century BCE to the early fifth century CE. This study defines the north-western provinces as comprising an area within the borders of these modern nation states: the United Kingdom, France, Belgium, Luxembourg, the Netherlands, and Germany. Selected data from other areas of the Roman Empire, especially Austria, Switzerland, and Hungary, are included for the purposes of comparison.

The scope of this project is, therefore, wide-ranging, so it might be useful at this point to explain what it does not entail. Many aspects of actual Roman footwear are not considered in detail, because they have been studied at length by Carol van Driel-Murray and many other scholars (see Chapter 2). Nor does it research in depth anatomical foot-shaped votives to do with healing, since this aspect has been covered by other researchers, such as Chiarini (2017). It will not investigate the significance of images of sandals on mosaics, especially those found in baths, which Dunbabin (1990) discusses in detail. Likewise, the prospect of concealed shoes is not considered here.

Although every effort has been made to ensure that this research is as thorough as possible, a few texts, such as von Mercklin's *Römische Klappmessergriffe* (1940), and Guarducci's *Le impronte del 'Quo vadis' e monumenti affini, figurati ed epigrafici* (1943), proved unobtainable. Publishing bias should also be taken into consideration, since small finds, especially metal ones, are much less well published in Spain, Italy and eastern Europe (Eckardt 2022: personal comment). It is therefore inevitable that some foot- and shoe-shaped artefacts have been overlooked.

1.5 The significance of feet in other cultures

Meanings of feet and footwear are not unique to the Romans. In order to begin to examine the special ideology of feet in the Roman world, this section summarizes some of these by dint of comparison. This will only be a brief overview, since this topic could form an entire book on its own.

Some cultural meanings of feet and footwear do coincide with Roman ideology. The funerary use of feet and shoes occurs in Ancient Egypt, where sandals were provided for the deceased (Achrati 2003: 486). Foot-shaped vessels were also used in some burials in Ancient Greece (Smith 2018: 203), and in other areas of Europe in the Iron Age (Forrer 1942: 50; Kohle 2013: 53). Shoes and foot-shaped artefacts are common in Roman burials.

The Roman idea of feet as *pars pro toto*, that is, representative of a whole being, can also be seen in other cultures. The footprints of the Buddha are venerated throughout the Buddhist world (Strong 2007: 86). Islam acknowledges the footprints of Adam on a mountain in Sri Lanka (Galavaris 2006: 43), the footprints of Abraham in the Kaaba, Mecca, and those of the Prophet in the Dome of the Rock in Jerusalem (Achrati 2003: 488). The idea of feet representing a whole being continues. A commemorative sculpture installed in 2005 on the banks of the Danube in Budapest (Yad Vashem 2021) depicts 60 pairs of iron shoes as a memorial to Hungarian Jews shot in 1944–1945.

Feet as symbols of power is another recurring motif. The sandals and footstools of Egyptian pharaohs were decorated with images of their bound and prone enemies so that they symbolically trampled the foes of Egypt (van Driel-Murray 1999a: 131). Carved footprints at Dunadd fort, Scotland, and the Broch of Clickimin, on Shetland, are associated with kingship and inauguration rites (Thomas 1879: 28; Historic Environment Scotland 2021a and 2021b).

There are, however, associations of the foot that are not seen in the Roman world. These brief examples show that feet have many different meanings across the world and across time, and how they fit with Roman ideology. In Asian and Islamic countries, showing the sole of your foot is considered impolite. The foot is the lowest part of the body, in contact with the ground, making it the epitome of dirty (Bishop 2012). Thus, in Iraq, shoes can be used to show extreme disrespect (Weeks 2003), for example, a shoe was thrown at US President Bush by an Iraqi journalist in 2008 (Asser 2008), and statues of Saddam Hussein were beaten with shoes after his fall (BBC News 2003).

Feet can also have erotic connotations. In Ancient Greece, the foot was considered a symbol of the penis (Levine 2005: 59; 68). Feet are also used as euphemisms for the genitals in the Bible (Gravett *et al.* 2008: 170), for example, Isaiah 6:2 and 7:20; Ezekiel 16:25. While it is possible that the foot symbolised the penis to the Romans (Goh 2017: 14), this study found no clear examples of this. This aspect would, however, add another layer to the evidence for feet having an apotropaic role in Roman times.

Freud took up the idea of the feet symbolising the penis in 1905 (Brill 1938: 375) and included it in his theory of foot fetishism (Brill 1938: 567). An example of supposed foot fetishism is Chinese foot-binding, which was imbued with erotic overtones (Foreman 2015). The painful process, which involved breaking a girl's feet and binding them with a silk strip, was widespread for a long time, lasting into the twentieth century (Bossen and Gates 2017: 2). Girls were commonly told that the resulting 'lotus' feet were a passport to a more prestigious marriage and a better way of life (Bossen and Gates 2017: 8). However, it has also been suggested that foot-binding was adopted as an expression of Han Chinese identity (Foreman 2015; Bossen and Gates 2017: 6). Recent research suggests that foot-binding, which limited mobility, ensured young girls sat still and worked at tasks like spinning (Bossen and Gates 2017: 10), that contributed to the household economy (Bossen and Gates 2017: 25). This is a non-Roman example of feet being polysemous.

1.6 Conclusions

Through its analysis of a wide-ranging corpus of 1,492 foot- and shoe-shaped artefacts, and its structure, this study aims to build up an evidentiary picture of the social significance of representations of feet and footwear in the north-western provinces of the Roman Empire. It begins with some background information about actual Roman footwear and discusses ancient attitudes and more recent studies. The significance of Roman hobnailing is also considered. In order to establish some connotations of Roman shoes, their deposition in Roman era graves and wells is considered, before moving on to a series of case studies that looks at twelve different categories of foot- and shoe- shaped artefacts.

Overall, it argues that feet and footwear held a special place in the ideology of the Roman world, with meanings ranging from witty, novelty objects, through fashionable items, to artefacts appropriate for religious, funerary, and other ritual activities. Feet could stand in place of a person, act as a signature, and be symbols of power and status. They were also used apotropaically, especially on a journey, whether that be actual travel, the journey through life, or to the Underworld.

2

Ancient and modern attitudes to Roman feet and footwear

Feet and shoes were important in the Roman world as a primary means of transport and formed a direct connection with the environment. Across the empire Romans wore shoes, and footwear is well represented in Roman art and literature, yet this area of Roman culture remains under-researched. Where studies of Roman footwear and its representations are published, they are almost invariably in book chapters or articles, some of them running to just a few pages.

Roman footwear is worthy of discussion because it encapsulates an enormous reservoir of technological, chronological and social information (van Driel-Murray 1987: 32). It provides insights into aspects of identity such as gender, and economic status. Shoes reflect Roman ideas of class, rank, and profession (Goldman 2002: 101). Since the default position is barefoot, wearing shoes is culturally conditioned: they are a symbol of status and prosperity rather than a basic necessity (van Driel-Murray 2011a: 360). There are portraits of Emperors with bare feet, such as Augustus Prima Porta, since being barefoot in statues often signified that the person was divine, pious or a hero (Croom 2010: 74). *Caligae* (strappy army boots) immediately identified their wearers as soldiers. Differences in the style and ornamentation of *calcei* (closed shoes) worn with the toga showed elite social status. All sorts of Romans wore shoes, so footwear may give us access to the lives of the frequently invisible members of Roman society: non-elite men, women, children, and slaves.

The focus of Roman footwear studies has changed over time, along with attitudes to the past and the theories behind them, from describing shoes using art and literature as evidence, to analysing the cosmological symbolism in hobnailing patterns.

This chapter gives an overview of these changes and highlights the prevalent themes in Roman calceology (the study of footwear). It begins with a basic introduction to Roman footwear, then examines what Roman authors wrote about the significance of footwear. Next it considers the art-historical approach to Roman shoes, and critiques antiquarian approaches. It discusses some mid-twentieth-century influential Roman calceologists, before moving on to review more recent research. Once work on Roman footwear has been dealt with, the chapter moves on to consider Roman representations of feet and footwear.

2.1 Background to Roman footwear

As an organic substance, leather needs very specific environments to survive archaeologically. Waterlogged sites provide anaerobic conditions. Roman footwear has been found in riverbanks, (for example London), wells (the Saalburg), and ditches (Vindolanda). Hot, arid climates (for example Egypt and Syria) preserve leather by drying it. This means that extant footwear tends to come from the edges of the Roman Empire, with very little found in Italy, Spain or southern France (Goldman 2001: 109; van Driel-Murray 2016: 149).

Some examples of Iron Age shoes survive preserved in bogs or salt mines. Iron-Age leather was oiled or smoked to preserve it, and shoes were even made of rawhide (van Driel-Murray 2009a: 485), none of which lasted very long. Such shoes would have rotted on the feet. Prehistoric shoes were made in one piece, and not specifically for left or right feet but moulded with wear to the shape of the wearer's foot.

Roman shoes were radically different (van Driel-Murray 2016: 141). The main technologies introduced to the north-western provinces by the Romans were vegetable tanning, which preserved the leather, hobnailing (see Chapter 3), which attached the soles to the uppers on most types of Roman footwear and protected the soles from wear, and shoes made expressly for left and right feet (chirality).

Roman leather was treated with tannins extracted from tree bark or oak galls (van Driel-Murray 2009a: 485). Analysis has shown that the Romans used mostly fir-tree bark, but also oak and elm (Göpfrich 1986: 10). Tanning made the shoes more durable and therefore better value. This technology disappeared from the northwestern provinces as Roman influence decreased in the fourth century (van Driel-Murray 2016: 138). Other Roman footwear innovations included a greater variety of colour and ornamentation. Shoes were cut out according to fairly standard cutting patterns and stitched together. However, a basic closed shoe could be transformed into a luxury product (van Driel-Murray 2011a: 342) by cutting out shapes from the leather to produce a fishnet effect (Figure 2.1). Such shoes may have had coloured linings or been

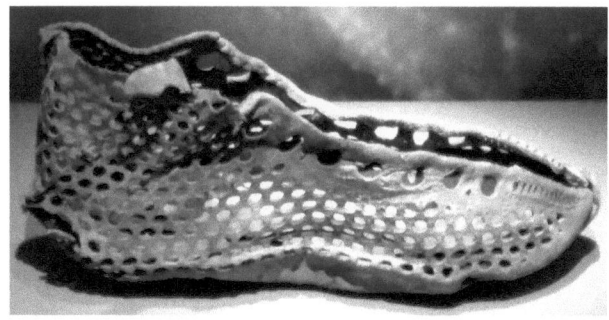

Figure 2.1: 'Fishnet' shoe, Vindolanda Trust (Photo: Author's own).

worn with bright socks (Goldman 2002: 121; van Driel-Murray 2011a: 342). They were expensive due to the time-consuming process of cutting out the leather (Greene 2014: 32). Economic status was shown by the quality of the workmanship, the materials used, and the decoration. These advances in footwear technology produced an unprecedented choice of attractive novelties (van Driel-Murray 2016: 141) which gave people of modest means a way to exhibit individuality, taste, and style (van Driel-Murray 2016: 133).

2.1.1 Classifying Roman footwear

Roman authors used a number of different words for types of footwear, but these are hard to identify, since we no longer know to what these terms refer. Diocletian's *Maximum Prices Edict* lists a number of types of footwear (IX.1-25), only some of which correspond to known shoes. Meanings of words will have changed over time as shoe fashions moved on (van Driel-Murray 2011a: 347). Therefore, scholars have developed Roman shoe typologies, often based on methods of construction, such as nailed or sewn together, or cut in one piece. This study uses the standard archaeological typology for Roman shoes:

Carbatinae

These are un-nailed shoes, cut in one piece and stitched (Figure 2.2). The cut and fit of some *carbatinae* show they were made by skilled shoemakers (Busch 1965: 166). This is confirmed by Rhodes (1980: 127). (See also section 2:4).

Caligae

These sandal-like military boots came in two varieties: high, which came above the ankle (see Figure 6.24), and low, which stopped below the ankle. They consisted of three main pieces of leather: a sole, an insole, and a middle section cut in one piece to include the strapwork (van Driel-Murray 2011a: 362), fastened together with hobnails, which also made the boots last longer, gave more grip, and supported the foot (Bishop and Coulston 2006: 112). *Caligae* were well suited to their purpose (van Driel-Murray 2011a: 362). Openwork uppers helped to prevent trench foot and the straps allowed the boots to fit an individual's foot without rubbing (Bishop and Coulston 2006: 112-113). However, cold may have been a problem when wearing *caligae*. There is artistic evidence that a kind of sock or foot-wrapping was worn with them (van Driel-Murray 2011a: 363; Göpfrich 1986: 19).

Given that a soldier might have expected three pairs of *caligae* per year (van Driel-Murray 2011a: 340), it is perhaps surprising that more have not been excavated. However, to date almost none have been found in the centre of empire due to the very specific conditions needed for leather to survive. *Caligae* disappear from the archaeological record by the end of the first century CE, (van Driel-Murray 2011a: 345). However, the *caliga* continues much later in iconography. *Caligae* are visible on the Column of Marcus Aurelius, completed by 193 CE, and the *Portonaccio Sarcophagus*, of a similar date. Some can even be seen on the Arch of Septimius Severus, dedicated in 203.

Calcei

There is general scholarly agreement that *calcei* are closed shoes or shoeboots (Goldman 2001: 116). *Calcei* were made from several pieces of leather and had nailed soles. They show change over time, coming higher or lower up the foot (Figure 2.3; see also Figure 9.3). Many shoeboots have been excavated, including those that replaced the *caliga*. However, not all types of *calceus* survive archaeologically; those worn with the toga were made from such fine leather that the shape of the wearer's toes was visible. While many portraits of Roman men wearing such boots exist, none have been excavated (see section 2:3).

Soleae

These sandals resemble modern flip-flops (Figure 2.4). Sandals were worn indoors by everyone (Goldman 2002: 109) but, in the first century CE, were deemed inappropriate for elite men to wear outside (Gell.*NA*.XIII.22; Olson 2017: 86). It was, however, customary for higher-status men to wear sandals when dining. These were removed for reclining, and sent for when it was time to leave (Olson 2017: 86). In the second half of the third and early fourth centuries, wide sandals became fashionable for men (Figure 2.5).

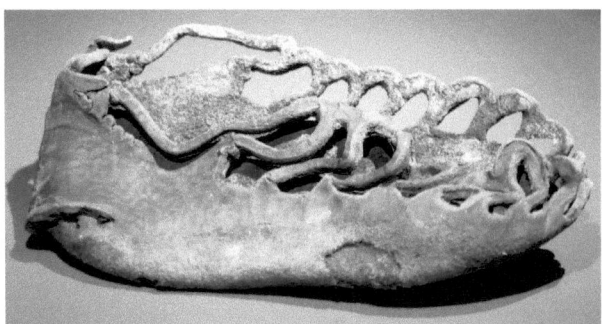

Figure 2.2: A child's carbatina, Vindolanda Trust (Photo: Author's own).

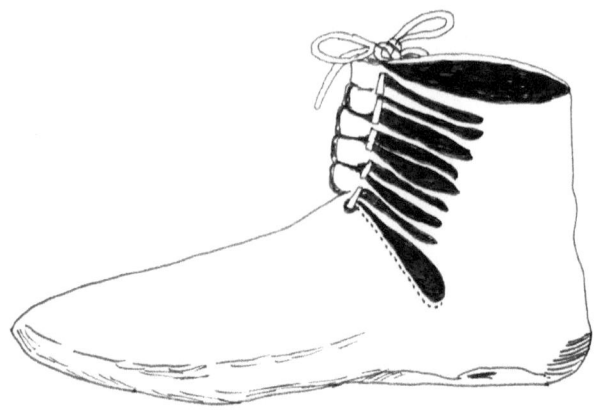

Figure 2.3: Mainz calceus. (Author's drawing).

Ancient and modern attitudes to Roman feet and footwear

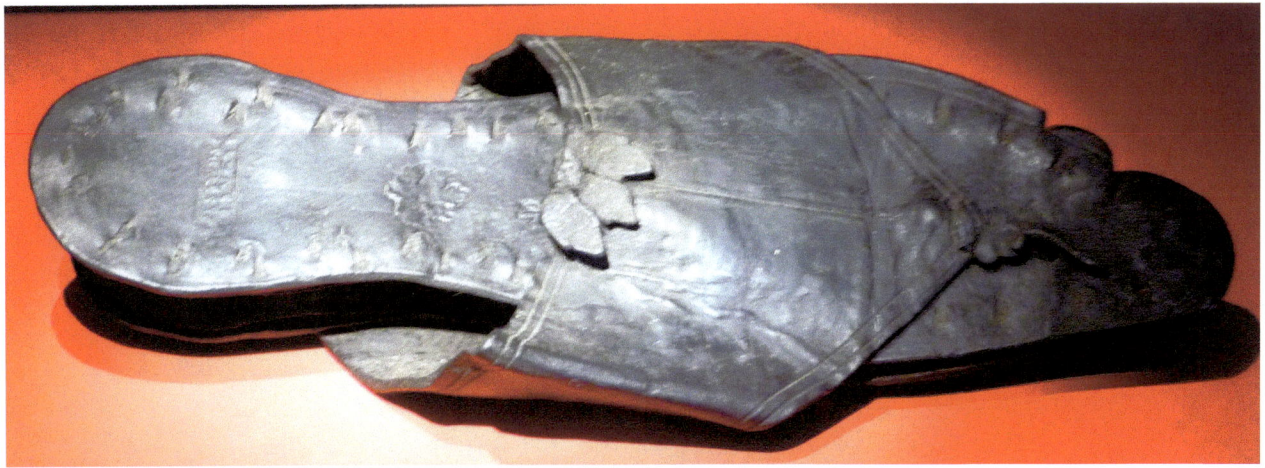

Figure 2.4: 'Lepidina's' sandal, Vindolanda Trust. (Photo: Author's own).

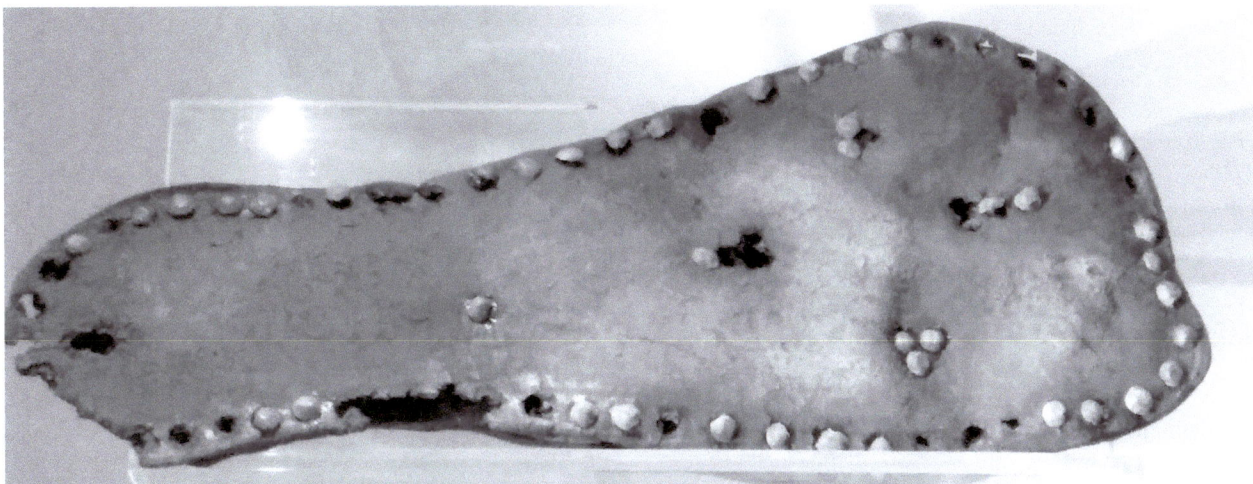

Figure 2.5: Man's wide sandal sole, Vindolanda Trust. (Photo: Author's own).

Socci

These were un-nailed house-shoes made from separate soles and uppers. Most surviving examples are from Egypt.

Sculponeae

These could be fine wooden shoes worn to protect the feet from hot floors in the baths (see Figure 3.1), and rougher ones worn by agricultural workers (see section 4.1). They were held onto the feet with leather straps. The wooden soles were sometimes nailed.

Other Roman footwear

There are depictions of some types of footwear that are not found in the archaeological record and which may be artistic inventions. One example is a kind of ornate boot surmounted with feline heads (Goldman 2001: 123; Goette 1988: 403). These appear on statues of emperors, heroes and some deities, for instance the emperor Antoninus Pius (National Archaeological Museum, Naples: Inv. No. 6078), Antinous as Bacchus (National Archaeological Museum, Naples: Inv. No. 6314), and the Farnese Lar (Figure 2.6) (National Archaeological Museum, Naples: Inv. No. 5975).

Another example is the type of sandal often known as *crepidae*, an ancient Greek style seen on Roman statues of philosophers (Olson 2017: 87) and healers, for example, a statue of Aesculapius (Figure 2.7) (National Archaeological Museum, Naples, Inv. no. 6360).

Fine leather tends to decay, and what usually remains of Roman shoes is the sole (Rhodes 1980: 100), so we cannot rule out the possibility that such styles did not exist. Indeed, Roman authors describe people as wearing sandals called *crepidae* (for example, Cicero *Pro Rabirio Postumo* 10.27; Livy 29.19.12; Suetonius *Tiberius* 13; Horace *Satires* 1.3.127). However, there is no guarantee that what these ancient authors meant by *crepidae* is what we understand by the term today (Driel-Murray 2011a: 347; Goldman 2001: 109). For the sake of convenience and consistency, this study uses *crepida* to denote a Greek style of sandal with fairly ornate straps.

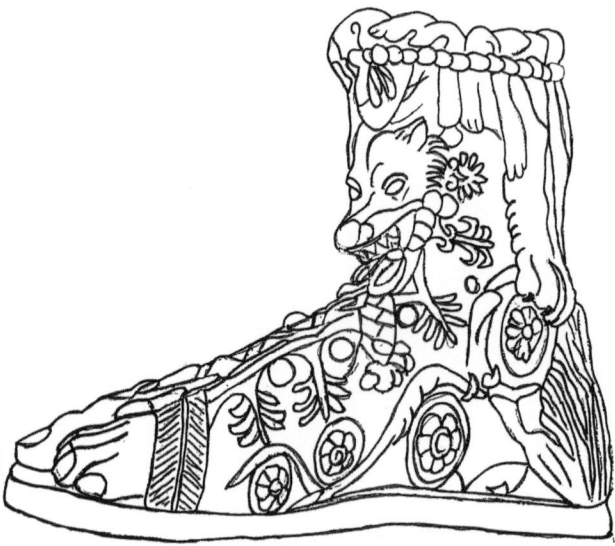

Figure 2.6: 'Hero' boot on the Farnese Lar.

2.1.2 Roman footwear fashion

Roman footwear exhibits change over time stylistically and technologically: *caligae* are replaced by more closed boots; sandal-soles change shape; *calcei* uppers become higher or lower. Due to her extensive study of Roman footwear from across the empire, van Driel-Murray (2016: 143) has observed that changes in footwear often follow classic fashion cycles. The different styles cluster within well-defined chronological limits (van Driel-Murray 2001a: 187; van Driel-Murray 2011a: 344). Footwear fashions appear at the same time in the extremities of the Roman Empire so, despite a lack of comparable examples from Italy and southern Gaul, it seems reasonable to assume that trends run throughout the empire (van Driel-Murray 2011a: 342). Because of these recognisable trends, Roman footwear can be used as dating evidence (van Driel-Murray 2001a: 191).

2.2 What the ancient Romans wrote

Footwear was socially significant in Roman life. Ancient authors' criticisms of prominent men for wearing inappropriate footwear show that ideas of the wearer's identity in terms of rank, status, and gender were conveyed by shoes. Suetonius criticized the emperor Gaius because 'In his clothing, his shoes, and the rest of his attire he did not follow the usage of his country and his fellow citizens' (Suet.*Calig*.52). By wearing the kinds of footwear that were appropriate for his bodyguard or for women (Suet.*Calig*.52), Caligula was not conforming to elite expectations of how an emperor should dress. Suetonius also censured Nero for similar footwear misdemeanours (Suet.*Nero*.51), whereas he praised Augustus for always having the appropriate footwear to hand (Suet.*Aug*.73). Martial comments on a former slave wearing high-status shoes to which he was not entitled (Mart.2.29). Even leaving aside considerations of elite male bias in Latin literature, ideas about status and beliefs bound up in

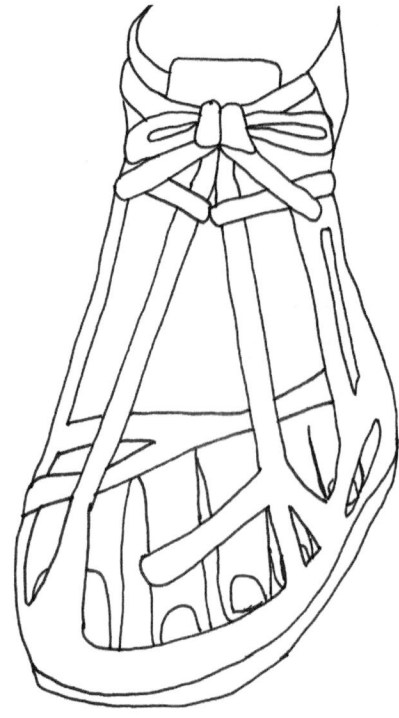

Figure 2.7: Crepida on a statue of Aesculapius.

Roman feet and shoes must have been sufficiently widely understood for the authors' points to have been grasped.

A number of Roman metaphors involving footwear also demonstrate its social consequence. To call for one's shoes after dining out (*calceos poscere*) signified the intention of leaving (Plin.*Ep*.9.17.3), while richer men called for their sandals (*soleas poscere*) (Hor.*Sat*.2.8.77). Footwear also played a metaphorical role in rites of passage and changes of status, for example, becoming a senator was described as 'to change one's shoes' (*calceos mutare*) (Cic.*Phil*.13.13.28). The colour of footwear could also show a change of status: for example, brides seem to have worn yellow shoes (Catull.61.160; *Aldobrandini Wedding*, Vatican Museums Inv. No. 79631). Such changes of clothing are not unusual in rites of passage (for example, van Gennep 1960: 130). The use of metaphors involving footwear is a further indication of its position in the Roman psyche.

There is some evidence in ancient texts for the idea that feet were a proxy for a whole being, often divine. This concept of *pars pro toto* can be seen in Apuleius' *Metamorphoses*. In 11.17, Apuleius describes the crowd at the end of the Isis festival kissing the '*vestigia*' of the goddess which are made of silver and stand on the temple steps. This is usually taken to refer to a silver statue, but the Latin is more appropriate for the footprints of the goddess (Dunbabin 1990: 96). The feet of the statue are mentioned again in *Metamorphoses* 11.23, where the protagonist, Lucius, is taken back to the temple and placed 'right in front of the goddess's feet', a singular honour. The Latin word used for feet here is, again, '*vestigia*'. The word '*vestigia*' is used a third time for the feet of the goddess in *Metamorphoses*

11.24, where Lucius describes prostrating himself before the goddess and wiping her feet with his face. Chapter 8 of this study explores carved footprints, many of which are attributed to Isis, and some of which came from Rome, so the translation of '*vestigia*' as footprints in this instance seems valid. One could argue, as Dunbabin has, that Apuleius is writing not about a whole statue, but about the footprints of Isis(1990:96).

Latin texts also attest to Roman superstitions involving feet and shoes. It was considered unpropitious to start a journey with the left foot (Apul.*Met*.1.5) or even to put on the left shoe first (Plin.*HN*.2.24). On the other hand, the right foot was considered lucky (Sil.*Pun*.7.172), so much so that Vitruvius advocated odd numbers of temple steps: 'For, since the first step is ascended on the right foot, the right foot must also be set on the top of the temple steps' (*De arch*.3.4.4). Testing whether this advice was followed proved difficult, due to the lack of surviving Roman temple steps. However, a survey of 18 Roman temples that still have steps shows that these all had odd numbers (Table 2.1)

Such beliefs were not just linked to the more general issue with the left in Roman superstition. A Catullus poem speaks of the 'good omen' of lifting the bride's feet across the threshold (Catull.61.159). The foot was also used in wishing good luck, '*i pede fausto*' (Hor.*Epist*.2.2.37) or, more literally, 'Go with your lucky foot'. Cicero hints at other bad omens surrounding the foot, 'we had better look out when we stumble, or break a shoe-string, or sneeze!' (*Div*.2.84).

Thus, the material cultural embodiment of a cosmology involving feet and footwear must have been important in elite Roman society. There is, however, little written evidence to show what the people who lived in the north-western provinces might have thought.

2.3 An art-based approach

The earliest studies of Roman shoes were based on art and literature, an art-historical, antiquarian approach to Roman dress, for example, *Gallus; or, Roman scenes of the time of Augustus* (Becker 1838: 424–428). Another work which uses a similar approach is the *Histoire de la chaussure, depuis l'antiquité la plus reculée jusqu'à nos jours* (Lacroix and Duchesne 1852). This describes the appearance of Roman footwear (with illustrations) based mainly on Roman sculpture, but with some reference to Latin texts.

Mommsen (1888: 891 note 1) used ancient texts to reconstruct the kind of boot worn with the toga (Figure 2.8). In fairness, toga *calcei* do not survive in the archaeological record, so literature and art are the only sources for this

Table 2.1: Numbers of surviving steps on Roman temples.

Temple	Location	No. of steps
Maison Carrée	Nîmes, France	15
Temple of Portunus, Forum Boarium	Rome, Italy	11
Temple of Antoninus Pius and Faustina	Rome, Italy	21
Capitolium (Capitoline Triad)	Ostia, Italy	21
Temple of Mars Ultor	Rome, Italy	17
Pantheon	Rome, Italy	5
Roman temple	Alcántara, Spain	7
Temple of Apollo	Pompeii, Italy	9
Temple of Augustus and Livia	Vienne, France	13
Temple of Juno Caelestis	Dougga, Tunisia	11
Temple of Bacchus	Baalbek, Lebanon	13
Temple of Minerva	Sbeitla, Tunisia	9
Temple A, Largo di Torre Argentina	Rome, Italy	7
Temple B, Largo di Torre Argentina	Rome, Italy	9
Temple C, Largo di Torre Argentina	Rome, Italy	7
Temple D, Largo di Torre Argentina	Rome, Italy	7
Piazzale delle Corporazioni temple	Ostia, Italy	13
Roman temple	Cordoba, Spain	15

footwear. The textual evidence is, however, contradictory. The details about which rank was signified by how many straps, and exactly what colour the footwear was, are very much open to debate. The picture becomes even more confused when sculpture is added to the mix. For example, Isidore of Seville (34.4) writes that patricians' shoes had four straps tied in two knots. Goette (1988: 450; see also 251, figure 35) argues that togate portrait statues show two further arrangements of straps: one with a single knot, and one of very fine leather with no straps or knots.

Although some Roman footwear was found at Whitley Castle fort as early as 1825, during the digging of a drain (Sopwith 1833: 39), and shoes were excavated in Mainz in 1857 (Göpfrich 1986: 5), and at the Saalburg in 1870 (Busch 1965: 158), this appears to have been ignored by works such as the *Dictionnaire des antiquités grecques et romaines* (Daremberg and Saglio), published in ten volumes between 1877 and 1919. There is some reference to archaeological evidence in the later volumes, for example the entry for *solea* (1877: 1387-1390), but most antiquarian studies of Roman shoes are based on art.

Some, more recent, scholars also rely heavily on Roman art, with little reference to actual archaeological shoes. In the case of Goette, this is because he is writing about the forms of footwear that appear on elite Roman statues, for example, the kind of ornate boot worn by the *Farnese Lar* (see Figure 2.6). There is no archaeological evidence to show that such boots ever existed but this has not prevented research into such artistic representations because of the message they give about the wearer's identity.

One major problem with this approach to Roman footwear studies is that art does not necessarily portray footwear accurately, since early imperial Roman art is traditional and conventional, and tends to show people dressed in formal clothing (Olson 2008: 141), rather than everyday wear. Another difficulty is that, because of the bias of Roman art and literature towards the elite, scholars have tended to focus on prestigious footwear and ignore what most people of the Roman Empire may have worn on their feet.

2.4 Antiquarian footwear finds

Along with the nineteenth century finds of Roman footwear from Whitley Castle, Mainz and the Saalburg, shoes were also excavated in the late nineteenth and early twentieth centuries at Birdoswald, Bar Hill, and Newstead forts, and Cologne.

In 1898 Haverfield reported a one-piece Roman shoe from outside Birdoswald fort on Hadrian's Wall. He mentions that other Roman shoes had been found in England (but does not say where), some of them presumably from Birdoswald, and 'in various other countries' (Haverfield 1898: 142). He identifies the shoe as a *carbatina*, quoting Catullus 98.4, which is a possibly a misnomer, as Catullus uses '*carpatinas*'. Haverfield draws an analogy between

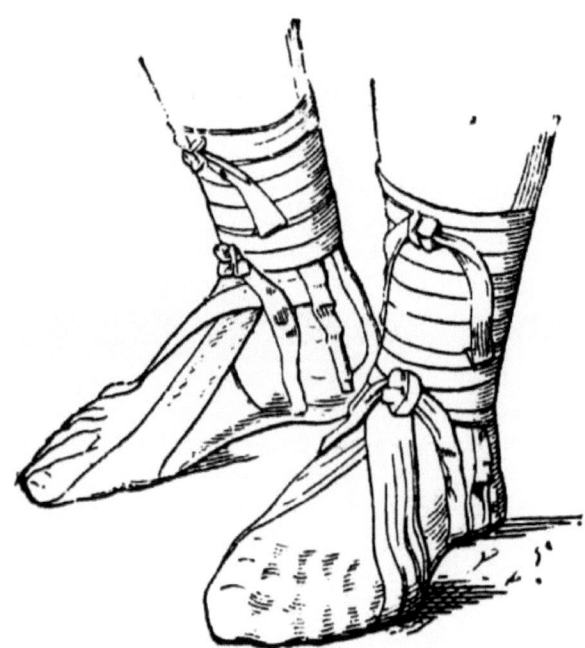

Figure 2.8: Toga calcei (Daremberg et Saglio vol. 1 1877: 817 fig. 1016)

this 'class of shoes which are distinct from the *calcei, caligae*, etc., of literature' and a kind of nineteenth century shoe worn by 'peasants' (1898: 142). An art-historical approach would not help because, despite the complexity and ornateness of some *carbatinae*, and their apparent popularity, at least across the north-western provinces, Roman art only ever seems to show this type of shoe in the context of defeated 'barbarians' (for example, on the *Portonaccio Sarcophagus*, and *Trajan's Column*). However, later scholars acknowledge that *carbatinae* show almost limitless variations on a basic pattern, and are subject to fashion influences (van Driel-Murray 2011a: 353, especially fig. 24). The wearer's status could be shown by quality (Greene 2014: 32) and yet, although Haverfield remarks on the ornamentation of the Birdoswald shoe (1898: 142), he assumes it is low status. Despite writing a year later than Jacobi, Haverfield appears to cling to the antiquarian, art historical approach.

Jacobi, on the other hand, recorded the Roman finds from the Saalburg in 1897 from an archaeological perspective. He points out that shoe forms were only known from art and that it was the footwear assemblage from Mainz that first brought knowledge of Roman shoe technology (1897: 494). Unlike Haverfield's report, Jacobi's contains some surprisingly modern features, covering Roman tanning (1897: 492), shoe construction and nailing patterns (1897: 493). While Haverfield's only reference is to Catullus, almost in passing, Jacobi provides footnotes and a thorough bibliography (1897: XX–XXVI). Admittedly, this may be due to the difference in genres, Haverfield's being a short report in a journal, and Jacobi's part of a substantial archaeological report. Jacobi compares the types of shoes found at the Saalburg with the Mainz assemblage (1897: 494), which was the first time this had happened. He comments on shoe sizes being an indicator for the wearer's age and gender (Jacobi 1897: 498), which is one of the many aspects of Roman footwear studied by van Driel-Murray (1987; 1992). Jacobi (1897: 160; 495) also relates the quality and ornamentation of some of the Saalburg shoes to economic status, specifically a woman's sandal with gold decoration (1897: 497). However, he also describes *carbatinae* as peasants' shoes (1897: 497). Within the art-historical approach there appears to have been a kind of hierarchy of status in types of footwear.

MacDonald's account of the Roman shoe finds at Bar Hill, on the Antonine Wall, shares many features with Jacobi's. There is a comparison with other assemblages, in this case Birdoswald and the Saalburg, and some discussion of nailing patterns and the significance of shoe size with regard to gender (MacDonald 1906: 102; 104). What is different here, is that MacDonald begins to question the art-historical approach. He recognizes that the shoe types found at Bar Hill cannot be classified 'under their *proper* Latin names' (MacDonald 1906: 101), and that looking to art for evidence 'would not be reasonable' (MacDonald 1906: 101) because 'Rome and its neighbourhood naturally dominate the literary tradition' (MacDonald 1906: 101), likewise art, and the Bar Hill garrison was 'composed of Romanized provincials, not of Romans' (MacDonald 1906, 101). Unlike Jacobi and Haverfield, MacDonald does not assume that the *carbatinae* found at Bar Hill are peasants' shoes.

In recognizing that the cut of a shoe might express a social distinction (1906: 101), MacDonald also appears to be more aware of how Roman shoes reflect the status of their wearers, noting that the *calcei* found were probably worn by officers and the more well-to-do among the civilians (MacDonald 1906: 106). He comments, too, on decorative nailing patterns (MacDonald 1906: 104), which were not studied in much detail until the late twentieth century. He even remarks on evidence for disability from a child's shoe, which has an iron support 'to correct some slight lameness' (MacDonald 1906: 104). Footwear bearing possible indications of disability is not commented upon in any detail until Gansser-Burckhardt in 1942.

However, despite acknowledging that 'the remnants are so scanty that we cannot say … what the original appearance of the whole may have been' (1906: 106), MacDonald makes assumptions about some of the footwear. Based on the numbers found, he feels compelled to find the traditional Roman army boot among the shoes (MacDonald 1906: 106). This is unlikely, since the *caliga* disappears from the archaeological record by 100 CE (van Driel-Murray 2011a: 345), and even the early enclosure at Bar Hill is now widely considered an Antonine period temporary camp dating to after 140 CE (*The Antonine Wall*, 2017).

Curle's 1911 report on the excavation of Newstead Roman fort is largely similar in approach and findings to MacDonald's. In addition, Curle begins to demonstrate the importance of dating to footwear, identifying the single *caliga* found at Newstead as first century (Curle 1911: 151) and a *calceus* as second century (Curle 1911: 152), with which van Driel-Murray would agree (2001a: 188–189). On the other hand, Curle (1911: 151) does compare the Newstead *caliga* with those on monumental reliefs, so he has not moved away entirely from the art-historical tradition. This is also apparent in Curle's comparison of *carbatinae* with the shoes of 'barbarians' on Trajan's Column, although he tempers this by adding that the one-piece shoes from the Saalburg and Newstead provide 'examples of much more skilled leatherwork than in the simple *caligae* from Mainz' (Curle 1911: 151).

By 1926, the assumption that *carbatinae* are low-status footwear has dwindled. It is certainly absent from Fremersdorf's report on a 1924 find of Roman leather in Cologne. His report continues to make comparisons between footwear assemblages, specifically Mainz and the Saalburg (Fremersdorf 1926: 44; 46; 52). Fremersdorf says that the archaeologists hoped they would find some very early shoes (1926: 46), but that the dating evidence showed all the footwear came from a late second- to early third-century context (1926: 56). Nowadays, we know that the wide-soled sandals found in Cologne could be used to date the assemblage (van Driel-Murray 2001a: 193 fig. 3).

Fremersdorf does not use a traditional art-historical approach to his analysis of the Cologne footwear, although he does compare nailing patterns with those found on Roman lamps (Fremersdorf 1926: 46 fig.2). This may be justified, because there is a remarkable parallel between two of the lamps and actual nailing patterns (Fremersdorf 1926: 46 figs. 2.b and c). However, the other lamp uses a mock nailing pattern to spell out the maker's name (Fremersdorf 1926: 46 fig.2.a; 48). The most novel aspect of Fremersdorf's report is his comparison of decorative stamps on the leather with those from Mainz and the Saalburg, noting that some are very similar, and may be makers' marks (Fremersdorf 1926: 52). This kind of detail is not revisited until the 1980s (Rhodes 1980: 118–119), but becomes important as a sign of how far shoes were traded (van Driel-Murray 1997b: 56–57), and as a marker of wealth and status (van Driel-Murray 2001a: 192).

These early archaeological reports about Roman footwear already show some of the concerns of more recent calceologists: an interest in hobnailing patterns; aspects of the wearer's identity shown by the shoes, especially wealth, age and gender; stamps which show the spread of trading in shoes; and the dating of shoes, which can show fashion trends.

2.5 Some influential Roman calceologists

In the twentieth century, Roman footwear studies, which modern scholars still consult, began to be produced. In 1942, Gansser-Burckhardt published a summary of the leather found at the Roman fort of Vindonissa (Windisch in Switzerland). His research was influential because he asks whether the different sizes of shoes found on this military site are proof that women and children lived in the fort (Gansser-Burckhardt 1942: 67). Van Driel-Murray has since researched this question, noting that 'virtually the only kind of Roman clothing to survive intact—footwear—is also a relatively sensitive exponent of sexual dimorphism' (van Driel-Murray 1995: 4). Footwear therefore provides 'valuable evidence for the changing composition of the population in and around forts between the 1st and 3rd centuries' (van Driel-Murray 1987: 33). She concludes that, although it is generally accepted that there was a legal ban on the marriage of soldiers (van Driel-Murray 1995: 7), the evidence from footwear shows that Roman forts were never a male-only preserve (van Driel-Murray 2011a: 360).

Gansser-Burckhardt also investigated the significance of hobnailing patterns. Sadly, his conclusion that a circular nailing pattern on some *caligae* from Vindonissa was intended to correct mild club foot (Gansser-Burckhardt 1942: 68–73) is now widely discredited. Göpfrich (1986: 15) calls it a controversial theory, but suggests that some nailing may have been orthopaedic. Van Driel-Murray (1999b: 172) points out that, if Gansser-Burckhardt were correct, many soldiers in the garrisons of Velsen and Valkenburg, where *caligae* had similar nailing patterns, would have suffered from club foot. Groenman-van Waateringe (1974: 78) calculates that, according to Gansser-Burkhardt's theory, 27% of the *caligae* found at Valkenburg were nailed for club foot. It seems improbable that such a high level of affliction existed in the Roman army, and there are alternative theories for this nailing pattern. Rhodes (1980: 103) suggests that similarities between the Vindonissa *caligae* and some from Billingsgate may show that they were produced by the same workshop. Van Driel-Murray interprets the circles as good luck (1999a: 132) or sun symbols (2002a: 97). More recent work by Greene (2018a: 319) based on the Vindolanda assemblage shows that hobnailing at the heel may have been used to correct a slight over-pronation or supination, but there is no mention of club-foot.

In 1965, Busch revisited the Roman footwear from the Saalburg. Her report, running to fifty-two pages with forty tables of sketches, and a catalogue, is much more substantial than Jacobi's, with only eight pages. Busch's discussion of Roman footwear is very thorough, and has been cited by the majority of later Roman calceologists. An example of progress since Jacobi is Busch's discussion of *carbatinae*. There is no suggestion here that they were peasants' shoes, although they were among the cheaper footwear (Busch 1965: 166).

Perhaps the most original and influential section of this report is Busch's discussion (1965: 175) of change over time in shoe fashions. This was noticed in subsequent assemblages. Based on footwear finds from Vindolanda, where the dates are known from stratigraphy, van Driel-Murray (2016: 143) has argued that Roman shoes can be used as dating evidence.

Göpfrich's approach to the Roman footwear from Mainz is similar to Busch's. Among her contributions to Roman calceology are a comprehensive account of the substances used in Roman vegetable tanning and leather dying (Göpfrich 1986: 10). In her analysis of the Mainz *caligae* she also makes one of the few direct comparisons of Roman footwear with artistic representations (Göpfrich 1986: 17–18). She also shows an awareness that Roman footwear could be used to express social differences, but that this was done less through form than by the costliness of the decoration (Göpfrich 1986: 23).

Michael Rhodes's report on the footwear from Billingsgate Buildings, London, has also proved influential. He suggests seven reasons why uppers have not survived on shoes (Rhodes 1980: 100–101). His typology of hobnailing patterns (Rhodes 1980: 104–107) has since been adopted and extended by several scholars (van Driel-Murray 1983: 20–22; Mould 1997: 331–335; Burandt 2016: 9–12).

2.6 Recent Roman shoe research

Within the last twenty-four years, overviews of Roman footwear have been produced as chapters in books about Roman clothing. In her introduction, Croom (2010: 12) warns of the dangers of relying too heavily on art because it does not reflect everyday life and therefore tends to show only those wealthy enough to commission it (Croom 2010: 11). She gives a useful, clear description of the different types of Roman footwear, with some analysis of how shoes reflected status. Sadly, all of the illustrations come from artwork, despite Croom's cautions, and her geographical proximity to Vindolanda.

Goldman (2002) also provides a very detailed discussion of Roman footwear styles with illustrations. She uses evidence from a wide variety of sources, although few of these are archaeological. Clearly some scholars still use an art-historical approach to Roman footwear without reference to real shoes. Indeed, Goldman asks (2002: 109) what actual leather finds add to literary references and artistic representations. This question should surely be posed the other way around. However, we do have to rely on artistic sources for some forms of Roman footwear, because they do not survive archaeologically. While Goldman's chapter is a comprehensive and useful introduction to Roman footwear, it has been criticized for lacking an awareness of the anthropological and sociological literature on dress, remaining more descriptive than analytical (Edmondson and Keith 2008: 6).

Le Forestier (2013) examines some shoes found in burials in the Île de France from a different perspective. Uniquely, he combines anatomical details of feet with a study of Roman footwear. He suggests that it is possible to tell whether a corpse was buried wearing shoes from a careful examination of how the foot bones have fallen as bodies have decayed; feet encased in stiff leather do not exhibit a lateral rotation (le Forestier 2013: 180). This becomes even more significant in the case of some Gallo-

Roman graves where a pair of shoes was placed beside the body. Le Forestier (2013: 181) discusses the probability that shoes were deposited beside a corpse because the deceased was already wearing shoes which had left no archaeological trace. In some cases, there is evidence from nails that a corpse was buried wearing shoes (le Forestier 2013: 166). If the taphonomy of the feet in burials with no nails is examined carefully, it should be possible to establish whether the person was buried wearing shoes (le Forestier 2013: 181).

As to why people were buried with extra pairs of shoes, le Forestier (2013: 182) warns that interpreting Gallo-Roman grave goods is 'delicate', but suggests three possible reasons for shoes deposits: they reflected social status; they eased the journey into the afterlife; or they were simply a gift to the deceased. He wonders whether the deposits consisted of all the shoes the deceased possessed, just those which could not be re-used by the community, or a representative selection, noting that a much more thorough analysis of the data from many Gallo-Roman burials would be necessary to answer these questions (le Forestier 2013: 182).

2.7 Research into hobnailing

Hobnailing was part of Roman footwear construction, prevented wear and gave better grip on muddy ground. Le Forestier (2013: 164) points out that nails are often the only archaeological evidence for Roman shoes and that nails were not carefully excavated or documented until the late twentieth century. He commends lifting blocks of earth around nails which may indicate shoes and scanning them to obtain a three-dimensional image (le Forestier 2013: 178). Van Driel-Murray (1999a: 132) also laments the lack of care taken with hobnails and describes a similar methodology for recording them (van Driel-Murray 2011a: 352). Apart from the presence of shoes, Roman hobnails can also be used to help establish the gender of the wearer as, in the Île de France at least, more nails are found in men's graves than in women's (le Forestier 2013: 166), probably since men's feet tend to be larger.

Wearing more rigid, nailed shoes alters a person's stance and gait (van Driel-Murray 2011a: 350) and hence the drape of their clothing (van Driel-Murray 2001a: 195), affecting their *habitus*. It makes a difference to the feel (van Driel-Murray 2002b: 119) and sound (van Driel-Murray 2011a: 337) of walking, and left very characteristic footprints. As can be seen from some Roman tiles, nailing patterns became a sort of signature, a statement of personal identity (van Driel-Murray 1999a: 132). Nailing patterns could also be attractive, becoming a 'fashion accessory' (van Driel-Murray 1999a: 132).

Van Driel-Murray has researched some of the possible symbolism of Roman nailing patterns. Some appear to represent cosmological symbols (van Driel-Murray 2002a: 99) or commitment to a particular deity (van Driel-Murray 1999a: 132). Other motifs, such as circles and swastikas, may be general good luck symbols (van Driel-Murray 1999a: 132). Such apotropaic hobnailing designs would have made Roman footwear doubly protective, both physically and spiritually.

Nailing patterns are represented on the underside of foot-shaped lamps, some of which stood on a flat surface, where the pattern would not have been visible (Fremersdorf 1926: 46, fig. 2; Eckardt 2007: 229 fig. 13.5). Thus, hobnailing patterns may provide a key to some of the symbolism inherent in Roman footwear.

2.8 Spiritual shoes

Van Driel-Murray (1999a: 136) investigates other, spiritual, symbolism attached to Roman shoes. The sole of a shoe takes on the imprint of the wearer's foot, thus a shoe can function as 'a spiritual graffito' or signature. In this symbolic role, marking a physical presence and carrying the imprint of the owner's personality, footwear readily becomes a *pars pro toto*, substituting for that individual (van Driel-Murray 1999a: 136), hence its appearance on some Roman ceramic building materials.

Many Roman shoes in wells are part of the final fill of domestic refuse but, now that footwear can be dated independently, some shoes can be linked to ritual activity. According to van Driel-Murray (1999a: 137), some footwear found at the bottom of wells can be dated to the period of construction and therefore regarded as foundation offerings. Shoes have even been found behind the wooden construction of wells (van Driel-Murray 2011a: 337). Van Driel-Murray explains that, because they link people to the earth, 'shoes are ... appropriate offerings to chthonic forces, especially in ... commencement rituals for sources of water where a living sacrifice would be literally polluting' (van Driel-Murray 1999a: 137).

2.9 Other foot-related research

Tiles bearing footprints as a kind of signature have been mentioned above. Richlin (2014) discusses a tile from a temple in Pietrabbondante which carries the hobnailed footprints of two female slaves (or possibly freedwomen), accompanied by inscriptions in two languages, Oscan and Latin (Figure 8.31). This is rare evidence for Roman women, slaves, and literacy (Richlin 2014: 2). Wallace-Hadrill (2008: 90) points out that the tile was high in the temple roof, where nobody could see it. Imprinting tiles was one method by which ordinary people could stamp their identity on high-status buildings. There are many instances of intentional Roman footprints in roof tiles and concrete but little research into this phenomenon as yet (see Chapter 8).

The idea of the foot as a marker for identity extends into foot-shaped stamp matrices. Like prints in tiles, these copper alloy stamps from across the empire are under-researched, appearing merely in general discussions of this type of artefact.

Some research has been carried out into *planta pedis* carvings in Roman temples. Dunbabin (1990: 88) concludes that these marble 'footprints' can stand in place of the deity being worshipped or the worshipper. As in many cases, here the footprints stand *pars pro toto*, either for the human or for the divine (Dunbabin 1990: 86). Dunbabin (1990: 88) also alludes to the healing power of the divine foot.

Images of sandals occur in secular surroundings, for example on mosaics in Roman baths, where they bear a 'multivalent interpretation' (Dunbabin 1990: 101). They may be a reminder to wear sandals to protect the feet from hot floors (Dunbabin 1990: 101). They might convey the luxury and comfort associated with bathing (Dunbabin 1990: 101). They could even perform an apotropaic function (Dunbabin 1990: 101), especially when placed at the entrance (Dunbabin 1990: 102). Indeed, sandal images with this significance are found at entrances in buildings which have no connection with bathing or hypocausts (Dunbabin 1990: 102). However, like much research into Roman foot symbolism, the *planta pedis* phenomenon does not appear to have been linked to actual footprints in Roman tiles.

The sandal *fibula* (see Chapter 7) presents another version of nailed soles. These are the most common skeuomorphic design of Roman plate brooches, and the second most common design of plate brooches after the horse and rider (Croom 2018: 303). Research into these artefacts is mostly confined to catalogues of different brooch types from across the north-western provinces (for example: Feugère 1985: 376–380; Mackreth 2011: 167–168; 179).

Crummy (2007: 227) hypothesizes that sandal fibulae show an allegiance to Mercury and 'can be interpreted as the human, pedestrian form of his divine flying footwear'. Eckardt (2013: 221) agrees that there is a possible association with Mercury. Crummy (2007: 227) also comments that the popularity of shoe brooches may be because their simplicity made them cheaper to produce.

Eckardt discusses 63 shoe brooches known from Britain. She considers the possible symbolism of sandal *fibulae*, suggesting they may have been lucky charms, commemorated a journey or provided protection through the journey of life (Eckardt 2013: 217), but does not consider the possibilities of group identity, fashion or fun. Unusually, Eckardt (2013: 228–229) discusses some other shoe-shaped artefacts such as jugs and lamps, pointing out that no full survey of this material has been attempted (Eckardt 2013: 229). This study tries to rectify that.

Croom's chapter about the shoe brooch from Arbeia (2018) discusses their geographical and social distribution and their symbolism along similar lines to Eckardt. Since the right was considered lucky in the Roman world, one might expect a preference for right-footed shoe brooches. However, both Croom and Eckardt point out that there is no pronounced partiality for right or left feet (Eckardt 2013: 221; Croom 2018: 306).

2.10 Conclusions

This chapter presented and summarized a range of ancient written evidence for the significance of Roman footwear. It also examined scholarly studies of Roman shoes and artefacts representing feet and footwear, noting a paucity in this area of study. The main problem with research into the significance of Roman feet and footwear is that most studies only consider one side of the coin. The evidence for footwear tends to come either from art or from archaeology. As early as 1980, Rhodes commented:

'A more comprehensive and exacting reconsideration of the textual references and artistic representations of Roman footwear is necessary in the light of the growing number of shoe-finds from the northern Roman provinces.' (Rhodes 1980: 102)

Until very recently, this was not even attempted. Art can provide information on areas of footwear where gaps exist in the archaeological record (Harlow and Nosch 2014: 8) and gives at least some idea of what people wore (Larsson-Lovén 2014: 261). Archaeology can show what people really wore, but only in certain areas of the Roman Empire and not for all types of footwear. Both of these disciplines need to be considered together if we are to gain a more nuanced picture of shoes and status.

A similar dichotomy exists for related artefacts. There are many studies of Roman lamps and brooches, for example, yet specific studies of foot- or shoe-shaped artefacts are rare. Osteoarchaeologists have reported on skeletons, but studies of Roman feet that were buried in shoes are uncommon. Thus, we see that Roman calceology lacks a cohesive study which combines different aspects of the evidence to produce a comprehensive picture of the ideological significance of feet in the Roman world.

3

The point of Roman hobnailing

This chapter examines the significance of Roman hobnailing from different perspectives. It is included because of the symbolism found in actual Roman hobnailing patterns, and because representations of hobnailing are common on shoe-shaped artefacts, so it is necessary to establish their significance. The chapter considers what we can learn from Roman hobnailing and its categorisation, for example, the dating of footwear, and information about the wearer's age, gender and occupation. It also explores what Roman hobnailed footwear might have meant to the people who wore it, and how hobnailing was related to the construction and presentation of identities in the north-western provinces. The study will cover how hobnailing affected the wearer's gait, stance and *habitus*, and how it was used to express aspects of self-presentation, fashion and spiritual beliefs.

3.1 Background to Roman hobnailing

Hobnailing was one shoe-making technology that made Roman footwear very different from the footwear of Iron Age communities (van Driel-Murray 2016: 141). It was an intrinsic part of footwear construction, attaching the sole to the upper and, by protecting the sole from wear, prolonged the life of shoes (van Driel-Murray 2016:141), one of the qualities which may have made this new aspect of footwear popular across the north-western provinces.

Only certain types of Roman footwear had nailed soles: military boots, especially *caligae*; closed shoes, or *calcei*; and sandals. This method of manufacturing footwear was originally imported from the Mediterranean area and was probably spread across the north-western provinces by military shoemakers (van Driel-Murray 2016: 140). Some other types of Roman footwear have been found with nails, but this is exceptional. Shoes made from one piece of leather, *carbatinae*, are not usually nailed because they are constructed from a single piece of leather and have no layers of sole to protect the foot. Although a few examples have been reinforced with a nailed sole, it is not always clear if this is original or if an old nailed sole was used to repair a worn *carbatina* (van Driel-Murray 2011a: 352).

Wooden pattens found in the vicinity of a bathhouse, such as Heerlen in the Netherlands, the Saalburg (Busch 1965: plate 30), or Vindolanda (van Driel-Murray 1993: plate V), were intended to protect the feet from hot floors and are generally not nailed. These are often finely carved and some show depressions carved for the toes (Figure 3.1). However, nailed soles have been found on coarser wooden shoes which may have been worn by people who worked in dirty conditions (van Driel-Murray 2011a: 358) such as the farm labourers referred to by Cato (*Agr*.13.2).

Nailed Roman shoes are international in character (van Driel-Murray 2001a: 191) and show little regional variation in style (van Driel-Murray 2011a: 342). There are, however, some regional differences in hobnailing on Roman footwear. Although the archaeological evidence is poor, civilian footwear in the Mediterranean and Egypt seems to have been generally soft soled (van Driel-Murray 2011a: 345). There was a marked preference for one-piece shoes (*carbatinae*) in Germania (van Driel-Murray 2016: 132).

Not all kinds of heavy-duty footwear have nailed soles (van Driel-Murray 2016: 140–141). Hobnailing is absent on later military boots from Egypt because nailing was unsuitable for the environment, being awkward on rocky terrain (van Driel-Murray 1999b: 174). The consequences

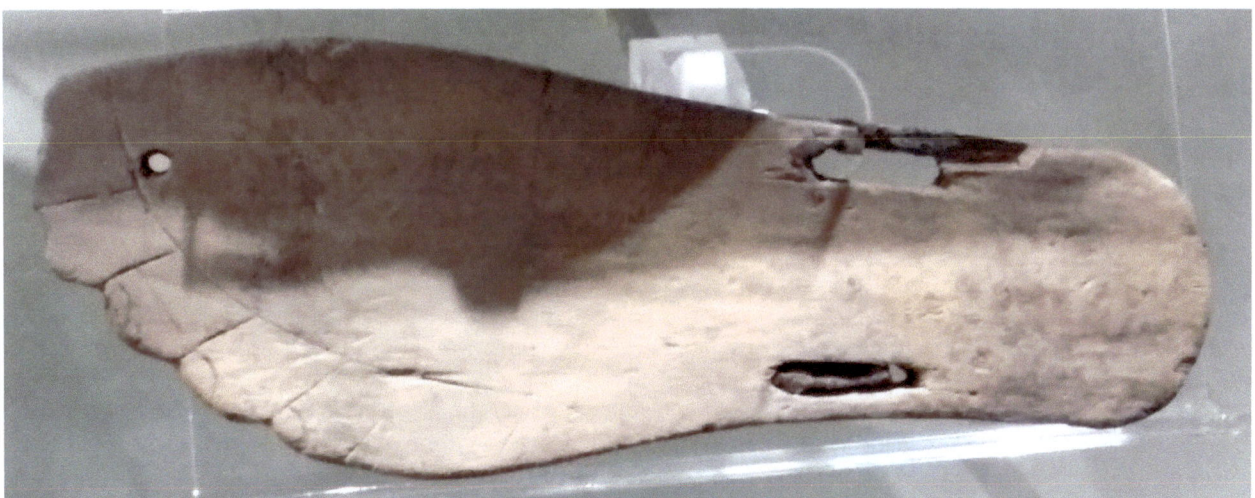

Figure 3.1: Sculponea from Vindolanda. (Photo: Author's own).

of *caliga* nails slipping on stone surfaces are reported by Josephus (*BJ*.6.1.8). Julianus, a centurion storming the temple in Jerusalem, slipped on the marble pavement because of his 'shoes thickly studded with sharp nails' and was killed. Nevertheless, north of the Alps, shoes and sandals with nailed soles are the norm (van Driel-Murray 2016: 141), possibly because the climate called for better grip, so the popularity of hobnailing might include an environmental factor.

Hobnails were available separately from shoes, as recorded on writing tablets from Vindolanda. One records 100 nails for boots (*caligares*) being supplied to one Gracilis at a cost of 2 asses (Tab.Vindol.II.186: 7–8). Another tablet documents nails supplied for different types of footwear: 350 boot-nails (*clavi caligares*) for Taurinus; 25 nails for the sandals (*calciamentis*) of Tetricus; 20 for some shoes (*galliculis*); and 30 for the *campagones* of Prudentius (Tab.Vindol.III.604). Taurinus is also named in Tab. Vindol.III.605 with regard to shoe nails and was, perhaps, a shoemaker. Diocletian's *Maximum prices edict* lists workmen's boots (IX.5a) and soldiers' boots (IX.6) without nails. So we see that the separate purchase of hobnails was necessary because some footwear was supplied without nails. Nails also worked loose and fell out due to wear, causing the footwear to need re-nailing (van Driel-Murray 1993: 33; see also 2011a: 365).

3.2 The significance of Roman hobnailing for archaeologists

Because of the specific environmental conditions needed for leather to survive archaeologically, hobnails are frequently all that remains of Roman footwear. Their presence shows that an item of Roman footwear was there and, as Burandt's research shows (2016: 15), may indicate which type of shoe it was. This is one reason why the careful recording and excavation of hobnails is advocated (le Forestier 2013: 164 and 178; van Driel-Murray 2011a: 352). This is demonstrated by the ornate nailing patterns shown up by the unpublished x-ray of a soil block containing hobnails from a burial, an image of which can be seen in the Museum of London (Figure 3.2). Another reason is that, in the absence of organic survivals, hobnails form the only evidence for the role of footwear in burial rituals (van Driel-Murray 1999a: 132). Lastly, the correlation between nailing and shoe-size, gives some indication of the age and gender of the wearer, and the wearer's occupation. Some scholars have also suggested that the size of nails used may be an indicator of gender, with finer nails being used for women's shoes (Gansser-Burckhardt 1942: 66; Fremersdorf 1926: 46). It is also possible, however, that different weights of nail were used for different types of footwear (for example Tab.Vindol. III.604). Göpfrich (1986: 15) comments that, on some of the finds from Mainz, two different sizes of nail were used on the same shoe, those used for construction being larger than those used to stud the sole. Van Driel-Murray (2002b: 119) also notes smaller nails in third-century elaborate nailing patterns.

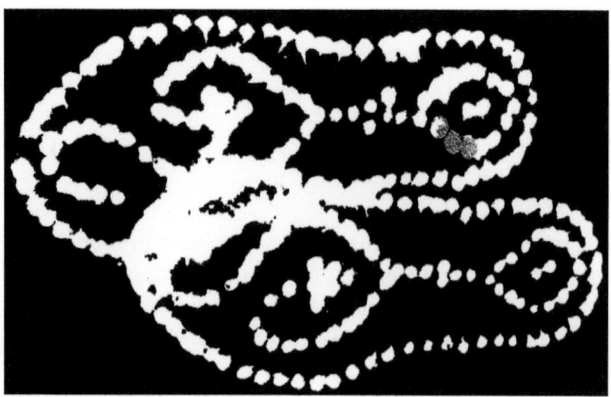

Figure 3.2: X-ray of hobnails. (Photo: Author's own).

Because the rapidity of change in Roman footwear fashions affects not just the uppers, but also the nailing patterns (van Driel-Murray 2002b: 116), these can be useful in dating shoes, and may therefore constitute valuable independent dating evidence (van Driel-Murray 1999a: 132). Circle and cross patterns occur with D-shapes on *caligae* from early sites, such as Kalkriese, Velsen, Valkenburg, Xanten, and even as footprints in the tiles made at Dormagen (van Driel-Murray 1999b: 171). However, *caligae* disappear from the archaeological record by about 100 CE (van Driel-Murray 2011a: 345) and different nailing patterns appear with the subsequent military footwear-styles (van Driel-Murray 1999b: 178). The diamond arrangement in the tread, the most common pattern in London but also found elsewhere, dates to the second century (Keily 2000: 4; Rhodes 1980: 107). The tendril pattern was popular mainly in the third century (van Driel-Murray 1987: 38). S-patterns occur after 190, big asymmetrical S-shapes around 220–30, while groups of triple nails are 'characteristic of the second half of the third and early fourth centuries' (van Driel-Murray 2016: 135–136). This timeline of Roman hobnailing patterns is based on extensive research by van Driel-Murray into Roman footwear found in dated contexts. The evidence provided by Roman hobnailing should therefore be regarded as important for archaeologists.

3.2.1 Hobnailing as evidence of the wearers

Hobnailing patterns provide some evidence for their wearers' occupations. Relatively dense nailing patterns indicate people doing heavy work, such as waggoners, farmers, or men pulling barges (Burandt 2016: 12). Military shoes tended to be heavily nailed too (Rhodes 1980: 107; Busch 1965: 172; Gansser-Burckhardt 1942: 59; Keily 2000: 2). Indeed, nailing patterns in *caligae* show similarities (van Driel-Murray 1999b: 171). Rhodes suggests that similarities between the nailing patterns of *caligae* may be an indication that these boots were produced by the same workshop (1980: 103). Another possibility is that soldiers were taught how to make *caligae* (Baratta 2006: 206–207; Olson 2012: 55) by a skilled shoemaker or *sutor institor caligarius* (CIL 9.3027), who may have passed on his nailing designs.

Gender may also be indicated by some nailing patterns. Busch suggests that an S-shaped pattern indicates a woman's shoe (1965: 194; 198–199). MacConnoran claims that there is a correlation between nailing patterns and shoe-size (1986: 218) and it is now widely recognised that shoe-size is a guide to the wearer's age and gender (van Driel-Murray 2011a: 360–361). Heavily nailed shoes tend to be at the upper end of the size range (MacConnoran 1986: 218) and, therefore, were worn mostly by men. This is supported by le Forestier, whose work on shoes from burials in the Île de France ascertained that more nails were found in men's graves than in women's (2013: 166). This may be due to men having larger feet on average, or may show that those men had occupations which required more grip in muddy conditions. Although van Driel-Murray suggests that the correlation between heavy nailing and foot size is only slight (2011a: 351), there is still a correlation.

Burandt suggests that hobnailing pattern types may indicate footwear type (2016: 9). The relationship between hobnailing pattern and shoe type was suggested earlier by Rhodes (1980: 114). This correlation could be useful for identifying the shoe style of a find that consists merely of a sole, or even of just the hobnails *in situ*. Burandt's type A certainly seems to correspond to sandals, and type E to *caligae* (2016: 15). For example, the nails alone can tell us that the shoes in Figure 3.2 date to around 220–230 CE because of the asymmetrical S pattern (van Driel-Murray 2016: 136) and, according to Burandt's theory (2016: 15), belonged to a pair of closed shoe-boots, or *calcei*. They are not heavily nailed, so were probably not worn for heavy work. Indeed, their presence in a burial suggests that they were smart shoes.

That hobnailing patterns can indicate the type of shoe they were attached to, the approximate date of the footwear, and give some information about the wearer's occupation, age, and gender, highlights the significance of Roman hobnailing to archaeologists and calceologists. But what can we learn about the meaning of hobnailing for the people who wore the nailed footwear?

3.3 The significance of hobnailing for people in the Roman Empire

3.3.1 Hobnailing and domination

In the early imperial period, hobnailing was synonymous with military identity. One of the signs of Roman might and military supremacy was the sound of hobnails, and many scholars have commented on the 'awesome effect of the sound of thousands of hobnailed feet marching over paved roads' (van Driel-Murray 2011a: 363; see also Goldman 2001: 122; Sumner 2009: 198; Haynes 2013: 262). A law banning Jews from wearing nailed shoes (*Shabbat* 6.2) continued in operation because the noise of hobnails warned of approaching Roman soldiers (Bishop and Coulston 2006: 113). Military monuments included depictions of the nailing on footwear, for instance, the Trajanic frieze on the Arch of Constantine's central passage (Figure 3.3).

By extension, hobnailing seems to have been associated with brutality and domination. In *Satire* 3, Juvenal complains about the difficulties of walking in Rome: 'Soon I'm trampled by mighty feet from every side and a soldier's hobnail sticks into my toe' (247–248). In *Satire* 16, on the subject of the advantages of military life, Juvenal says that if a civilian seeks redress for being beaten up by a soldier, 'he gets a hobnailed boot for a judge' (13–14) that is, he will be kicked by soldiers. Later in the same satire, Juvenal points out the consequences of offending 'all those heavy boots and all those thousands of hobnails' (16.22–25).

This association would not have been unusual. Metaphors for domination to do with trampling underfoot and disrespect occur in Dio Cassius' accounts of Cleopatra (50.24.3) and how Augustus should handle the law (52.34.8). The idea of the foot as the seat of power and submission persist in reports of later emperors, for example, kissing feet as a sign of obeisance (*SHA.Max.*8.7). Nine princes of different tribes prostrated themselves at Probus' feet (*SHA.Prob.*14) and he 'put down all barbarian nations under his feet' (*SHA.Prob.*20). Some care is needed when dealing with the *Scriptores Historiae Augustae*, due to the unreliability of its sources (Rohrbacher 2016: 149) but this aspect of feet and footwear is part of a much broader cultural notion and, in this instance, the evidence can be accepted.

3.3.2 Nailing and fashion

The great variety of ornamental nailing found on Roman footwear demonstrates a very different and more positive view. Far from expressing domination, Roman nailed footwear gave ordinary people a means to show their 'individuality, taste, and style' (van Driel-Murray 2016: 133) because nailing patterns vary, depending on the type of shoe, its purpose, and the taste of the buyer (Göpfrich 1986: 15). Roman footwear was regularly embellished

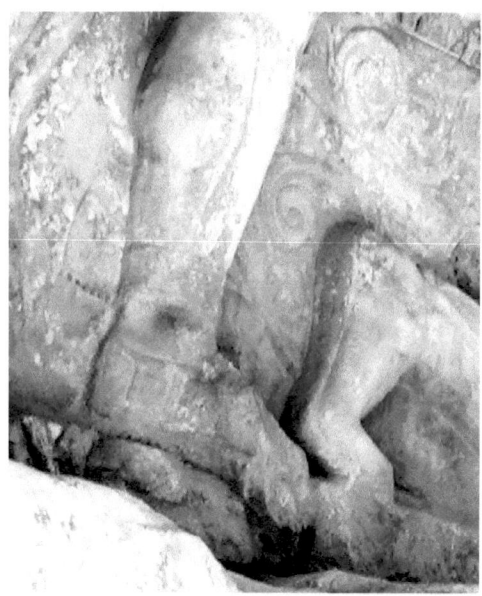

Figure 3.3: Hobnails depicted on the Arch of Constantine (Photo: Author's own.)

Roman Feet and Shoes

with elaborate, non-essential decorative patterns (van Driel-Murray 2016: 135) (see Figure 3.4). This was partly an expression of personal identity because the wearer would have been instantly identifiable by their distinctive footprints (van Driel-Murray 1999a: 132).

The popularity of the various designs changed over time and the patterns in which shoe nails are arranged are 'remarkable expressions of what might be called Zeitgeist' (van Driel-Murray 2016: 135) making nailing a fashion accessory (van Driel-Murray 1999a: 132). The possession of such fashionable goods would have given the owner a level of prestige thanks to the acquisition of cultural capital (Bourdieu 1995: 135).

Modish footwear was not confined to the better-off, urban dwellers: 'Even the workers at a remote upland cattle yard at Pontefract … aspired to fashionably pointed hobnailed boots' (van Driel-Murray 2016: 145; see also 2002b: 121 fig. 12). Fashionable hobnailing is evidence that ordinary people were prepared to spend money not just on essential items, but on 'ephemeral goods that added to the comfort of themselves and their family as well as enhancing their feelings of self-worth' (van Driel-Murray 2016: 149).

3.3.3 The cosmological side of hobnailing

The repetition of symbols in nailing patterns points to deeper personal concerns than mere fashionable decoration (van Driel Murray 1999a:138). Shoes protect travelling feet from harm, and this metaphor is extended to protection for the journey of life and into death (van Driel-Murray 1999a: 131). The idea that nailing patterns made footwear simultaneously physically and spiritually protective may be implicit in some designs. As mentioned earlier, swastikas and circles were good luck symbols (van Driel-Murray 1999a: 132). Swastikas occur fairly regularly in hobnailing patterns (van Driel-Murray 2016: 135). The Sanskrit word *svastika* translates as 'well-being, fortune, luck', and the swastika is a symbol of good fortune in Hinduism, Buddhism, and Jainism (Oxford University Press 1992). Some Latin words, such as '*ave*', have their origin in Sanskrit (Lewis and Short 1879), so some Roman ideas may have had similar origins. It is thought that a lozenge pattern with a single nail or cluster of nails inside (Figure 3.5) makes the design resemble an eye, adding an apotropaic symbol to the shoe to ward off the evil eye (Burandt 2016: 13–14). In the late third and fourth centuries, a trefoil pattern comprising groups of three nails

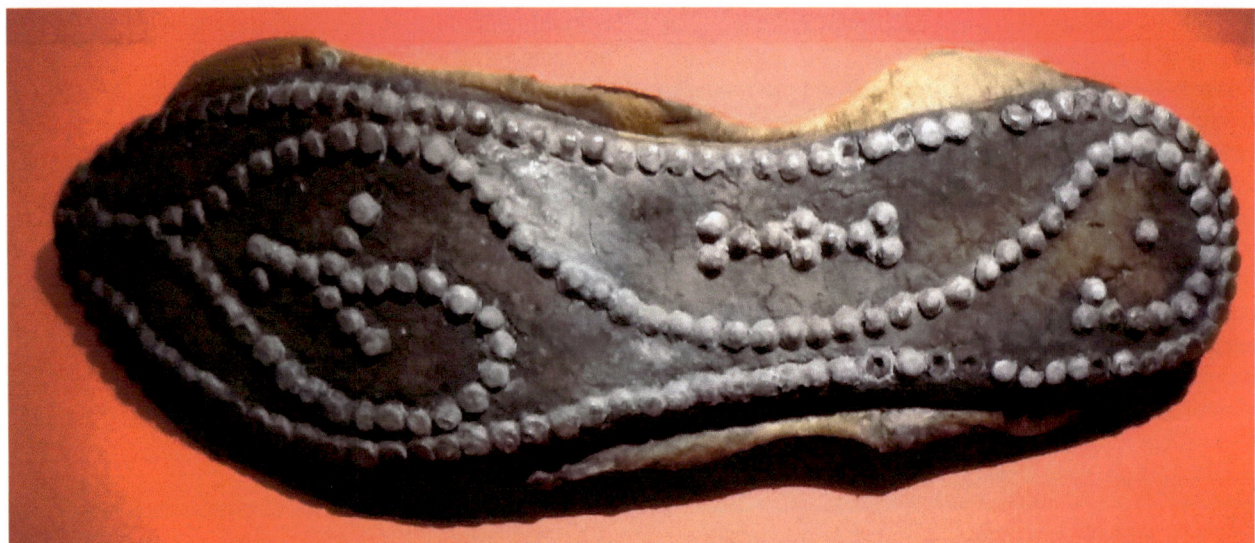

Figure 3.4: Shoe with ornate nailing pattern, Vindolanda Trust. (Photo: Author's own).

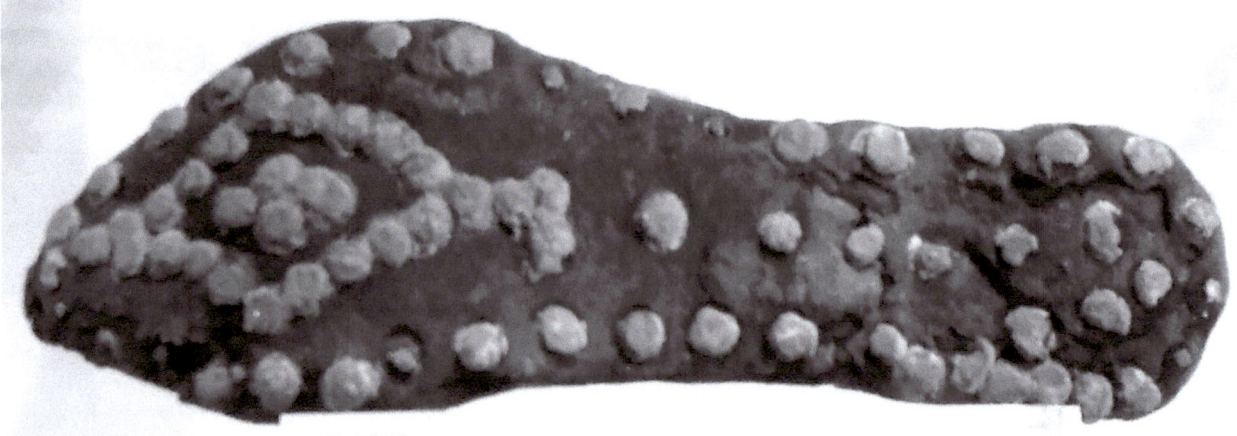

Figure 3.5: Shoe with lozenge nailing pattern, Vindolanda Trust. (Photo: Author's own).

occurs at military and civilian sites throughout the western Empire for a period of about 70 years (van Driel-Murray 2011b: 48). What the patterns signified is unknown, but the specific message communicated was evidently understood across a wide range of society (van Driel-Murray 2011b: 48), as indicated by the fact that the patterns have such general currency (van Driel-Murray 1999a: 132).

Through their nailed footprints, people could show that they were under the protection of, or committed to, a particular deity (van Driel-Murray 1999a: 132). Some Roman footwear has patterns which resemble cosmological symbols, particularly those of Pisces and Aquarius, considered to rule over the feet and legs (van Driel-Murray 2002a: 99). Sandals belonging to a third-century boatman whose ship sank are nailed with a trident for Neptune, possibly as a sign of the wearer's profession, or for 'better divine protection than they actually received' (van Driel-Murray 1999a: 132). Another symbolic association is with Mercury (van Driel-Murray 1999a: 134), who was patron of travellers (Crummy 2007: 226) and is linked with healing (Crummy 2007: 225). The relationship between nailing symbolism and protection on journeys seems entirely appropriate.

Mercury also fulfilled the role of psychopomp, guiding the souls of the dead into the Underworld. Nailed footwear is found in burials and the exact position of the nails shows whether the shoes were being worn by the deceased or were placed in the grave as a symbol of preparation for the afterlife (van Driel-Murray 2011a: 352). In the Île de France, a woman was buried with shoes by her right hip (le Forestier 2013: 171). The soles have S and lozenge nailing patterns (le Forestier 2013: 173 Figs. 9a and e), which may have been to protect her on her last journey. Thus, hobnails in Roman burials are to do with the spiritual preparedness of the dead (van Driel-Murray 1999a: 131).

3.4 Hobnailing and group identity

One of the major debates around Roman material culture in the north-western provinces is how far the use of Roman objects, including footwear, denotes acceptance of 'the full gamut of Roman values' (Webster 2001: 217). Because nailed footwear was a distinctly Roman product (van Driel-Murray 2002b: 119), it has been linked to defining a 'Roman' identity (van Driel-Murray 2011a: 360). Van Driel-Murray (2002a: 101) is 'increasingly sceptical of the tendency to regard Roman provincial culture as little more than a thin veneer, covering an essentially unchanged native society underneath' and considers Roman-style nailed footwear as a visible symbol of a 'personal commitment to the new order' (van Driel-Murray 2011a: 350).

Certainly, wearing close fitting, rigid shoes would have affected the person's stance and gait (van Driel-Murray 2002b: 119), which would have changed the wearer's *habitus*. Initially, walking on Roman nailed soles would have felt very different compared with wearing un-nailed Iron Age footwear, and would have taken some time to become accustomed to. However, this situation surely only applies to the first pair of nailed footwear that a person in a recently conquered province wore. By the second century, Roman-style nailed footwear must have become the norm and there may no longer have been any change in gait.

Van Driel-Murray (2016: 145) also argues that people chose their footwear for many different reasons and that this may rather illustrate a sense of community, within which personal display was negotiable. This is more in keeping with current ideas that provincial artefacts may appear Romanized but can, in certain contexts, likewise operate according to a 'different, indigenous, set of underlying rules' (Webster 2002: 219). It is now widely recognised that dress, including footwear, can express many facets of identity simultaneously and be actively manipulated 'to provide a unique insight into the complex cultural processes at work within a provincial population' (Rothe 2009: 2). We should be more alert to 'the potentially heterogeneous and discrepant local responses to imperial Roman domination' (Eckardt 2002: 26) and, rather than use terms such as 'Romanized', or 'indigenous', refer to local, regional, or provincial practices.

One example is a shoe (Figure 3.6) found in the *praetorium* at Vindolanda which has a nailed sole, although it belonged to a baby who was too young to walk (Greene 2014: 32). The infant needed neither the protection, nor the grip, provided by the hobnails, which suggests a deeper significance to hobnailing. How far the nailed shoe signals the child's *Romanitas* is difficult to judge. It is, however, a visual statement of its status as the child of a high-ranking officer, and suggests that the baby had a role in the public appearance of the family (Greene 2014: 32). Half the children's shoes excavated from this period at Vindolanda are plain *carbatinae* (Greene 2014: 32) so, given the cost of the shoe due to the amount of skill and labour necessary to produce the 'fishnet' upper (van Driel-Murray 2011a: 342), this tiny, nailed shoe probably stood more for rank and wealth than for Roman affiliation.

Barthes (1993: 13) says that dress signifies the extent to which the wearer (whether a group or individual) participates in the system and this must surely apply to fashionable Roman footwear. It is impossible to tell, however, whether this would mean participation in the Roman Empire and all it stood for, or participation in the local community and its values. Identity is a complex social construct which is significant at all scales of social organization (Collins 2008: 45) and Roman footwear can only show us aspects of identity which are evolving, complicated, and interwoven with local, regional and Empire-wide customs and practices (Eckardt 2014: 208). The answer probably lies somewhere different on the spectrum for each individual.

Roman Feet and Shoes

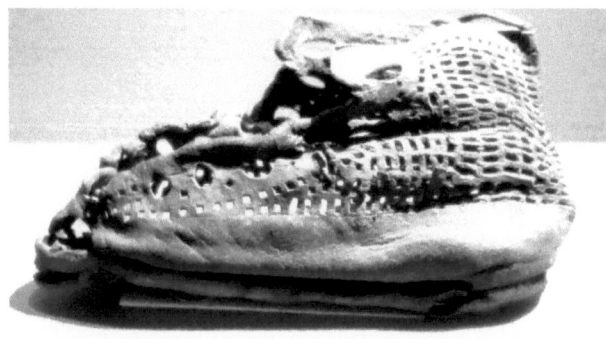

Figure 3.6: Baby's nailed shoe, Vindolanda Trust. (Photo: Author's own).

3.5 Hobnailing in iconography

A variety of ornamental objects includes depictions of Roman hobnailing which may point to its social and cosmological significance. As can be seen from hobnailed footprints on some Roman ceramic building materials (see Chapter 8), nailing patterns became a sort of signature, a statement of personal identity (van Driel-Murray 1999a: 132). Roman artefacts with hobnailing iconography may share similar meanings to actual footwear.

Roman lamps in the shape of feet wearing sandals often feature hobnailed soles, even those made to sit on a surface where the nailing pattern would not show. A Roman footlamp in the Museum of London has an ornate nailing design similar to that on real footwear (see Figures 6:29 and 6:30). Fremersdorf uses three examples of footlamps from Cologne (1926: 46 fig. 2) to illustrate hobnailing patterns. One of these (Figure 6.31) has the name of the maker, Vitalis, picked out in nails (van Driel-Murray 1999a: 133). A flask in the Louvre (MNB 468), sometimes described as a lamp (Forrer 1942: 86–87: van Driel-Murray 1999a: 133), has the Greek for 'follow me' on the sole in nails (Figure 3.7). A shoe-shaped lamp from Mainz has a similar hobnailed inscription (Bond 2014).

A pair of glass oil flasks (see Figure 5.29) in the shape of sandals, from a third-century woman's burial in Cologne, also features a row of hobnails around the rim of the soles. Again, this is only visible when the objects are being carried. Possibly the nailing had amuletic qualities. The artefacts are also symbols of the luxury and comfort associated with Roman bathing (Dunbabin 1990: 101), so we again see hobnailing coupled with statements of identity. That artefacts were produced with depictions of nails which could not be seen under normal circumstances, must at least demonstrate a fascination with Roman hobnailing, if not its ideological importance.

3.6 Conclusions

This chapter has highlighted the various significances of Roman hobnailing, including its archaeological importance, and its ancient symbolism. Roman hobnailing is important nowadays because it can provide us with information about the identity and beliefs of the person whose shoes it adorned, even when the leather footwear has decayed. It is doubly important because it can give us access to aspects of the lives of people who are otherwise invisible, such as women, children, and the less well-off.

Care should, of course, be taken with all studies of Roman material culture, and hobnailing is no exception, as Gansser-Burckhardt's now discredited identification of nailing patterns for club-feet demonstrates (1942: 68–73). We cannot know the actual meaning of the symbolism, or the methods by which this knowledge was communicated. Nailing patterns which depict cosmological symbols, such as Neptune's trident, are more easily interpreted than S-shaped patterns.

Nevertheless, it is clear that Roman hobnailing was used as a means of communication and the symbolism would have been generally accepted and recognized (van Driel-Murray 1999a: 132; Olson 2008: 6). Since nailing patterns left very characteristic footprints, they became a statement of personal identity, a sort of signature (van Driel-Murray 1999a: 132). The Romans appear to have been proud to be identified as individuals by their footprints (van Driel-Murray 199a:133). Shoes protect feet from harm and so, by extension, hobnailing patterns may have played an apotropaic role, even in artefacts. Wearing shoes with fashionable nailed designs would also have brought personal prestige and signalled membership of a particular circle. Hobnailing is certainly bound up with Roman military identity. All of these attributes show that hobnailing was socially and cosmologically very important in the Roman Empire. It is, therefore, unsurprising that many artefacts feature representations of hobnailing.

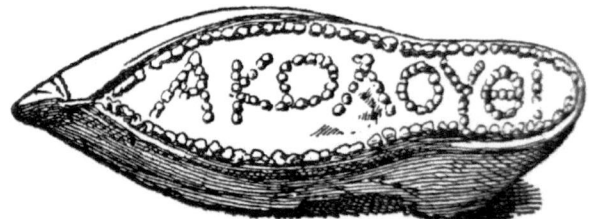

Figure 3.7: Flask or lamp with hobnailed inscription 'follow me' in Greek. (Forrer 1942: 86 fig.22).

4

The social significance of deposited Roman footwear

This chapter considers what the deposition of footwear in Roman graves and wells may tell us about its social significance, at least in the north-western provinces of the Roman Empire. This case study was chosen because it illustrates the various levels of meaning and symbolism attributed to actual Roman shoes, which it is necessary to establish before going on to discuss the social significance of Roman foot- and shoe-shaped artefacts.

One difficulty with investigating the deposition of footwear is evidentiary bias caused, above all, by problems of archaeological survival. Frequently the only evidence that remains of Roman footwear is fragments of leather or, more usually, hobnails. The lack of evidence is complicated by the fact that not all Roman footwear was nailed, and sewn footwear tends to decay without trace (Clarke 1979: 322; van Driel-Murray 1999a: 137; le Forestier 2013: 181). However, enough does survive to make this a worthwhile study.

A further problem is how to recognise ritual. While markers for ritual or structured deposition are discussed later in this chapter, it would be useful to have some kind of overall definition to work with. Merrifield (1987: 6) describes ritual as:

> Prescribed or customary behaviour that may be religious, if it is intended to placate or win the favour of supernatural beings, magical if it is intended to operate through impersonal forces of sympathy or by controlling supernatural beings, or social, if its purpose is to reinforce a social organisation or facilitate social intercourse.

This is not a very recent definition of ritual, but these are difficult to find. Some later scholars claim that it is impossible to devise a satisfactory universal definition of ritual (Hill 1995: 101; Brück 1999: 314) and hence do not. Others cite Merrifield's (Fulford 2001: 200; Cool and Richardson 2013: 191). This, therefore, seems a reasonable starting point, as it identifies and defines three possible strands of ritual behaviour.

Ritualised activity is fairly obvious in Roman funerary customs, but much more difficult to identify in the fill of wells. This chapter will therefore begin by considering the evidence for funerary ritual involving the deposition of shoes and what this may have signified. It argues that Roman footwear may have been chosen as grave furniture because it displays the identity and social standing of the deceased and their mourners. It will also demonstrate that Roman shoes had a spiritual dimension: the protection offered to the feet by shoes became a metaphor for other kinds of protection, and the fact that worn Roman footwear retained the imprint of its wearer's foot made it an appropriate substitute for the person (van Driel-Murray 1999a: 136).

Another setting in which Roman footwear is deposited is the fill of wells. The interpretation of this phenomenon is complicated. However, this section considers how common the phenomenon of Roman footwear deposited in wells is. It then discusses 'structured' or 'ritual' deposits, and whether and how we can distinguish ritual deposition from rubbish. It explores how far the deposition of Roman shoes in wells can be interpreted as having some ritual significance. The lifecycle of Roman wells (van Haasteren and Groot 2013) is associated with ritual practice, and footwear with a different date from a well's backfill may form part of the same ritual activity as the more obvious ritual items (van Driel-Murray 1999a: 137). The chapter goes on to investigate the votive use of footwear in wells, and tests the theory that it was mainly left shoes that were used for this purpose. Finally, there is a discussion of why shoes were considered appropriate ritual deposits.

This study expects to identify different ritual settings for the deposition of shoes, social, religious and apotropaic, or 'magic'. It also expects to find that not all footwear deposits were ritual in nature, and that individual beliefs probably varied.

4.1 The deposition of Roman footwear in graves

Shoes in Roman burials undoubtedly form part of rituals surrounding the treatment of the dead. Footwear worn by the deceased can be regarded as ritual because there is no necessity to dress a corpse. There is also much evidence of shoes having been placed in and around the tomb, rather than being worn by the deceased.

As with the evidence for Roman shoes elsewhere, it is usually only the ironwork that survives (Pearce 2016: 458), be it hobnails or shoe cleats, although some leather footwear has been found in burials with the right environmental conditions, for example, at Boscombe Down (Wessex Archaeology 2018). The lack of evidence for footwear in graves does not mean that the deceased were not wearing shoes: not all Roman footwear was nailed, and sewn leather footwear usually leaves no easily discernible archaeological trace (Paresys et al. 2016: 30, note 6; Clarke 1979: 322). However a dark soil stain in grave 12111 at Pepper Hill, Kent, may be the decayed remains of unnailed shoes (Biddulph and Booth 2006: 47), and similar staining is noted at Butt Road, Colchester (Crummy et al. 1993: 129). It has been argued by some

French scholars that the way in which the foot-bones fall in the grave is affected if the deceased was wearing shoes (le Forestier 2013: 182; Gaultier *et al.* 2009: 84). Le Forestier (2013: 182) recommends a careful taphonomic analysis in order to understand the relationships between the subject's foot and shoe during their decomposition. This only helps to identify footwear in Roman graves if the deceased was wearing the shoes.

In order to examine the proportion of Roman burials with shoes, whether the shoes were worn or placed, and to what extent the practice changed over time, this study conducted a statistical analysis of 186 funerary sites with a total of 18,465 graves where a known amount of footwear was found. The data were obtained from the Rural Settlement of Roman Britain project (RSRB), from Philpott's study in cases where his data could be verified, from reports such as Clarke's and Booth's works on the Roman cemeteries at Lankhills, and from le Forestier's report on the Île de France. The data were checked carefully to ensure that the evidence of footwear was in the burials and not in other features on the same site. Of the 18,465 burials, 1,756 (9.5%) contained evidence of footwear. This is an average; percentages vary across the time periods when the cemeteries were in use (Table 4.1; see also Figure 4.2).

The 186 sites are not exhaustive: Pearce found 1112 Romano-British burial sites recorded between 1921 and 2010 (2016: 448 table 2); the 186 Romano-British burial sites with evidence of footwear known to this study represent 15% of Pearce's total. Philpott includes 60 more British sites with 64 graves, le Forestier an additional 26 French sites, and Gaultier *et al.* a further 36 French sites with 192 graves. These have not been included in the statistical analysis because the data were incomplete or could not be verified by this study.

In cremation burials hobnails are sometimes included with pyre debris, and sometimes come from placed shoes. In the case of hobnails mixed in with ashes, it is unclear whether or not the hobnails were included deliberately (Philpott 1991: 166). It is possible that a few nails were placed in a grave as a symbol of a pair of shoes (Turner 1990: 76). Shoes could be placed anywhere in a cremation grave, for example, at Skeleton Green, some of the footwear was found next to the flagon and urn (BXIII, Partridge 1981: 259 fig. 99), either side of the urn (BXXIX, Partridge 1981: 260 fig. 100), and on top of a Samian dish (BXXXV, Partridge 1981: 262 fig.101). The provision of intact shoes in cremations with other furniture shows footwear was considered a desirable grave offering (Philpott 1991: 166).

In many instances the hobnails discovered in inhumations were found near the feet, but not necessarily on the feet, meaning that, in many Roman inhumations, shoes were placed rather than worn (Philpott 1991: 168; Böhme 1974: 131; Stead *et al.* 2006: 95). Occasionally footwear was deposited in unusual places, for instance, the cemetery at Kelvedon (Rodwell 1988: microfiche 1.A4), and the peripheral cemetery at Poundbury (Farwell *et al.* 1993: 99 table 9.7), each contain a burial with hobnails by the deceased's head. Marsh Leys burial G83 has evidence of 3 groups of hobnails near the skull (Luke and Preece 2011a: 55). In grave one at Mucking cemetery 1b, the shoes were placed above the knees on top of the coffin (Evans and Lucy 2008). There are instances of more than one pair of shoes being deposited in some graves: grave 277 at Butt Road, Colchester contained two pairs (Crummy 1983: 42), as did grave 39 at Kelvedon (Rodwell 1988: 73). There is even evidence of single shoes being placed in graves. At least four graves at Pepper Hill, Kent, only yielded enough hobnails to represent one shoe, and it is suggested these were offerings from mourners (Biddulph and Booth 2006: 59). The excavation in Bonneuil-en-France of a group of eight Gallo-Roman graves dating to the third century revealed one where five shoes were tucked down by a woman's right hip (le Forestier 2013: 170). Five is a strange number for shoes, which are usually worn in pairs, and le Forestier (2013: 170) suggests that originally six were deposited, but one may have been removed while stripping the levels. Le Forestier (2013: 174) claims that there are two pairs of shoes in this grave, and this is possible considering the similarity in styles. However, although the hobnailing patterns for shoes C and D match, there is a marked difference between shoes A (Figure 4.1a), with an S-pattern, and E (Figure 4.1b), which has a diamond design (le Forestier 2013: 173. fig. 9), making it unlikely that this was a pair, as hobnailing patterns seem to have been produced in pairs (see Figure 3.2), and making it more likely that D was a single shoe. This may be a version of the votive use of single shoes seen in Roman wells.

Table 4.1: The percentage of Roman graves containing footwear for each time period.

Period cemeteries active	C1-C1	C1-C2	C1-C3	C1-C4	C1-C5	C2-C2	C2-C3	C2-C4	C2-C5	C3-C3	C3-C4	C3-C5	C4-C4	C4-C5
Total no. graves	186	500	372	2302	1002	8	1034	7454	91	79	3018	91	1999	279
No. graves with footwear	4	83	56	169	89	3	168	298	53	11	302	16	451	53
% graves with footwear	2.2	16.6	15	7.34	8.88	37.5	16.25	4	58.24	13.92	10	17.6	22.6	19.2

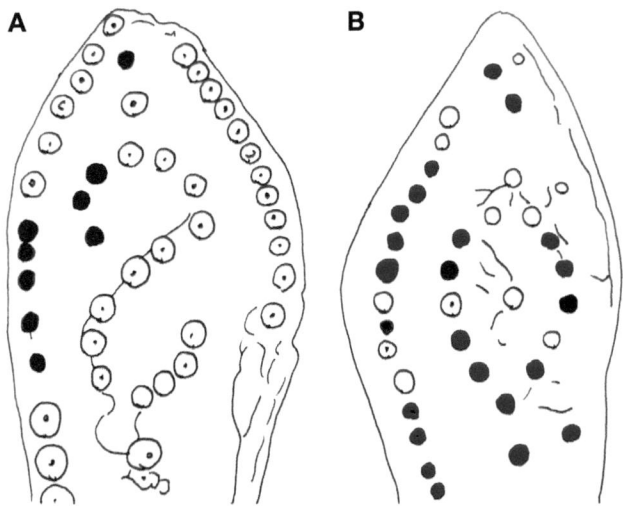

Figure 4.1: a) Bonneuil-en-France shoe A; b) Bonneuil-en-France shoe E.

The 186 funerary sites in this study show a continuation of the Roman practice of depositing shoes in graves from the first century to the fifth (Figure 4.2). The earliest known examples of Romano-British cremation burials with hobnails come from King Harry Lane, Verulamium, and date to 40–60 CE (Philpott 1991: 165). Early Romano-British inhumations with footwear are Sutton Poyntz, Dorset, found with mid first- to early second-century pottery (Philpott 1991: 167). Other early sites with evidence of shoes include two Durotrigan burials at Alington Avenue, Dorchester, dated 75–125 CE (Davies *et al.* 2002: 124) and Neatham, dated 50–100 CE (Philpott 1991: 165). Inhumations with Roman footwear become more frequent in the second and third centuries (Philpott 1991: 167) and the practice peaks in the fourth century before declining (Armour *et al.* 2007: 102: van Driel-Murray 2011a: 345). This may be due to a change in burial practices, or to a change in footwear fashion where fewer nailed shoes were worn (van Driel-Murray 2011a: 345).

In terms of regionality (Figure 4.3), the prevailing view seems to be that the deposition of footwear in Roman period graves was a custom of Iron Age origin. Leech *et al.* (1981: 199) argue that, because the deposition of shoes apparently does not occur in Mediterranean lands, it could be associated with burial customs 'exclusive to the Celtic world'. Watts (1993: 197) is of the same opinion. While Philpott (1991: 170) cites Leech *et al.*, he points out that, in addition to the burials with shoes found in France, Germany, Belgium, and the Netherlands, there is evidence of the practice from ancient Greece. It is possible that footwear does not show archaeologically in the Mediterranean area of the Roman Empire because hobnailing was less prevalent there (van Driel-Murray 2016: 140–141).

However, this study has found evidence of nailed footwear deposited in Roman graves in Italy, for example at Vagnari in Puglia (Prowse and Small 2009: 7, Table 1). There are also records of hobnails found in Roman burials in Milan (Palumbo 2001: 130). Finds of hobnails in Roman graves are quite common in Italy's alpine area, and there have been some from the south of Italy (Palumbo 2001: 131). This implies that the practice of depositing shoes in Roman burials was not limited to the north-western provinces and, therefore, may have been a Roman phenomenon that spread, like Roman footwear.

4.1.1 Why deposit shoes in graves?

The answer to this question may simply be that their owner liked them (Clarke 1979: 407). The shoes may have been chosen by mourners as a display of the deceased's and their own social standing. Some shoes in burials appear to show high status. A stone coffin found at Boscombe Down, Amesbury, contained two people who were both wearing expensive shoes. The woman's slippers had cork insoles, a fur lining and are described as luxury shoes imported from the Mediterranean. The child's shoes were calf-skin

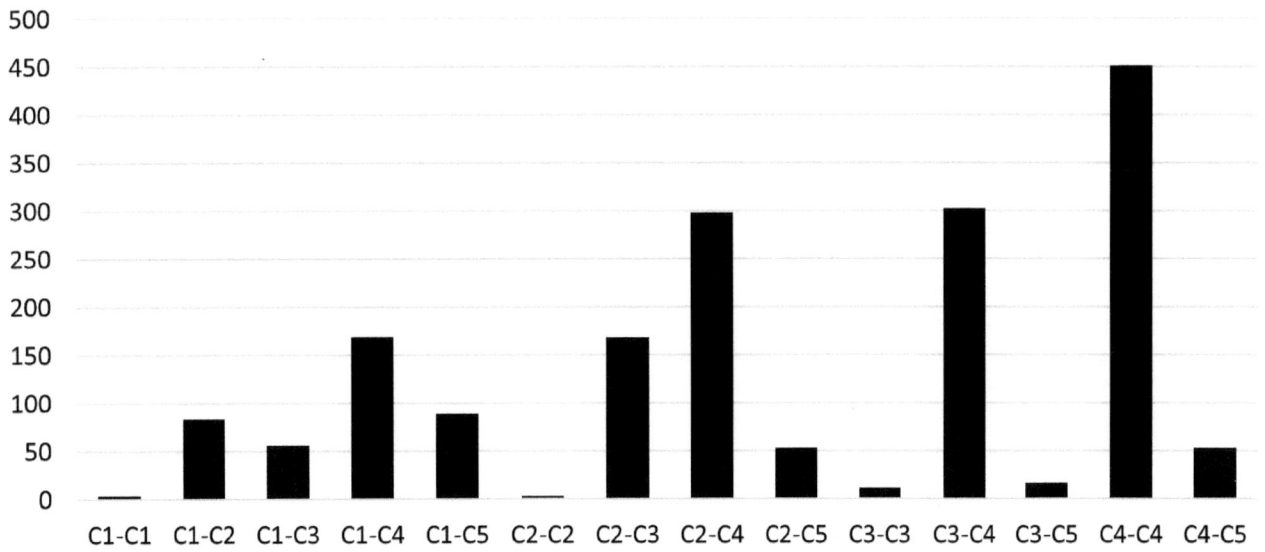

Figure 4.2: Graph to show the chronological distribution of footwear in 1,756 Roman graves.

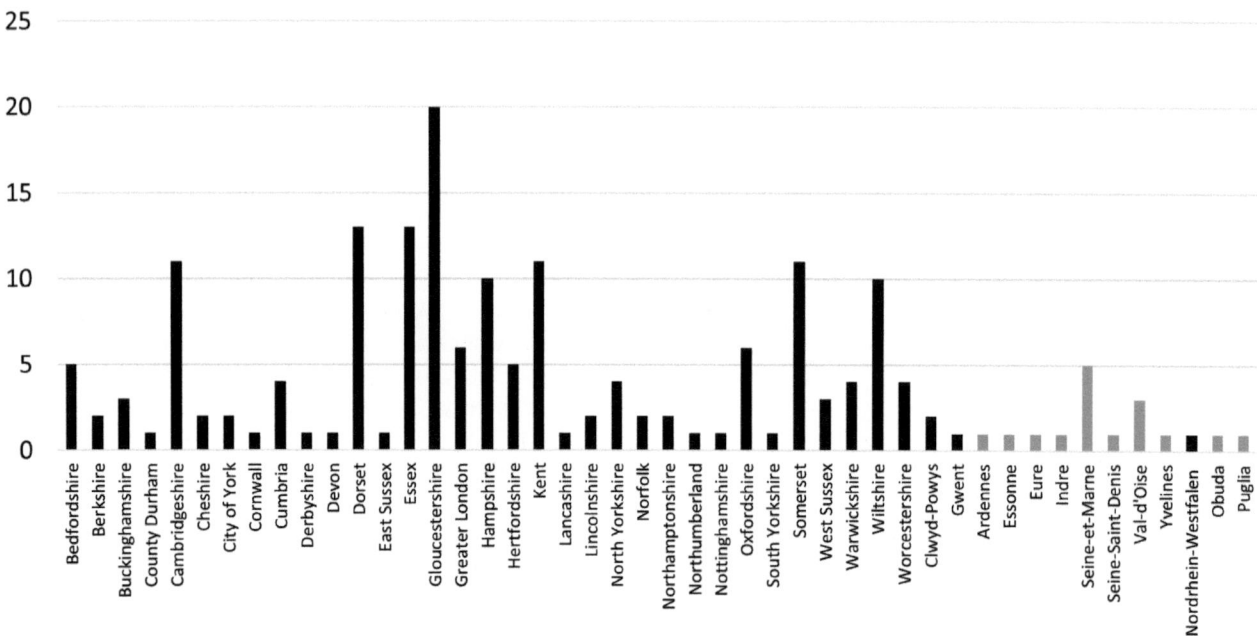

Figure 4.3: Chart to show Roman funerary sites with footwear by region.

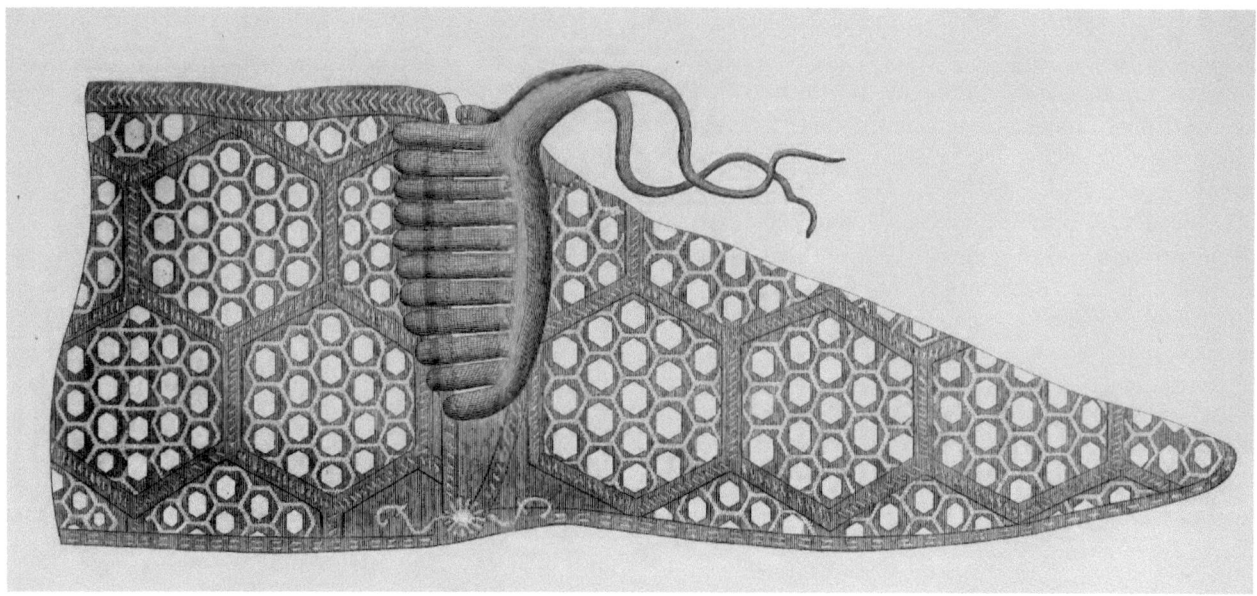

Figure 4.4: Purple and gold shoe from Southfleet. (Rashleigh, P. 1803: Pl. 39).

and unique in Britain (Wessex Archaeology 2018). A pair of shoes in a second- to third-century girl's burial at Southfleet, Kent (Figure 4.4), was purple with gold thread (van Driel-Murray 2011a: 340) and had an openwork, and therefore expensive, design (Greene 2014: 32). Slippers found in *Aquincum*, Hungary, were embossed with gold sheet depicting Medusa's head (Topál 2003: 58). These are all examples of the creation of an image of 'the 'beautiful' dead that extended aristocratic self-presentation through dress ... to the grave' (Pearce 2013: 458). The deceased's mourners were showing that they could afford to put these valuable items in the ground.

Philpott (1991: 172) argues that there is some evidence that burials with hobnails are of middle-ranking individuals due to the kind of grave furniture found with them. On the other hand, the occurrence of hobnails in Romano-British cremations is almost ubiquitous (Turner 1990:76). Hobnails are often found in burials where there are few other grave goods, for example at Clos au Duc, Evreux, where 5.8% of burials were furnished and many tombs contained isolated hobnails (Pluton *et al.* 2008: 220), and at Kelvedon, where footwear was the most common grave furniture after pottery vessels (Rodwell 1988: 47). Wait (1985: 244) suggests that lower-value offerings such as shoes may represent the activities of family-sized groups. It is therefore likely that footwear was one of the things that less-wealthy people could afford to deposit in their loved-ones' graves, as it was available to almost all social classes (van Driel-Murray 2016:132).

The number of hobnails may be a sign of the deceased's gender. Women's graves tend to contain fewer hobnails than men's (le Forestier 2013: 166; Armour *et al.* 2007: 61), possibly because women have smaller feet on average, or because men tended to have occupations which required more grip in muddy conditions.

Some children's graves contain adult-sized shoes (Philpott 1991:173), for example, the purple shoes from Southfleet (Figure 4.4). Although there are none in the late Roman cemetery at Lankhills, many children were buried with adult-sized shoes (Booth 2010: 314). At Butt Road, Colchester, no clear distinction as to age was determined for footwear in graves (Biddulph and Booth 2006: 39), although children's graves containing shoes were identified (Biddulph and Booth 2006: 40, table 2.11). This practice may be because the grieving families were expressing a wish that their child had died as an adult, or a belief that the child would enter the afterlife fully grown. It has been noted that children's graves are rarely provided with nailed footwear (le Forestier 2013: 181: Philpott 1991:167) but this does not necessarily mean that children had no deposited shoes. Unnailed *carbatinae* were popular for children (Greene 2014: 32) as they incorporated room for growth.

To examine how sex and age influenced burial with footwear, data from the Late Roman cemetery at Lankhills were used. Of 314 graves, both inhumation and cremation, 139 (44%) contained evidence of shoes. Among the inhumations, there was an equal number of adult males and females (Booth 2010: 345) but the numbers for burial with footwear are not so even: only 40 (probable) female graves contained shoes compared with 54 (probable) males. There were also 23 children and 22 indeterminate burials with footwear (Figure 4.5). Age does not appear to be a significant factor. The data also show that 38% of the burials with footwear at Lankhills did not contain any other grave goods while others contained coins, pottery, items of personal adornment and evidence of feasting.

As well as a display of identity, Roman burial practice had a strong religious component and rites were centred around a belief in the afterlife (Philpott 1991: 235). The most common interpretation for the deposition of footwear in Roman graves is as a provision for the journey to the Underworld (Philpott 1991: 238; van Driel-Murray 1999a: 131; Booth 2010: 336; Watts 1993: 211; Clarke 1979:407: Biddulph and Booth 2006: 59; Barber and Bowsher 2000:137) and this seems to be the most likely. There are, however, very few Romano-British graves that contain both shoes and coins to pay the ferryman. Only twelve cemeteries in the dataset of 186 with evidence of footwear have graves that also contain coins (Philpott 1991: 364–369). With the exception of Lankhills, the greatest number of graves with shoes and coins is four (Stanton Harcourt, Oxfordshire; Ilchester, Somerset; Woodyates, Dorset; and Infirmary Field, Chester). In Lankhills late Roman cemetery, 126 out of 332 graves contained shoes, of which only 12 had coins too (Booth 2010) while, in the earlier cemetery, just 13 out of the 151 graves with footwear also contained coins. So there appears to be no correlation between footwear provided for the journey and money to pay the fare.

Roman footwear has been linked to Mercury (Crummy 2007: 225) and his role as the protector of travellers. The deposition of footwear in burials may also be linked to Mercury in his role as psychopomp, which is bound up with ideas of a journey. However, van Driel-Murray (1999a: 132; see also Biddulph and Booth 2006: 59) reminds us that we do not know the direction of the journey and deposited shoes may have enabled the deceased to return from the world of the dead. Philpott (1991: 237) suggests that, in the early Roman period, it was believed that the dead continued to live in the tomb and therefore needed footwear. A further possibility is that shoes were placed to remind the deceased to set off on their journey (Merrifield 1987: 75) so that their shades did not disturb the living (Biddulph and Booth 2006: 59; Clarke 1979:407; Philpott 1991: 86). One final suggestion is that, in the context of graves, single shoes may have

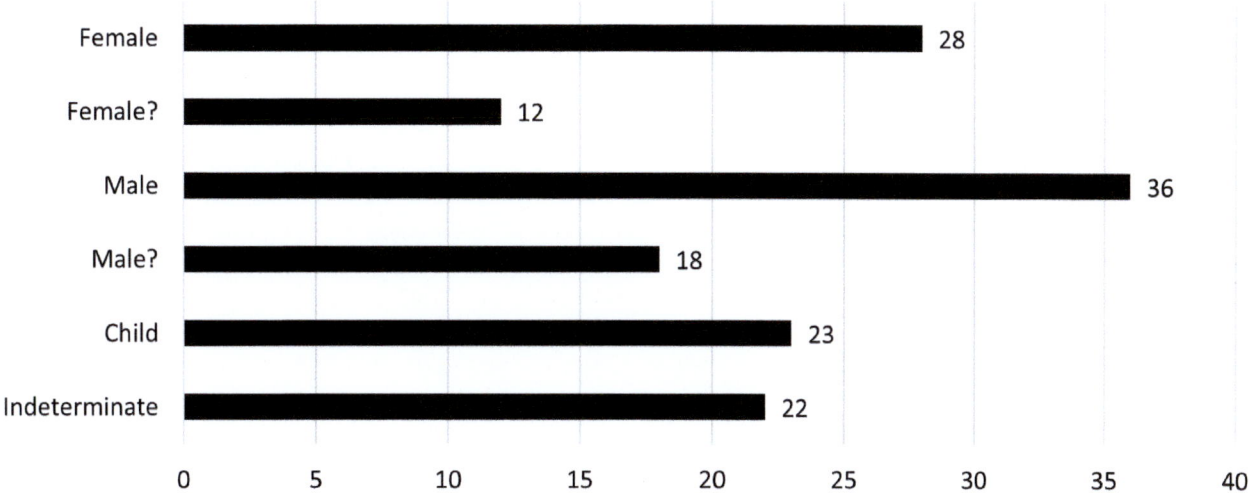

Figure 4.5: Chart to show the sex and approximate age of 139 people buried with shoes in Lankhills Late Roman cemetery.

'represented the living person in the realm of the dead, accompanying the deceased and connecting both worlds' (Biddulph and Booth 2006: 59). Roman footwear as *pars pro toto* is a common aspect of their meaning. Whatever the reason for depositing shoes in graves, they are clearly of ritual significance in this context. So, is this the case for footwear deposited in Roman wells?

4.2 The deposition of Roman footwear in wells

If the practice of depositing Roman footwear in wells were not common, it would have little social significance. One of the first tasks, therefore, was to determine how widespread this phenomenon is. There is not sufficient space here to explore the data from all excavated Roman wells, so this study took a sample based on the catalogue from Albrecht's database (2014: 227ff), which includes information from 492 wells. The remaining wells from the Saalburg were added: Albrecht records only 60 out of the 99 wells excavated (Busch, 1965: 161). A further thirteen wells from Rainau-Bruch, Germany, which are also not in Albrecht's dataset were included, as was a well in Geldermalsen-Hondsgemet, in the Netherlands (van Driel-Murray 2009b: 854). This gives a total of 545 wells from *Upper Germania* and *Raetia*, of which 81 contained shoes (14.9%). In addition, an advanced search on the RSRB website revealed data for 411 wells in England and Wales, 169 of which contained leather shoes, hobnails or both (41%). The RSRB data for the 411 wells were checked carefully to eliminate any sites with 'well' in the place name or references to horseshoes.

Because this dataset lacked examples from an urban setting, Roman wells from London were investigated. A search for Roman wells in the London Archaeological Archive and Research Centre (LAARC) online catalogue produced 393 results; 37 of these were removed because their data are included in this study within the relevant county information, for example Perry Oaks/Heathrow Terminal 5 was in both the LAARC and RSRB databases.

This gives a total of 356 Roman wells in London, of which 64 were found to have contained leather shoes or hobnails (16.3%). The study also located eight further wells containing shoes which did not come from any of the aforementioned databases, six from military settings, one from a town, and one from a rural site. This provides a total dataset of 1,311 excavated Roman wells from different regions and different settlement types, 322 (25%) of which contained evidence of shoes (Figure 4.6).

There are inevitably some problems with the data. Because there was neither the room, nor the time, to research every excavated Roman well, it was necessary to choose a sample, and any sample runs the risk of being statistically unrepresentative. Although Germany, England and Wales are well represented, the sample includes only a modicum of data from Scotland, France, or the Netherlands, so the evidence for the north-western provinces is not completely firm. On the other hand, it does contain data for more than the 350 Romano-British wells identified by Burgers (2001: 46), and might therefore be taken as a fair indication of the deposition of footwear in Roman wells in England and Wales. In terms of site type, there is very little variation in the numbers of wells containing shoes among rural sites (31%), towns including *Londinium* (28%) or military sites (28%). What the RSRB terms 'nucleated' sites—small, unwalled towns or villages—makes up 10%, while 'religious, ritual and funerary' sites, those with shrines, temples or cemeteries, account for the remaining three percent (Figure 4.7). Therefore, this sample does appear to represent a reasonable cross-section of site types and is largely in line with Fulford's findings (2001: 215), in that 'patterns of structured behaviour in relation to pits and wells can be seen across the spectrum'.

The number of Roman wells containing shoes varies according to region. In Germany, the state of Hesse produced records for 57 wells containing shoes, while Bavaria only produced one. This data is probably biased due to the concentration of wells along the *Limes*, especially at the Saalburg, but may also be affected by lack of shoe

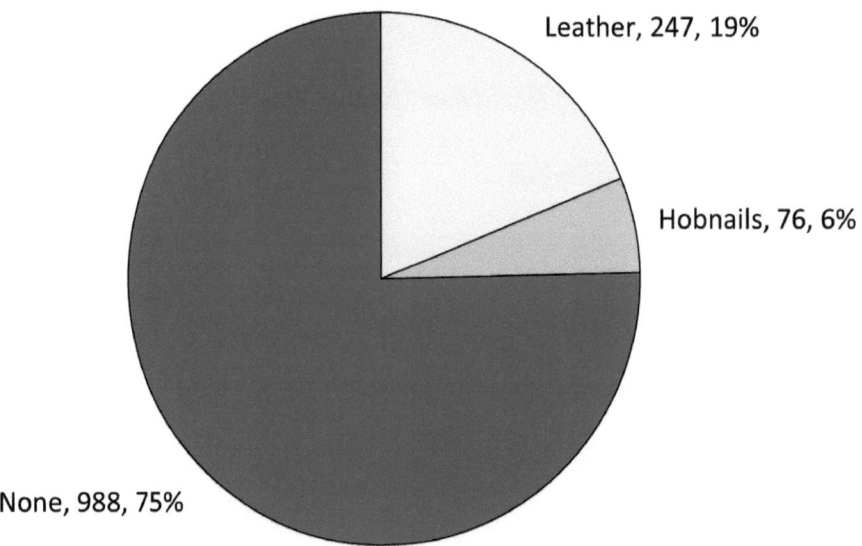

Figure 4.6: Chart to show the proportion of 1,311 Roman wells containing evidence of shoes.

survival or lack of detailed records. With the exception of *Londinium*, which boasts 71 Roman wells containing footwear, probably due to the size of its population, the largest numbers of Romano-British wells with shoes are found in Gloucestershire (13), Cambridgeshire (11) and Essex (10). On the other hand, there were few results for some counties, for example East Sussex, and no results for others, for example Suffolk and Greater Manchester (Figure 4.8). There are many possible explanations for this, apart from the deposition of footwear not happening in Roman wells in these areas. It may be that any Roman sites in such counties were not rural in character and therefore did not appear in the RSRB database. Roman wells may not have been excavated in these areas. These counties may have incomplete records of wells with shoes, or no Roman footwear evidence survived there.

The number of Roman wells containing evidence of shoes tails off over time, being more common in first- and second-century wells (Figure 4.9). This may be due to the non-survival of stitched, rather than nailed, footwear, which often leaves no archaeological trace. Certainly, footwear finds from the fourth century are rare (van Driel-Murray 2011a: 345) and nailed footwear appears to decline rapidly from the middle of that century (van Driel-Murray 2011a: 345). Dating evidence for the deposits may be lacking. It is also possible that the practice of depositing shoes in wells became less frequent in the later Roman period. Nevertheless, even taking into account the lack of survival, change over time, and any problems with the data, it does appear that the deposition of footwear in Roman wells was a reasonably common phenomenon in the north-western provinces.

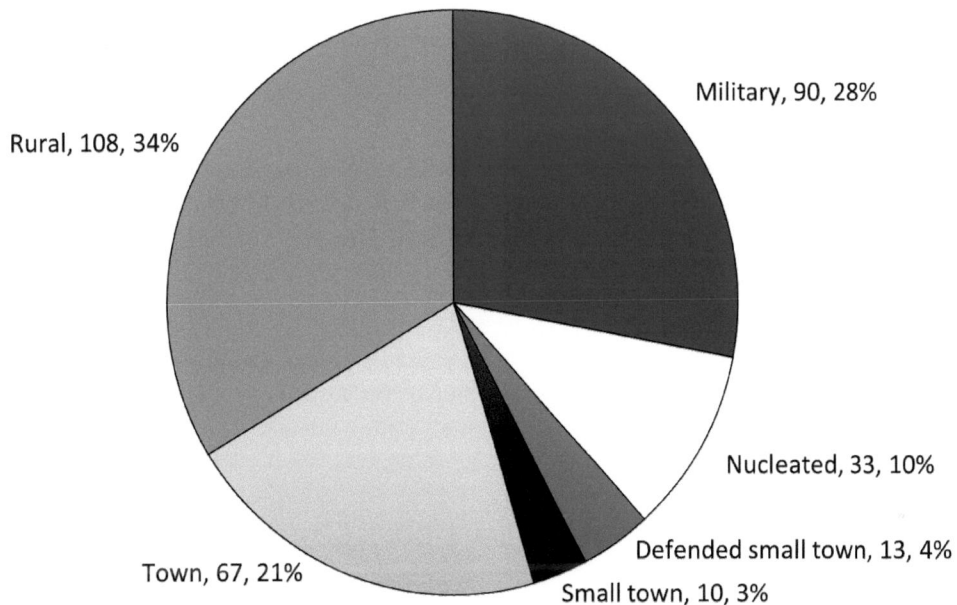

Figure 4.7: Chart to show the proportions of 321 Roman wells containing shoes according to site type.

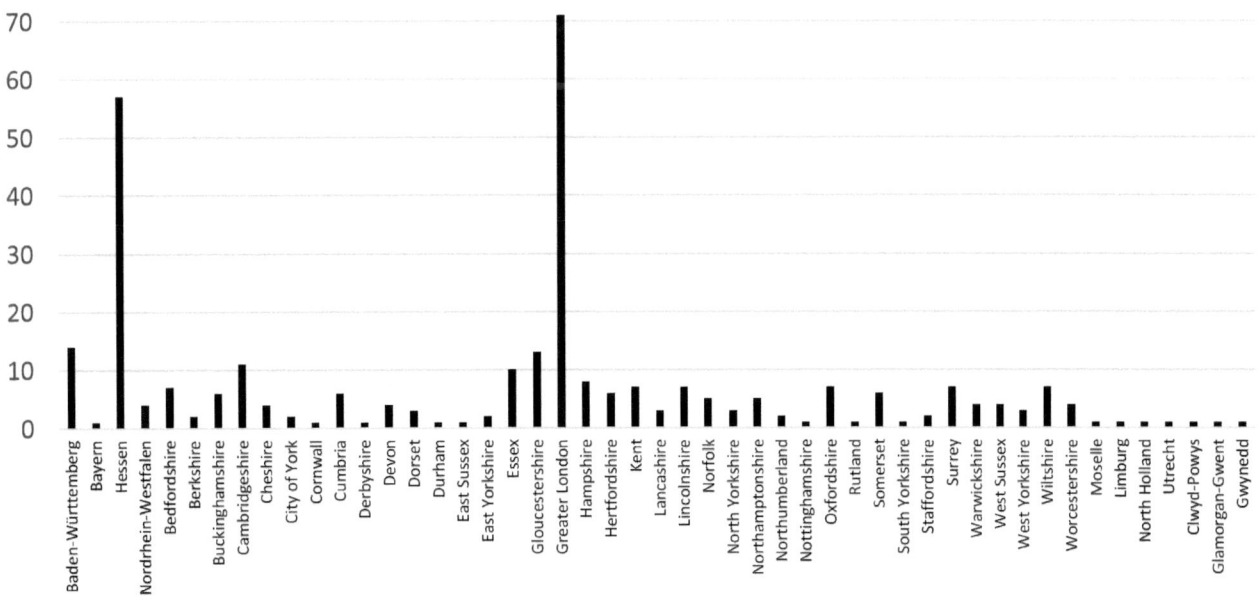

Figure 4.8: Chart to show the number of Roman wells with shoes by county/region.

Roman Feet and Shoes

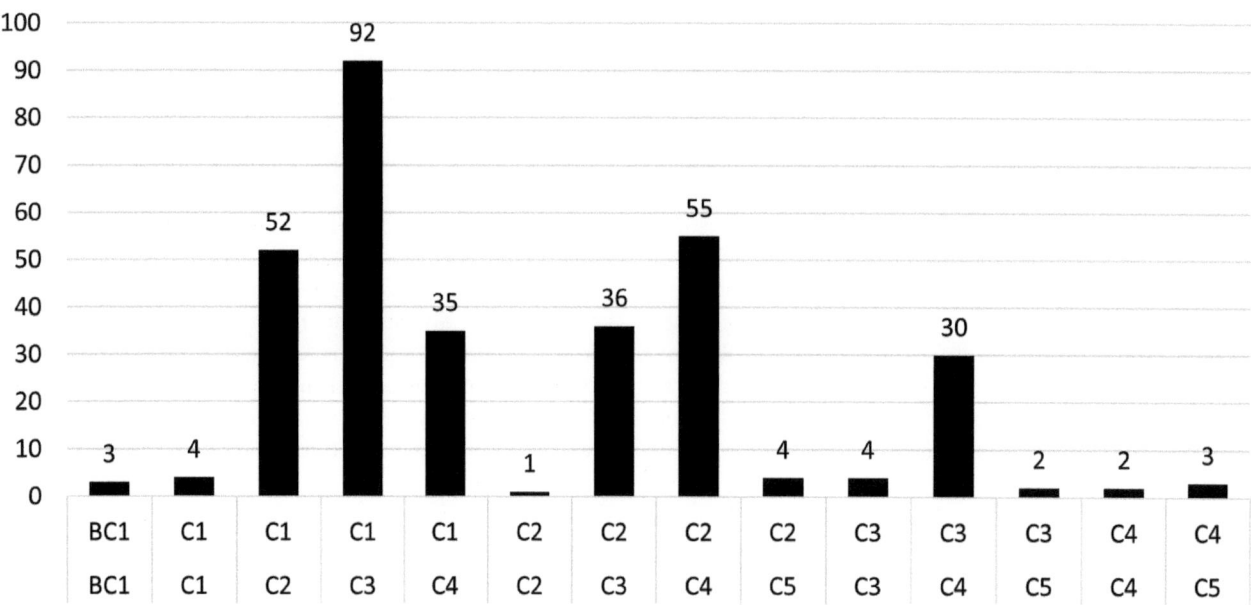

Figure 4.9: Chart to show the chronological distribution of 323 Roman wells containing footwear according to date of construction and decommission.

The dataset also considers the numbers of shoes found in each well. Some wells may contain very few: only one in a number of cases; two shoes were found in well one at Scole, Norfolk (Adams 1977: 207; 209). Others contain larger numbers: 32 came from well 14 at the Saalburg (Busch 1965: 162) and 74 complete shoes were found in well one at Welzheim (van Driel-Murray 2011a: 342). Hundreds of Roman shoes can come from one site with multiple wells: for example, the 99 Saalburg wells produced a total of 252 leather shoes and six wooden pattens (Busch 1965: 161). These unusually high or low numbers of shoes may constitute odd deposits, and could therefore indicate ritual activity.

4.2.1 Distinguishing deposits

Unlike Roman shoes in graves, there is a major problem with interpreting the deposition of footwear in Roman wells. It is very difficult to distinguish whether shoes were thrown away because they were worn out and the well, which had fallen out of use, was a convenient rubbish bin, or if footwear was placed in the fill of the well for a particular purpose that could be described as 'special' or 'ritual'. Haynes (2013: 198) argues that some Romano-British wells seem to have been filled with special deposits but apparently back-filled afterwards with site debris. This could imply that Roman ritual activities were not separate from everyday life, so the ritual use of such quotidian items as footwear should not be surprising. It is therefore perfectly possible for Roman wells to contain both structured deposits and rubbish dumps simultaneously. This section considers the problem and suggests some possible answers.

In the last thirty years or so, archaeological finds previously seen as rubbish have increasingly been identified as deliberately placed (Cool and Richardson 2013: 191). The difficulty lies in the extent to which we can distinguish items that have been deposited as part of a religious or symbolic rite. Hill's 1995 study of Iron Age Wessex is regarded as the seminal work. He was interested in how 'ritual' could be seen in material culture (Garrow 2012: 98) but also recognised that 'discovering significant degrees of structure and symbolism in archaeological deposits is not a secure basis for their interpretation as ritual deposits' (Hill 1995: 4). Hill (1995: 34) developed the concept of an average pit fill in order to be able to identify 'special' deposits. He was influenced by the work of Richards and Thomas (1984), who first coined the term 'structured deposit'. Earlier works, such as Merrifield's 1987 *The archaeology of ritual and magic*, and Ross's 1968 'Shafts, pits, wells—sanctuaries of the Belgic Britons?', were also influential in developing how to identify 'ritual' deposits.

More recently, Garrow has seen 'structured' deposition as a spectrum of behaviours which has 'odd deposits' at one end and 'material culture patterning' at the other (Garrow 2012: 94). Bell, who influenced Garrow, suggests that ritual is not a clearly defined category, but a relational and context-specific concept that derives from 'ritualization' practices. According to her, odd deposits should be considered the result of clearly ritualized practices because they were made consciously 'different' from others (Bell 1992: 74). Brück (1999: 329) has pointed out that what might seem 'odd deposits' to us may have been completely normal to people in the past. It is also the case that patterns can occur which may look like 'odd deposits' to an archaeologist (Garrow 2012: 109). Garrow (2012: 110–111) cites the example of material deposited in Merseyside recycling centres in the financial year 2010–2011. Some of the patterns of deposition observable here can be explained as seasonal; others are not so easy to account for (Garrow 2012: 111). What Garrow (2012: 111) does point out, however, is that suggesting these patterns of deposition were in no way a meaningful reflection of ideology or symbolism would be a mistake.

Many terms have been coined to describe the idea of patterned, or structured, deposits. Among them are: 'ceremonial, deliberate, formal, intentional, non-utilitarian, odd, peculiar, placed, ritual, selected, special, symbolic, token and unusual' (Garrow 2012: 93; Roskams *et al.* 2013: 3). However, what these words mean varies according to who is using them (Garrow 2012: 94). While Garrow (2012: 93) describes the terms as interchangeable, they have been interpreted as running together three separate concepts: the social context of an activity; related human actions guided by motives; and the character of artefacts which might be used to commemorate such contexts and actions (Roskams *et al.* 2013: 3–4). It is thus difficult either to distinguish or to define ritual practices.

However, certain objects found in Roman wells are thought to be indicative of structured deposits (Cool and Richardson 2013: 208; Fleming 2021: 110). Wait's statistical analysis aiming to find recurring patterns to distinguish ritual contexts from more commonplace functions showed that, during the Iron Age in southern England, the fills of wells and pits tended to contain deliberate layers comprising a number of indicators. These include human and animal bones, pottery vessels, weapons, querns, leather (especially footwear) and ash (Wait 1985: 52–53). It is generally acknowledged that such practices continued into the Roman period, becoming more widespread (Timby *et al.* 1998: 388; Fulford 2001: 213) with a greater variety of items, and less human bone and ash (Woodward 1992: 53). Human remains, especially skulls found as part of the backfill of a well, are indicative of ritual activity (Hill 1995: 100). Skulls have a symbolic significance in both the Iron Age and Roman worlds, as the head was believed to be the residence of the soul or spirit and may have served as a *pars pro toto* (Clarke 1996: 75).

Animal bone groups are also indicative of structured deposition, possibly to mark a change in use of the well (Merrifield 1987: 32). Of particular significance are horses, dogs, animal skulls, or whole bodies (Morris 2008: 9). Parts of deer are rare in Romano-British faunal assemblages (Cool 2006b: 112) and their occurrence in Roman wells suggests that deer played an essential role in the rites undertaken on decommissioning a well (Gerrard forthcoming: 13).

Another marker for possible ritual activity is the presence of querns (Hill 1995: 55; Merrifield 1987: 33; Garrow 2012: 105). Clarke (1997: 75) suggests that, in addition to their association with successful harvests, rotary querns perhaps symbolised the sun. Brück (2006: 304) describes the practice of depositing querns as 'redolent with the symbolism of death and rebirth' because the act of grinding grain sustains life through the production of food and is closely associated with the process of transformation. While Brück's description relates to the late Bronze Age, the continuation of quern deposition in wells has been noted (Merrifield 1987: 24). It does not seem to signify whether the querns are complete or merely fragments. Fragmentary artefacts may have served as offerings (Clarke 1997: 75). There may be an element of synecdoche in the deposition of fragments (Croxford 2003: 92).

Altars and figurines of deities may also be indicative of ritual activity if found deposited in wells, although it has been suggested that altars found in wells in military settings might simply have been disposed of during the abandonment process (Douglas 2015: 7). The disposal of such cult objects without ceremony might seem unlikely, although there is quite a history of reuse of altars in the Roman period for example in post pits at Maryport (Haynes 2020b: 217-218).

Finds of complete, or almost complete, pottery or glass vessels may be signs of structured deposition (Cool and Richardson 2013: 191) as they carry implications of plenty (Clarke 1997: 75), although this should not be taken for granted. As Cool and Richardson (2013: 192) point out, such complete vessels may have been dropped while collecting water and did not break, as their descent was cushioned. Nevertheless, pottery has been found in layers with other markers for structured deposits and the multiplication of such evidence becomes convincing (Merrifield 1987: 133).

Wait points out that none of these categories on its own is enough to identify a well or shaft's contents as of ritual origin (1985: 53) and stresses that the most important characteristic of ritual deposition is the deliberate organisation and placement of objects in layers, or in a single layer (1985: 54). Therefore, when assessing the potentially ritual nature of footwear deposits in Roman wells, it is essential to consider not only the shoes, but also the other artefacts that were found with them in the same stratigraphic context.

Although it contained no footwear, the deliberate organisation of objects in a Roman well is visible in the *fons Annae Perennae* in Rome, which provides a useful comparison with those from the north-western provinces. The reservoir was found to contain a number of deliberately deposited items including 549 coins, 74 lamps, some of them with *defixiones* inside, and complete vessels (which occur in the above list of ritual indicators). Some of these were religious offerings to the deity and her nymphs, while others were 'magic' (Piranomonte and Simón 2008: 3), in that they were curses intended to convince the supernatural patrons of the well to inflict punishments. All the deposits were of a ritual nature, showing a link between wells and ritual activity. Roman wells, or at least some of them, could therefore be regarded as potential *loci* for ritual practices.

4.2.2 Evidence for the ritual deposition of Roman shoes in wells

As we have discovered, it is difficult to distinguish whether Roman footwear was thrown away or placed symbolically in wells. However, if found in layers with groups of the above assemblage categories, it could be deemed part of such structured deposits. Indeed, Wait (1985: 53) includes leather, especially shoes and sandals, as his eighteenth category of evidence. Unfortunately, the level at which footwear is found in wells is not documented consistently, for example, Busch (1965: 161) comments that it is not always possible to give a find setting for the Saalburg shoes as they were not always recorded clearly. The data may be biased, as the leather from shoes deposited in the higher levels of wells is less likely to have survived because the environment is too dry; hobnails may be found, but unnailed footwear usually leaves no trace when it decays. Certainly, the 258 shoes from the Saalburg were all found in the deeper layers of the wells (Busch 1965: 161). It is not always clear from excavation reports which artefact assemblages were found with the footwear.

This study, however, examined the data for 42 wells (Figure 4.10) which all exhibit layering and at least three more of Wait's categories of ritual deposits, with the exception of the praetorium well at Vindolanda. This yielded 10 ox skulls with the shoes; the only other object found with them was a cabbage stalk (Birley 1977: 89). This compares unfavourably with the number and range of artefacts deposited in the praetorium well at Bar Hill, which included two boots among the altars, pottery, antlers, weapons and so forth (MacDonald 1906: 133–134). It has, however, been argued that a lack of artefacts can also make a deposit special (van Haasteren and Groot 2013: 41). It would seem, then, that shoes can form part of special deposits in Roman wells.

4.2.3 Roman beliefs and water

One reason why structured deposits may occur in Roman wells is the association of wells and other watery settings with religious beliefs. Water has always been important to humans, being drunk for its life-sustaining properties, heated for cooking food, and used to wash dirt from the body (Graham 2020: 35). Springs appear to be associated with abundance that might be culturally connected with 'wealth, health, plenty, life, fertility' (Betts 2016: 73). A number of divinities are water personified, for example, Oceanus, and various river gods. Wells may have given access to chthonic deities (Ross 1967: 50; Ross and Feacham 1976: 230; Rattue 1995: 27; Fulford 2001: 216). Therefore, the 'practice of depositing valuables in watery places extends far back into the Bronze Age' (Merrifield 1987: 24). The earliest Roman ritual activities associated with water are usually signalled by ceramic and copper alloy offerings (Graham 2020: 168). Many other, later Roman objects are found deposited in watery places, as will be discussed in ensuing chapters. The deposition of footwear in Roman wells may reflect this aspect of religious practice.

Roman religious sites and water frequently occur together. According to Frontinus, springs in Rome were venerated, especially as sites for healing (*Aqueducts* 1.4). Temples are commonly associated with springs, for example the temples to Sulis Minerva in Bath and Arnemetia in Buxton. In Rome itself, the reservoir of the *fons Annae Perennae* was found to contain a number of deposited items including coins, lamps and vessels. Nîmes was named after *Nemausus*, the deity of one of its springs (Gros 1984: 129), around which a sanctuary dedicated to Augustus was built (Gros 1984: 129).

It is unsurprising, therefore, that many Romano-British wells are associated with shrines or temples, for example, the ritual complex at Springhead, Kent (RSRB 2018: 9020) and Coventina's well, Northumberland (Allason-Jones and McKay 1985). The nearby Mithraeum at Carrawburgh also had a temple well (Rattue 1995: 28). Such juxtapositions also occur in Germany and France.

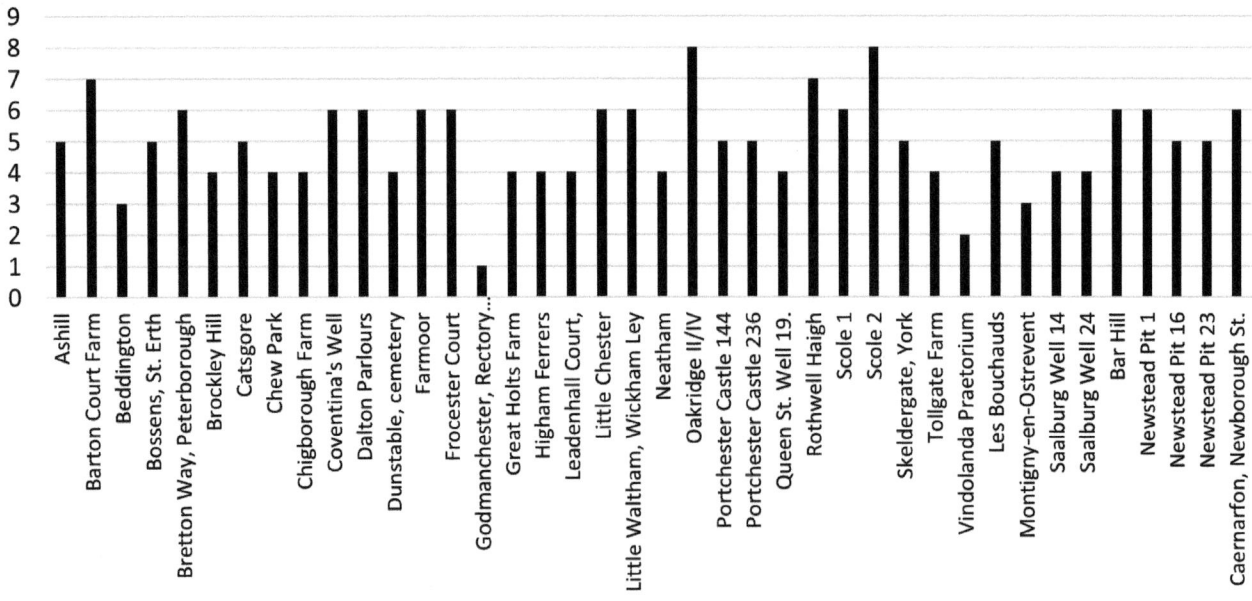

Figure 4.10: Chart to show the number of recognised ritual markers per site from 42 Roman wells with footwear.

Woodward (1992: 121–123) suggests that the practice of venerating wells continued into the medieval period and later with the phenomenon of holy wells. Certainly, well dressing can still be seen in the Peak District although, nowadays, this may have more to do with custom and tourism than belief. Rattue (1995: 27) sees Roman era attitudes to wells as more superstition than devotion, but superstition can still constitute belief. Indeed, people still throw coins into fountains and other water features for luck.

4.2.4 Footwear and rituals surrounding the biography of Roman wells

Structured deposits have been found that mark the commencement and end of the lives of Roman wells (Merrifield 1987: 48; Cool and Richardson 2013: 214; van Haasteren and Groot 2013: 27). Because of its recognisable fashions, Roman footwear can be dated independently (van Driel-Murray 2001). This dating evidence has enabled Roman footwear to be linked to the stages in the biography of wells, such as construction and abandonment, which seem to have been surrounded by rituals (Groot, 2009: 62), marked by deposition of one kind or another (Gerrard forthcoming: 5).

Footwear in the lowest layers of a Roman well is likely to be a deliberate deposit (van Haasteren and Groot 2013: 37) because, unlike brooches or hairpins, it is not easy to lose a shoe down a well accidentally. Shoes placed behind well linings can be interpreted as ritual markers for the construction stage in a well's lifecycle (van Driel-Murray 2011a: 337; van Haasteren and Groot 2013: 25). A high-quality sole with an ornate nailing pattern was found in the pit dug for the construction of a well in Venray, in the Netherlands (van Haasteren and Groot 2013: 25; van Driel-Murray 2011a: 337; see also 373 figure 82). A boy's sandal was found at the bottom of the well at Dalton Parlours, West Yorkshire (Mould 1990: 235; van Driel-Murray 1999a: 137) which, thanks to comparative studies of Roman footwear, can be dated to the third quarter of the third century, about a hundred years before the well went out of use (Mould 1990: 235). Another third-century sandal came from the base of a well at Katwijk, in the Netherlands, (van Driel-Murray 2011a: 373 figure 84), as did a shoe found in the Roman Well at Erps-Kwerps, Belgium (van Driel-Murray 2011a: 337, footnote 14). A set of hobnails was discovered in the backfill behind the lining of well 5 at Lower Slaughter, Gloucestershire (Timby et al. 1998: 386). While the style of this shoe is not available for dating purposes, the context points to this being a construction deposit. It seems that these shoes were deliberately placed at the beginning of the wells' biographies (van Driel-Murray 2011a: 337) and may therefore be regarded as ritual in character.

It has been suggested that shoes found higher up in a well's fill may be deposits linked to the abandonment of a well. Wells eventually fall out of use for several reasons: the well may have dried up or become polluted; the users could have moved away or the well might have collapsed (van Haasteren and Groot 2013: 32). Once a well is no longer used, it will fill up, which can happen in a variety of ways: naturally and slowly after abandonment; quickly to remove the hazards presented; or in order to prepare the site for reconstruction (Ross and Feacham 1976: 234; van Haasteren and Groot 2013: 32). The layers of material in a well's fill often reveal how this happened (van Haasteren and Groot 2013: 32). Items in the fill of a well could have been lost, thrown away or deliberately placed. The frequency with which waste (including leather) was dumped in wells, especially on the abandonment of a military site, makes the differentiation between ritual and quotidian deposition very difficult (Douglas 2015: 7).

Doubtless some deposits in wells are rubbish; a convenient way to dispose of old shoes and fill in a dangerous feature at the same time. Indeed, van Driel-Murray (1999a: 137) points out that Roman footwear was rarely repaired and easily discarded, and therefore most shoes in wells were probably refuse. The use of Roman footwear as part of the process of filling in and levelling out before reconstruction has been recorded at Vindolanda (van Driel-Murray 1993: 4) and in the fill of the Roman quay at St. Magnus House (MacConnoran 1986: 218). Nevertheless, van Driel-Murray (1999a: 137) admits that she used to assume, possibly wrongly, that shoes in wells were part of the final fill of domestic rubbish.

Van Haasteren and Groot (2013: 25) argue that a worn shoe sole found in the upper fill of the Roman well at Venray, which was originally interpreted as waste, was deliberately deposited during abandonment. They contend that the occurrence of two shoes in the well is not coincidental, that the second shoe is unlikely to have been refuse, since the fill contained few other finds, and that the choice of a worn shoe may have been deliberate, because the shoe, like the well, had reached the end of its life (van Haasteren and Groot 2013: 41). It is difficult to test this hypothesis since footwear does not usually survive in the upper layers of wells. However, well 266 at Brockley Hill contained part of a bottle 'unique to Britain, and possibly to the continent', which may have been deposited when the well was decommissioned (Brady et al. 2005: 32) and the remains of five leather shoes found with it are thought to strengthen the argument that this formed part of a rite of termination (Cool 2005: 51). Shoes may have been a particularly appropriate component of this ritual, since it could be described as being 'essentially a funeral for a place' (Fleming 2021: 77) and the funerary use of Roman footwear has been shown to be widespread.

4.2.5 The ritual importance of left and right

Apart from the inclusion of footwear in the lifecycle of Roman wells, it is thought that single shoes were occasionally deposited in wells as *ex voto* offerings of thanks or as the mark of a contractual obligation to a deity (van Driel-Murray 1999a: 136). Van Driel-Murray's (1999a: 136) suggestion that, from the Neolithic onwards, there was a preference for depositing the left shoe, while retaining the right shoe as a reminder of the vow has been widely accepted by scholars (for example, Cool and Richardson 2013:192; Houlbrook 2017: 268). One of the problems with this theory is that we can never know what happened to the other shoe. Another is that it may represent a statistically unsound group (van Driel-Murray 1999a: 136).

In order to test the theory, this study looked for a number of Roman wells which exhibited some of the characteristics of ritual deposition (see above) and also contained footwear found in layers with the other markers. There is insufficient space here to investigate whether all the wells in the earlier sample showed signs of structured, or even ritual, deposition, so a set of 42 wells was identified for a case study to look at numbers of shoes and the proportions of left versus right. Many of the wells researched were attached to shrines or funerary settings. These steps are intended to counter the argument that the shoe deposits in these wells were just domestic refuse. This dataset does not include wells where the evidence of shoes comes from hobnails or cleats, because the number of these per shoes is variable.

Of the sample of 42 'ritual' wells, three contained unknown numbers of shoes, because this had not been recorded in the antiquarian excavation reports; 14 did not record any numbers for left or right shoes, possibly because the footwear was too fragmentary to tell, or because chirality (whether a shoe is left or right) was considered unimportant by the author concerned. Of the 282 shoes that were numbered, 141 were not recorded as either left or right and are labelled here as 'unidentifiable'. These represent half of the sample (Figure 4.11). Of the shoes with known chirality, 76 were identifiable as left (27%) and 65 as right (23%). There is a preference for left shoes over right, but it is not very marked. However, we cannot know the chirality of the unidentifiable, fragmentary footwear which forms the greater part of the case study shoes.

Next, the unidentifiable footwear was taken out of the equation, leaving a total of 141 shoes, of which 76 (54%) were for the left foot and 65 (46%) for the right. Again, this shows a slight preference for the left foot. Some of the wells do have exclusively left shoes, such as Saalburg well 24 (Busch 1965) which held five shoes, four of which were for the left foot and one too fragmentary to tell, or Portchester Castle well 144, where all three were left shoes (Ambrose 1977: 247–262). Some wells contained a majority of left shoes, for example, Coventina's well, which yielded three left shoes and one right (Allason-Jones and McKay 1985: 37), and the well at Bretton Way, Peterborough, which yielded seven left and two right, although in this instance a further seven shoes were unidentifiable (Mould 2013: 54). In some cases, there was an equal number of each, for instance, at Farmoor, Oxfordshire, well F43 contained two of each. Wells with a majority of right shoes are Saalburg well 14 (Busch 1965) and Portchester Castle well 236 (Ambrose 1977: 247–262), although these also held unidentifiable fragments. Leadenhall Court well N15 contained two exclusively right shoes (Pritchard 1993: 78). Of course, this is only a small sample and a different set of wells might produce a different set of data. However, according to Greene (2018b), the result is in line with similar, recent research.

While the preference for left shoes in votive settings seems weak, what is striking is the number of single shoes that occur in Roman wells. Indeed, Jacobi (1897: 495) states that no pairs were found among the shoes from the Saalburg and Busch (1965: 161), writing nearly seventy years later, observes that, among the 341 shoes catalogued from the forts at the Saalburg, Zugmantel and Kleiner Feldberg, there are only 17 known pairs, most of which come from the baths at Kleiner Feldberg. Of the sample of 1,311 Roman wells discussed above, 102 were identified as containing one shoe. If the eleven wells which also contained additional fragments are removed, that gives a total of 91 wells containing a single shoe out of 247 wells with shoes (36.8%). It seems that single shoes were used in votive practices to do with Roman wells and that the choice of which foot was probably left to personal preference.

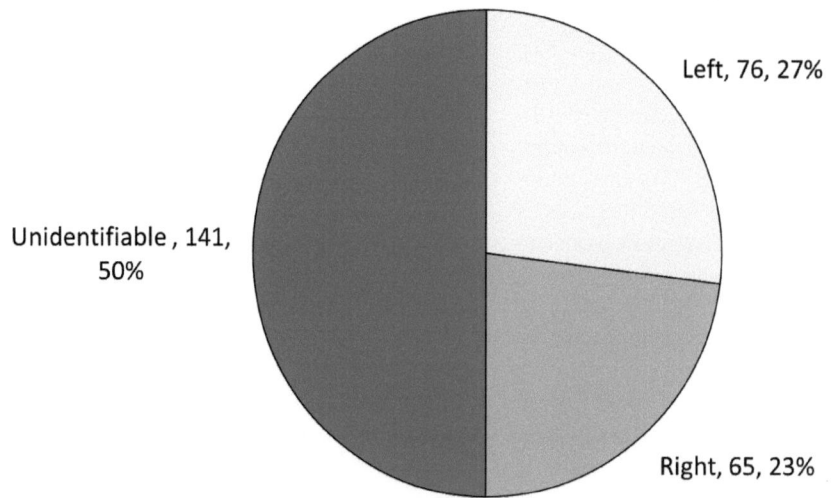

Figure 4.11: Chart to show the proportions of chirality in Roman shoes found in 42 wells with ritual associations.

4.3 Why were shoes thought to be appropriate ritual deposits?

Roman shoes are bound up with ideas of social status and identity. Grave markers feature men in togas with the appropriate boots (for example, Harl and Harl 2018a) or soldiers in *caligae* (Harl and Harl 2018b). Some later women's memorials feature sandals as a mark of their femininity (for example, *Corpus Inscriptionum Latinarum* (CIL) 9.3826). It appears that the association of footwear with the commemoration of the dead, extended across the empire. Actual footwear is also used in burials to display status.

Roman footwear also demonstrates a religious or spiritual element. It is thought that, in the Iron Age, pits, shafts, and wells were considered as entrances to the underworld (Ross 1967: 50; Ross and Feacham 1976: 230; Rattue 1995: 27) and well deposits may have been made in order to 'propitiate chthonic deities' (Fulford 2001: 216). Van Driel-Murray (1999a: 137) suggests that, because shoes connect humans to the earth, they were seen as particularly appropriate offerings to chthonic forces, making them appropriate for graves as well. Indeed, in London, Roman wells are often associated with funerary and religious practices (Gerrard 2011: 560).

Roman hobnails may have made the footwear particularly appropriate as part of funerary rites. Dungworth (1998: 153) has argued for the magico-religious symbolism of nails, especially to 'fix the dead', that is, to ensure that they stay dead. Bent nails, which are interpreted as apotropaic, are sometimes found in Roman burials and, since hobnails are bent as part of the shoe construction process, they may have been used for this purpose (Egging-Dinwiddy 2007: 9). This may explain some of the occurrences of single or small numbers of nails in some burials.

Shoes have a particularly intimate association with their wearers (Merrifield 1987: 134) because footwear retains the imprint of its wearer's sole (van Driel-Murray 1999a: 136). Since shoes are such highly personal items, they are inextricably connected with an individual's identity (Biddulph and Booth 2006: 59) and can take on the aspect of a *pars pro toto*, representing their owner (van Driel-Murray 1999a: 136; le Forestier 2013: 182; Dunbabin 1990: 86). It has therefore been suggested that footwear may be a substitute for human sacrifice (van Driel-Murray 1999a: 136–137), which would pollute a well, as would animal sacrifice. Because of their synecdochical quality, it is important that shoes used for a ritual purpose are worn, not new (van Driel-Murray 1999a: 137). This may mean that worn footwear deposited ritually in wells has been misinterpreted as refuse (van Haasteren and Groot 2013: 41). MacConnoran (1982: 61) describes the shoes from the Queen Street wells as the result of domestic dumping because of their worn condition even though they were found with acknowledged ritual markers. The ritual or rubbish question is also hard to answer at Tollgate Farm (Mould 2018: 165). The well at Rothwell Haigh contains markers of structured deposition (Cool and Richardson 2013: 208), but the shoes have been categorised as rubbish (van Driel-Murray 2011a: 51), despite their being atypical of the normal range of rubbish in the locality (Cool and Richardson 2013: 212) and having an unusually small size range (van Driel-Murray 2011a: 51). Perhaps the significance of the deposition of Roman footwear in wells needs to be reconsidered.

It is very difficult to tell whether shoes in burials were new or used because of the lack of leather survival. It is problematic to record how worn the hobnails from Roman burials are and, therefore, very rarely done. Unless the shoes were found on the individual's feet, it is also very difficult to tell whether the shoes belonged to the deceased or to a depositor. The footwear deposited in graves may therefore have represented the living friends and family of the dead. Nevertheless, shoes were deemed suitable grave goods throughout the Roman period.

4.4 Conclusions

This chapter has argued that Roman footwear is socially significant because it was thought appropriate for use in ritual activities, especially since it takes on the imprint of its wearer and was, therefore, thought to embody them. In Roman burials, shoes could be used to display identity and status. Footwear was certainly depicted on tombstones as a marker of Roman citizenship, military status, or female virtue. Roman footwear is connected to age, gender and occupation, so the type of footwear deposited may be a symbol of this. Expensive footwear in graves certainly shows the socio-economic status, not necessarily of the deceased, but of their family and social circle.

That shoes were placed, not just worn, in Roman graves shows that beliefs were attached to them that went above and beyond dress and fashion. What the beliefs about the deposited footwear were to the people who left it probably varied. It may have been apotropaic, to protect the deceased on their journey to the afterlife; it may have been comforting to know that something as personal as their footwear would accompany the dead as a reminder of those left behind; it may have been to prevent the deceased returning as a ghost; footwear may have been an offering to Mercury, or other chthonic deities, for the safe conduct of the dead.

Despite the complexities of distinguishing rubbish and ritual, this study has established, thanks to the stratigraphic context of footwear deposition and the patterns of assemblages with which it was found, that many deposits of footwear in Roman wells are of a ritual nature. The custom of placing shoes in wells appears to have persisted throughout the Roman period across the north-western provinces. Roman shoes may have been deposited as part of the rites accompanying the construction or decommissioning of a well, or have been *ex voto* offerings, possibly to chthonic deities. It has been shown that the votive deposition of footwear in wells was only slightly more likely to be left shoes than right.

Deliberately deposited Roman footwear gives us access to some of the shared beliefs of ordinary people in the north-western province of the Roman empire. Of course, not all footwear would have held the same significances for all people all of the time. Notwithstanding, whatever the beliefs of the Roman shoe-depositors, that footwear was considered an appropriate ritual deposit must speak volumes about its social significance.

5

The ubiquity of Roman foot- and shoe-shaped artefacts

This chapter aims to demonstrate that there is a variety of artefacts in the shape of shod or bare human feet which were ubiquitous and polysemous in Roman life. This chapter will discuss the social significance of a selection of 216 Roman small finds: amulets, finger rings, jugs whose handles terminate in feet, knife or razor handles formed like lower legs with feet, furniture feet, and oil flasks or *balsamaria*. Each of these sets of artefacts will be considered in a discreet portion of this chapter, and the conclusions section will give an overall view.

The artefacts were chosen because they depict feet and footwear. They also demonstrate themes of significance which run throughout this work: foot-shaped objects as novelty items, the apotropaic use of images of feet; feet in a religious, votive role; burial rites involving footwear; the significance of chirality and hobnailing; the foot as *pars pro toto*; and the idea of the foot as the seat of power and status.

5.1 Foot-shaped amulets

Amulets in the shape of feet or footwear were not a Roman innovation. There are examples from a wide range of pre-Roman settings. Nevertheless, certain distinctive Roman-period forms can be observed. This section examines the amuletic use of Roman foot-shaped pendants and finger rings with a view to emphasizing their apotropaic role. It considers the forerunners of Roman talismanic charms in the form of feet, and also why this shape may have been considered apotropaic.

Amuletic charms were ubiquitous in ancient daily life for medical, social, and religious reasons (Dasen 2015: 177). They are small items, sometimes in the shape of a foot (Perego 2010: 76) that are worn on the body as a defence against malevolent supernatural forces such as the evil eye (Perego 2010: 67). Foot-shaped amulets may also have been intended to protect or heal the relevant body part (Perego 2010: 76).

Amulets in the shape of feet or footwear pre-date the Roman era. An amulet in the form of a miniature gold sandal from Egypt, in the Museo Arqueológico Nacional, Madrid, (inventory number 15151) dates from 1539 to 1077 BCE (Figure 5.1a). Amulets representing a foot, either bare or wearing a boot, appear in La Tène A and in the Golasecca culture, Northern Italy, from the fifth century BCE (Feugère 1998: 23). Examples of such amulets (Figure 5.1b) have been found in sanctuaries and tombs (Feugère 1998: 23), including an amber bead from the 'Tomb of the Princess', Bliesbrück-Reinheim (Lourdaux 1999: 25). The electrostatic properties of amber made it appropriate for creating magical amulets (Davis 2018: 72).

The use of foot-shaped amulets, whether bare or shod, continued into the Roman period. The metaphorical protection provided by Roman feet and footwear is a theme which runs throughout this work. The foot is a liminal part of the body, forming the boundary between a person and the ground, and also between clean and dirty, a point through which harm can enter the body. Shoes protect feet

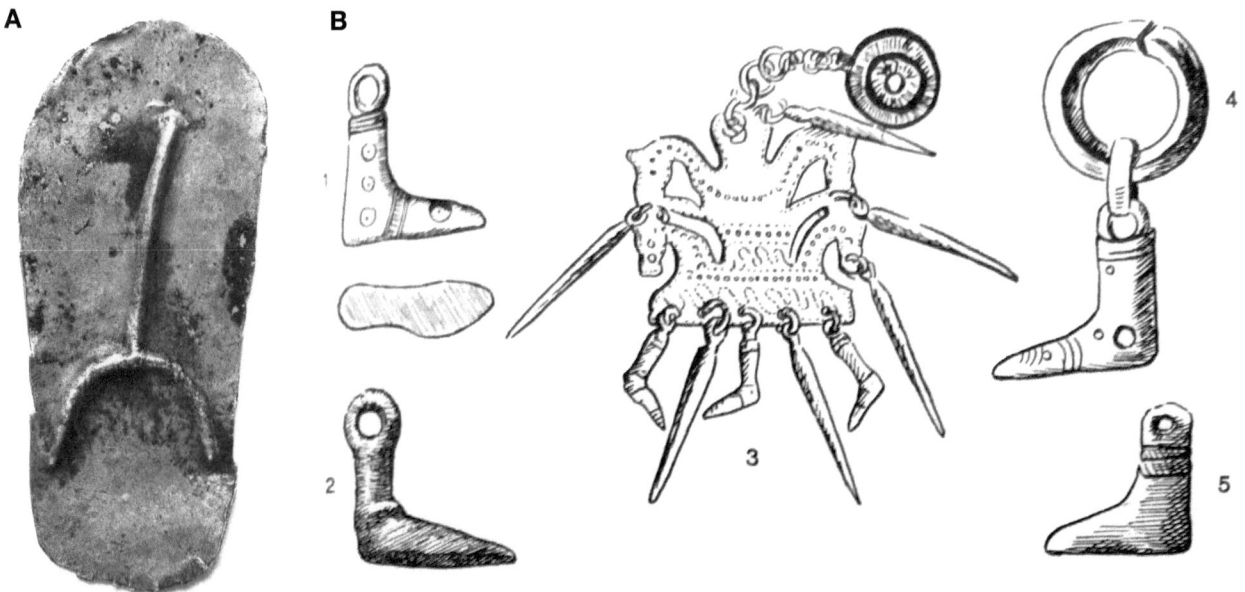

Figure 5.1: a) Egyptian sandal amulet, MAN Madrid. (Photo: Author's own). b) Iron Age foot-shaped amulets. (Forrer 1942 Pl. 9).

from cold, thorns, snakebite, and other harms (Forrer 1942: 77; van Driel-Murray 1999a: 131) and may, therefore, protect against evil influences (Forrer 1942: 78; Eckardt 2013: 231).

A right-footed copper alloy amulet (Figure 5.2a) was found in Tongeren (Faider-Feytmans 1979: 159). The foot is bare, which could mean that it represents the foot of a deity (Croom 2010: 74) which might have further strengthened its magical effects. Unfortunately, no details for its find setting are given (Faider-Feytmans 1979: 159).

A Roman charm in the form of a golden boot (Figure 5.2b) came from Italy, and is now in the British Museum (1872,0604.859). It dates to the first or second century, is 20mm tall, and portrays a left foot, with a message marked out in hobnails on the sole in Greek: 'be trodden on' (British Museum 2021). Trampling on something was a sign of power over it (Dasen 2015: 184), so this may have given the amulet more potency.

A jet amulet from Vindolanda also depicts a left foot, bare in this case (Figure 5.2c), so may represent a deity. Like amber, jet has electrostatic properties (Allason-Jones and Jones 1994: 272), and was thought to have both medicinal and apotropaic qualities (Parker 2016: 109). This may have doubled the protective effect of this amulet. What is unusual about this left foot is that it appears to have only four toes (Birley 2020). This foot may have been for healing purposes (Birley 2020), possibly of the owner's left foot, or because the left brought healing and restorative qualities (Smith 2018: 206). An oval amulet in the Thorvaldsens Museum, Copenhagen (inventory number H2221) also depicts a bare left foot (Figure 5.3). These amulets show that it was not only the right foot that was considered to have apotropaic properties.

Amuletic gems sometimes show feet as an attribute of a deity. A sard gem (British Museum 1814,0704.1471) is engraved with a winged foot of Mercury, *caduceus* and a butterfly. The foot is bare and left, which would have produced the impression of a right foot if used as a seal. Mercury was patron of travellers (Crummy 2007: 226), so this gem may have given protection on journeys, and is linked with healing (Crummy 2007: 225). Mercury also guided the souls of the departed into the Underworld (Crummy 2007: 227). The footprints of gods are evidence of divine presence (van Driel-Murray 1999a: 135).

A green jasper gem in the British Museum is engraved with a cockerel, a bare foot, a cornucopia, an ear of corn, and a term of Priapus (inv. no. 1923,0401.332). This combines the apotropaic properties of the foot with a phallic symbol, a well-known Roman talisman.

Serapis is also a deity represented by feet (Dow and Upson 1944: 58). His cult is linked to ideas of fertility, healing, power, and death (Nicgorski 2014: 154). A magical gem in the National Archaeological Museum, Florence features a bust of Serapis on a foot (Mastrocinque 2007: 40). Such amulets combine religious ideas intended to placate or win the favour of supernatural beings with magic, operating by controlling supernatural beings (Merrifield 1987: 6).

Roman finger rings with bezels in the shape of sandal soles may also have been considered apotropaic. They depict pairs or single feet, both left and right, and can show the nailed sole or the view from the top of the sandal. There are three examples showing the tops of sandals on the Portable Antiquities of the Netherlands (PAN) database, all of them found near the military site of Vechten (Figure 5.4). A copper alloy example shows a pair of feet (PAN-00035412), while the other two, made of gold, were found twisted together (PAN-00035415) forming a pair. The rings were found by metal detectorists, and there are no precise details of their find settings. However, the gold rings were broken by something sharp, which may be post-deposit damage, but could also indicate their use as votive objects, since these are often deliberately bent or broken in order to put them out of common use (Nickel 2011: 150) as part of a 'ritual killing' (Walton 2021: 58).

A pair of copper alloy rings in the form of feet wearing sandals was found at the sanctuary of Les Bolards, Nuits-Saint-Georges (Guiraud 1989: 210–211). It is, again, unclear exactly where on the site they were found but, like

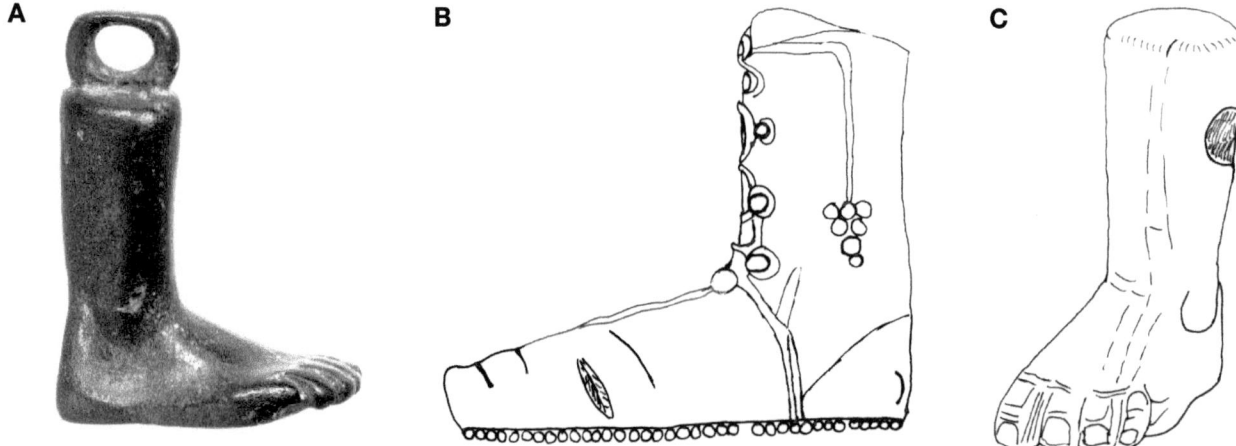

Figure 5.2: a) Tongeren foot amulet. (KIK-IRPA N002194). b) Gold boot charm. c) Jet foot amulet. Vindolanda Trust.

The ubiquity of Roman foot- and shoe-shaped artefacts

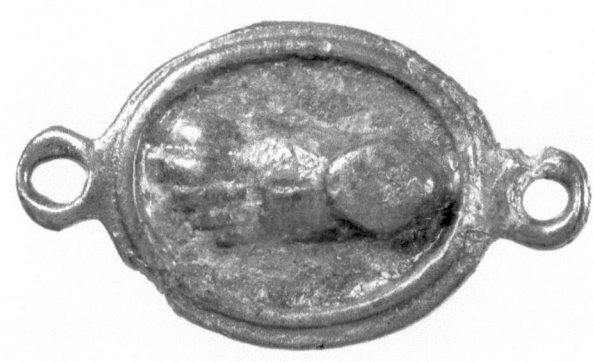

Figure 5.3: Left foot amulet (Photo: Thorvaldsens Museum, Copenhagen).

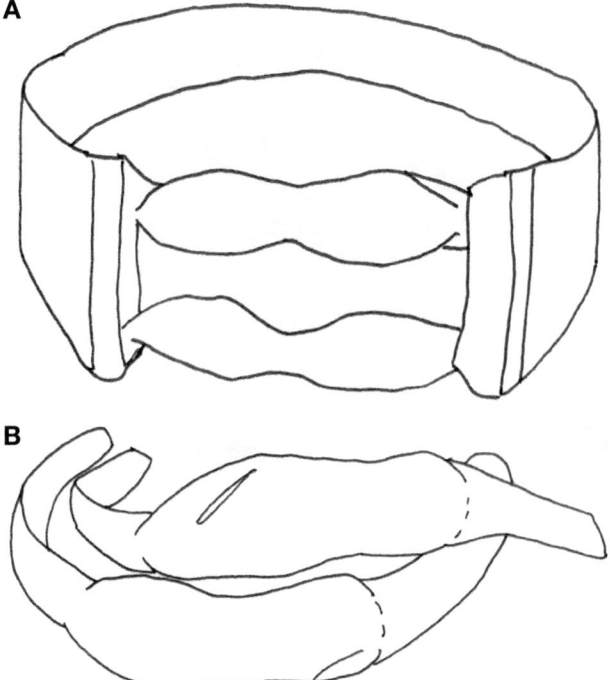

Figure 5.4: 'Sandal' rings from near Bunnik-Vechten.

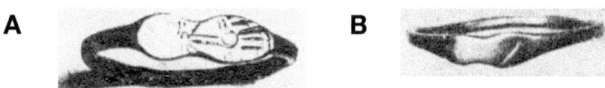

Figure 5.5: 'Sandal' rings from Vindonissa and RGM, Cologne (Henkel 1913: Plates 3.53 and 3.52).

the twisted rings from Vechten, they are broken, so these may have been votive deposits too.

Henkel gives two examples of sandal rings (Figure 5.5). One was found in the fort at Vindonissa and depicts a left sandal (1913: 9 and Plate 3.53). The other has a much less clear depiction of footwear (Henkel 1913: 9 and Plate 3.52), and it is unclear where it was found, although it is now in the Römisch-Germanisches Museum, Cologne.

The apotropaic use of Roman hobnailing may be indicated in a ring from Pommerœul, Belgium (Figure 5.6a). It depicts a pair of pointed soles with nails, and the bezel is plated with gold leaf (Cattelain *et al.* 2012: 152). A gold ring with a single, nailed, left sole may also be apotropaic (Figure 5.6b). Unfortunately, it was auctioned by Berganza and there are no archaeological details for this ring.

A final example of shoe-shaped rings is in the British Museum (AF.207). This depicts a sole and bears Christian symbols, two crosses, on either side of a set of three initials (Figure 5.6c). This early Christian ring would have shown its owner's religious beliefs, and placed them under the protection of Christ.

Thus we have seen the Roman use of pendants, gems, and rings in the shape of feet and footwear as amulets. We have also encountered the recurring themes of their votive and religious roles. This amuletic jewellery also illustrates the themes of the foot as *pars pro toto* for a deity, the apotropaic role of hobnailing, and the significance of chirality.

5.2 Jugs with handles ending in feet

Some Roman jugs sport a representation of feet and footwear where the handle meets the body. This is rather different from many Roman jug handles that feature divine, human, or animal heads. Indeed, research into the relative numbers shows that those with humanoid heads are more common than those with feet (Figure 5.7). This section aims to provide background information on such jugs and to examine their social significance. In order to achieve this, a corpus of 82 jugs with handles ending in human feet, or handles detached from such jugs, was assembled, beginning with the 40 in Tassinari's study

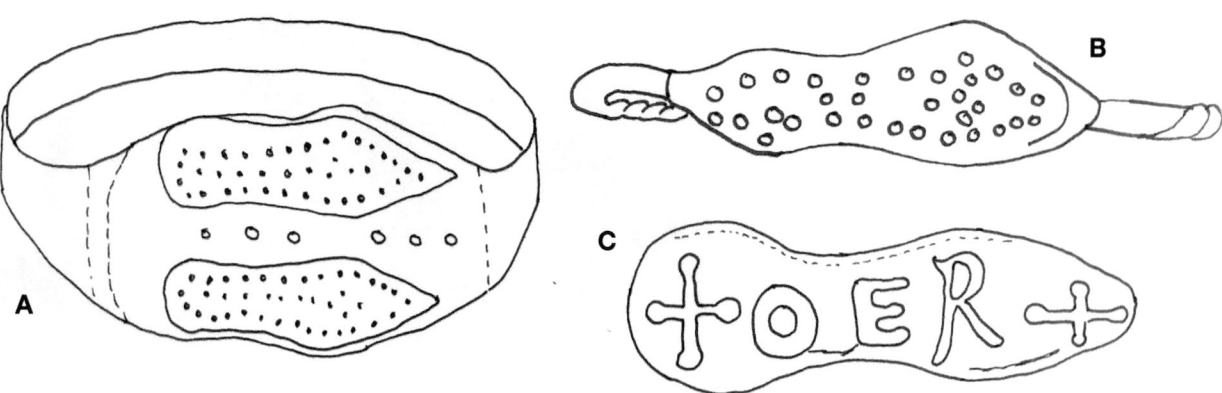

Figure 5.6: a) Hobnailed ring from Pommerœul. b) Hobnailed sandal ring: Berganza. c) Shoe-sole ring with Christian symbols.

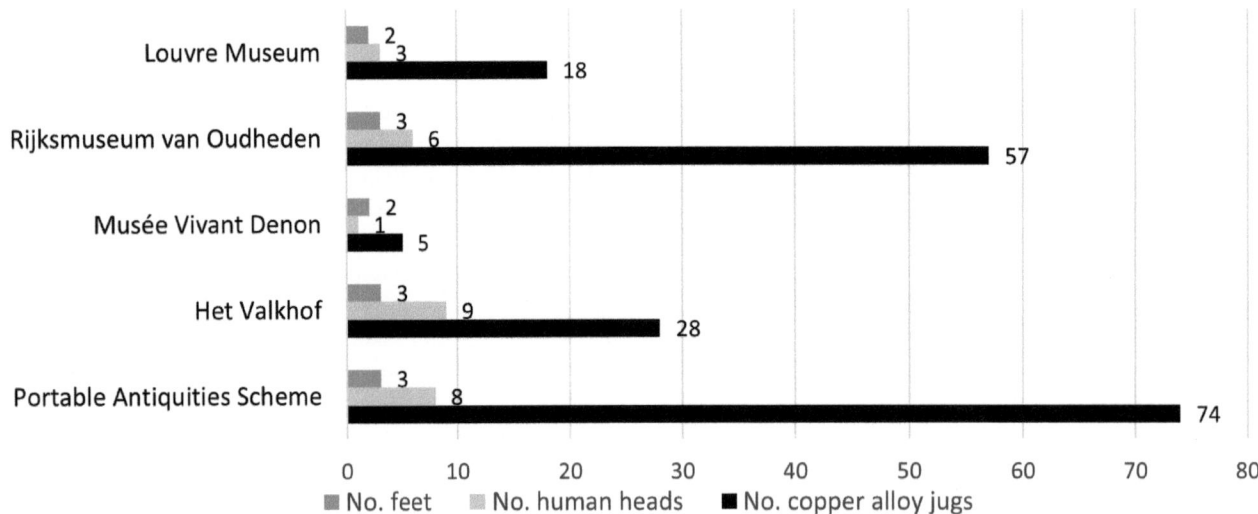

Figure 5.7: Chart to show the relative numbers of Roman copper-alloy jugs with handles terminating in human heads or feet.

(1973). To this was added information from various museum catalogues (Radnóti 1938; den Boesterd 1956; Menzel 1966; Fiumi 1977; Faider-Feytmans 1979; Szabó 1981; Kohlert-Németh 1990; Nenova-Merdjanova 1998; Sedlmayer 1999; Pozo-Rodríguez 2001; Mustaţă 2017), archaeological reports (Forster and Knowles 1913; Liversidge 1958; Vanvinckenroye 1984; Pirling and Siepen 2006; Crummy 2011; Crummy 2015; Hoss 2020), other studies (Barthel and Kapf 1907; Nagy 1945; Bonnamour 1977; Sanie et al. 1980; Ruprechtsberger 1985; Spânu et al. 2016), the Portable Antiquities Scheme (PAS) online database, and the *Artefacts* online encyclopaedia.

The foot-handled jugs date from the late first to the third centuries CE (Figure 5.8; Hoss 2020: 67) and are made of copper alloy, with the exception of one ceramic example from the Roman potteries in Berg en Dal, Netherlands (Tassinari 1973: 139). The metal jugs were beaten from sheet copper alloy (Szabó 1981: 57), and a separately cast handle was soldered on (Mustaţă 2017: 120; Hoss 2020:66). Handle moulds were found in a metal-worker's workshop in Tartus, Syria (Héron de Villefosse 1900: 318). Detached handles represent 26 of the 82 examples.

The jugs come in two slightly different shapes (Tassinari 1973: 135). The western group is tall and slender, with an extended cylindrical lower body, while the body of the eastern variety is ovoid (Figure 5.9; Crummy 2015). All the western type are very similar in size and shape, with the only differences being the chirality and footwear-type of the feet (Radnóti 1938: 167; Tassinari 1973: 136).

It is unclear exactly where jugs with a handle ending in a human foot were manufactured, apart from the evidence of handle-moulds from Syria. Scholars acknowledge that the problem is complex (Radnóti 1938: 168; Tassinari 1973: 139; Crummy 2006: 32). Nagy suggests that the jugs were produced in the Rhineland or upper Gaul (1945: 526). Szabó believes the western type was probably first produced in Gaul in the late first century, with production

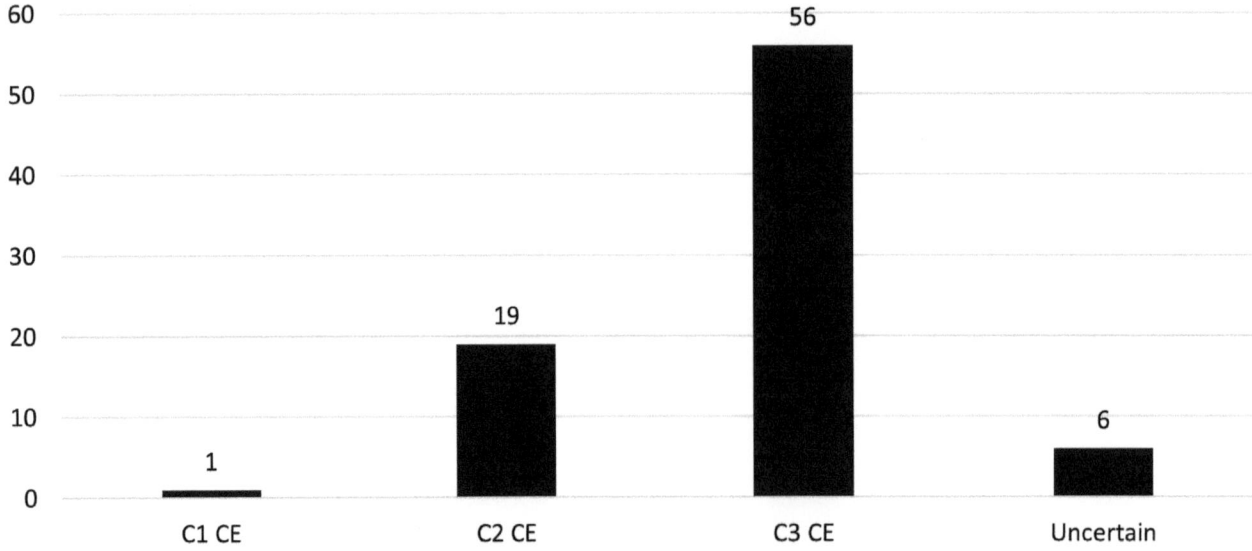

Figure 5.8: Chart to show the date of 82 Roman jugs with handles ending in feet.

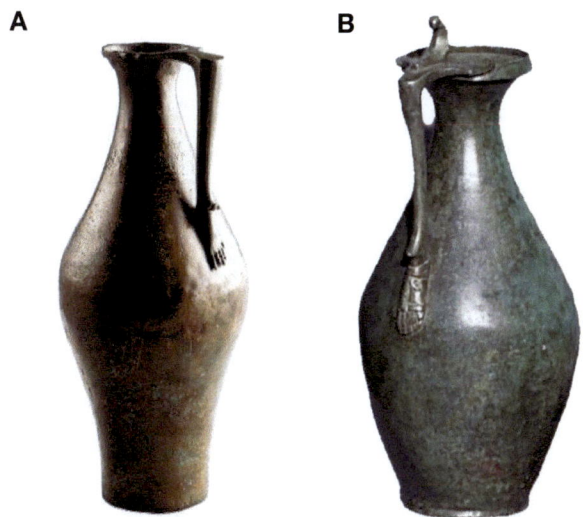

Figure 5.9: a) Western type jug from Gallo-Romeins Museum, Tongeren (74.A.53). b) Eastern type jug from Weißenburg. (Photo Author's own).

spreading to the Danube in the second (1983: 91–92). Sedlmayer argues that the more-widely-dispersed eastern type was produced in the Rhine-Danube area, principally for the export market (1999: 18), and that the design was probably transported east by military units (1999: 19). While this is possible, data for this study show that 10 of the 82 jugs were found on military sites, so their association with the army does not appear to be very close (Figure 5.10). More foot-handled jugs come from urban (29) and even rural sites (24). However, 19 are from an unknown site type, so a link to the army is still possible. We can say that jugs with handles ending in feet were probably manufactured in several provinces (Crummy 2015).

Foot-handled jugs have a wide distribution across the Empire from Syria to Britain, but are mostly found in the northern provinces of *Gallia Belgica*, *Germania*, and *Pannonia*, where they seem to follow the Rhine - Danube trade routes, and in southern Gaul along the valleys of the Saône and Rhône (Sedlmayer 1999: 20; Crummy 2015). The geographical distribution (Figure 5.11) of foot-handled jug finds is, however, not as straight forward as the western/eastern typology might suggest (Crummy 2006: 5). Eastern types have been found in Lux, Boyer (Bonnamour 1977: 22-23), Epfig (Tassinari 1973: 137), and Narbonne, France (*Artefacts* 2021 CRU-4044), and as far west as Tarragona and Garcíez-Jimena in Spain (Pozo-Rodríguez 2001: 176). Western types have been found in Bistrița, Romania (Mustață 2017: 120-122), Igar, Budafok-Háros and Székesfehérvár, Hungary (Szabó 1981: 54), and Ustikolina, Bosnia and Herzegovina. In addition, three jugs in the corpus were found beyond the Limes, two in Romania, at Muncelu de Sus and Mălăieștii de Jos (Spânu *et al.* 2016: 244), and one in a grave in Bitgum, Netherlands.

Tassinari found no Italian examples of (1973: 135) but Fiumi catalogues a foot-jug in the Museo Etrusco Guarnacci, Volterra, which was probably found nearby (1977: 135). There is also a detached handle ending in a left foot in the Vatican Museums (inv.65769). Crummy suggests that a jug found in Hauxton could be related back to early Italy (2015), and Szabó talks of Italian influence on the jugs (1983: 63).

Because of Roman ideas of the right being auspicious, the chirality of the feet on these jug-handles was examined (Figure 5.12). Most (40) are right feet, as might be expected. However, 23 of the jug-handles have left feet and 15 depict pairs. The chirality of the remaining four jugs is uncertain due to wear or lack of recording. Most of the feet (56) are bare and may, therefore, represent the feet of deities (Croom 2010: 74), whereas 19 wear sandals of a type that are seen on portraits of goddesses (Goldman 2001: 107). Although this might just be amusing ornamentation, the feet on these jugs could constitute another example of feet as synecdoche for deities, and therefore could be apotropaic, invoking divine protection. The footwear type on the other jugs is unclear, due to wear or fragmentation.

As part of a contextual archaeological approach for assessing their social significance patterns in the find

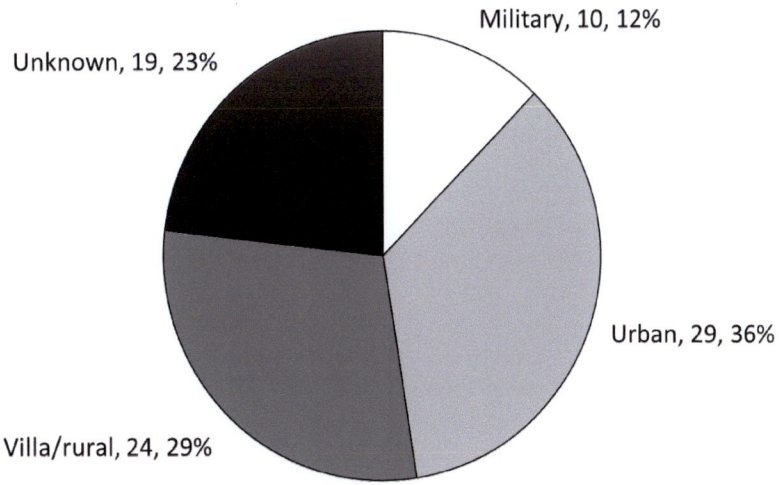

Figure 5.10: Chart to show the site type of 82 Roman jugs with handles ending in feet.

Roman Feet and Shoes

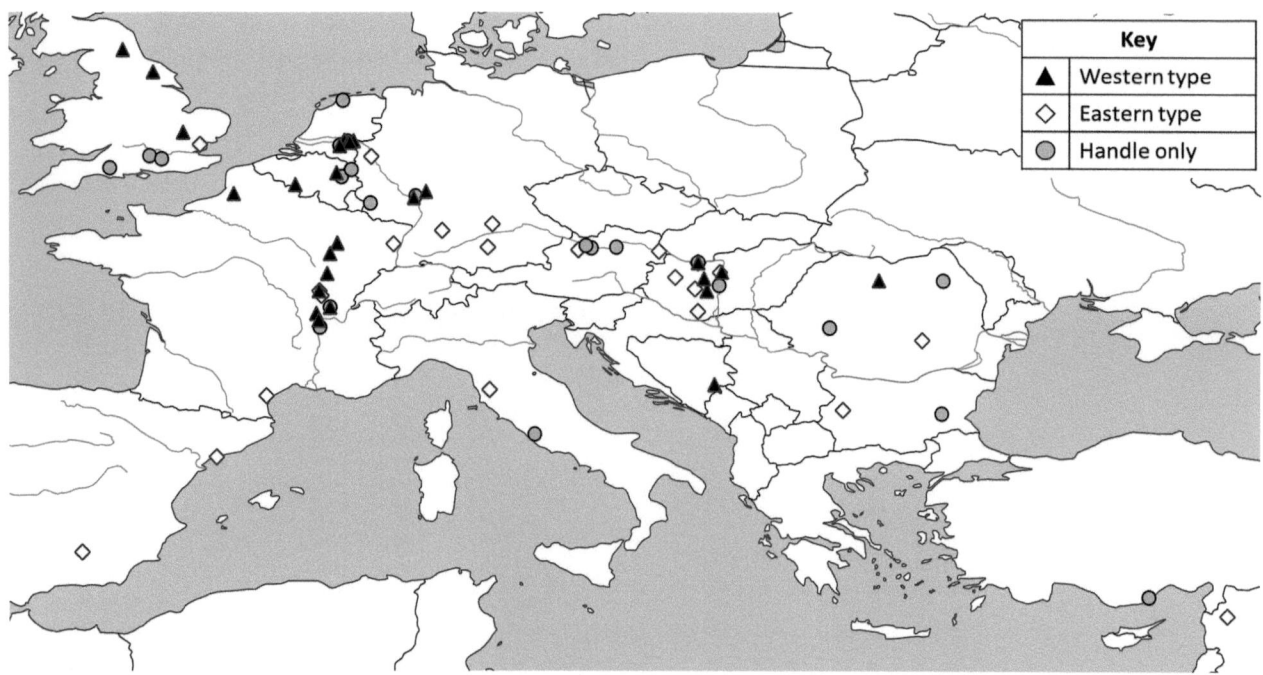

Figure 5.11: Map to show the geographical distribution of the different types of Roman foot-jug.

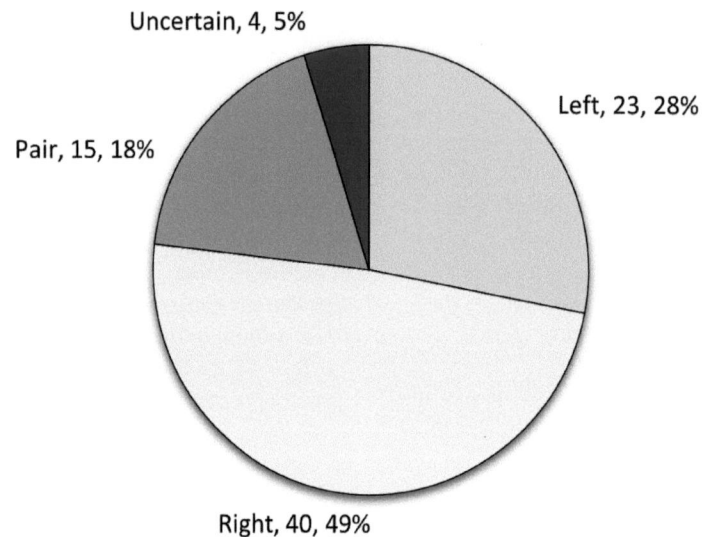

Figure 5.12: Chart to show the chirality of 82 Roman jugs with handles ending in feet.

settings of these foot-handled jugs were examined (Figure 5.13). The find setting of 29 jugs is unrecorded. Five are from religious settings, and 18 from watery contexts, eight of them on urban sites and 10 villa/rural. Funerary settings account for 14 foot-handled jugs, 10 western type and four eastern, 12 of them from graves. Eleven formed part of hoards. Jugs from 'other' find settings came from a sand quarry, a pottery, the Roman baths at Heerlen, and two from unspecified parts of military sites.

The inclusion of foot-handled jugs in funerary settings shows their significance as status markers, since many were found with other, expensive items. These are all examples of the creation of an image of 'the beautiful dead' (Pearce 2016: 458). The deceased's mourners were showing that they could afford to put these valuable items in the ground. The jug from grave 3 in Wehringen Roman cemetery, Germany, was found with a copper alloy tripod, a four-legged table, seven further copper alloy jugs, three cups with ram's head handles, 40 pieces of pottery, including a red painted plate and bowl (Szabó 1981: 64). The foot-handled jug from the Roman cemetery at Krefeld-Gellep, Germany, recovered in association with cremation grave 5595, contained nine coins, the latest of which dates to 259 CE (Pirling and Siepen 2006: 311), and was found with other copper alloy, and some glass, vessels (Pirling 1993: 393-395). The foot-handled jug found in Nagytétény, Hungary, was in a chariot burial that also included a folding stool, a bucket-handle, a copper alloy patera with an ornate handle, various other vessels, and three strigils (Károly 1890: 107 and Plate II).

The ubiquity of Roman foot- and shoe-shaped artefacts

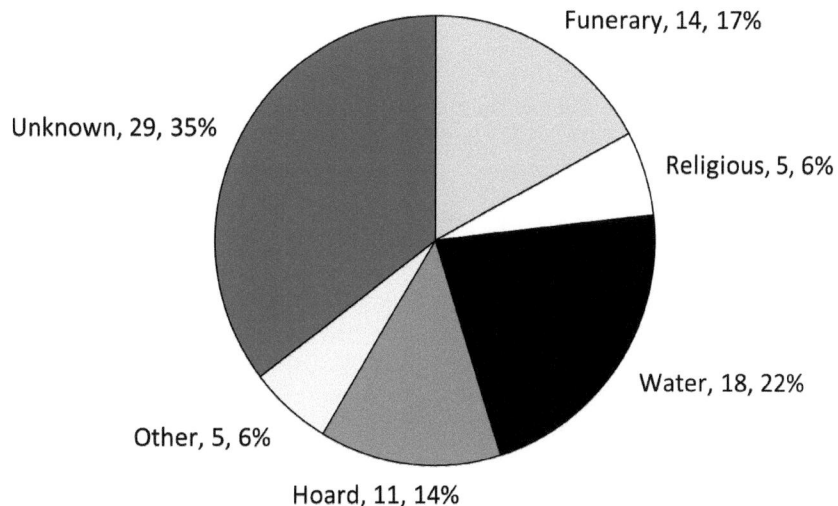

Figure 5.13: Chart to show the find settings of 82 Roman jugs with handles ending in feet.

A foot-handled jug from a Roman tomb in Ustikolina, Bosnia and Herzegovina, was found with an Eggers-Type 79 copper alloy bowl, a pan with a handle, a spear-shaped copper alloy object, and a copper alloy fibula (Szabó 1981: 64). The other foot-handled jug from a funerary site was found next to ritual hearth 2 in the south-western Roman cemetery, Tongeren, Belgium, along with three complete pottery vessels (Vanvinckenroye 1984: Plate 126). Judging by the grave furniture, these are high-status burials. The funerary use of foot-handled jugs may be linked to footwear in Roman burials. The depiction of the feet of deities on the handles would have made the jugs more protective. The jugs may also have been part of burial rituals to do with cleansing or feasting.

Three of the foot-handled jugs were found in, or near, religious sites. The Corbridge example was found at site 43, within the eastern military compound, near three temples, together with a bone plaque depicting a mother goddess (Forster and Knowles 1913: 235 and 276; Crummy 2015). This may be a votive deposit. Caution is needed, however, in associating this jug directly with the temples, as there is an intervening wall (Crummy 2015). The jug from Heybridge was found in a small pit next to the approach road to the site's temple precinct (Crummy 2015). Like the Corbridge example, no direct link can be established with the temple (Crummy 2015). However, a foot-handled jug from Igar, Hungary, was deposited in a sanctuary as part of a votive hoard containing a copper alloy *balsamarium* in the shape of a black African male head, a cauldron inscribed MANLVCI F, an umbo, a cup with a handle, and part of a buckle (Szabó 1981: 63). Szabó interprets this jug example as sanctuary equipment (1981: 63). It is worth noting that many Roman altars have jugs carved on the side (Henig 1984: 131: Mustață 2017: 45) as a symbol of the cleansing associated with religious ritual, for which the jugs may have been used.

Eighteen of the foot-handled jugs (22%) are from find settings involving water, such as rivers and wells. Eggers (1966: 100-110) provides some comparative data for the relative proportions of the find settings of Roman copper alloy jugs in general. He catalogues 23 from Britain, of which five are from hoards (22%), two are urban (8%), eight are from burials (35%), three are from wells (13%) and the find setting of two is unknown (9%). The remaining three (13%) are possibly from the river Granta near Hauxton Mill; one is foot-handled. A similar proportion of other types of Roman jug to foot-handled jugs are deposited in watery contexts.

Western-type jugs are often found in association with rivers, wells, and springs. Szabó (1981: 63) and Crummy (2011: 114) suggest they were purpose-made ritual, rather than domestic, vessels. Jugs from the corpus deposited in wells may support this argument. A well in Bad Cannstatt, Germany, contained two foot-handled jugs, one complete and the other fragmentary (Tassinari 1973: 136). A foot-handled jug was excavated with other copper alloy vessels from the Cartanyà well in the *colonia* forum in Tarragona (MNAT 2020). A jug from Grand, Vosges, was found in a well 12 metres down, along with other objects: two pans, a knife, a saw, some scissors, two padlocks, a copper alloy cauldron, and three ceramic vessels (Maxe-Werly 1871: 166-171). Slightly higher up in the fill were an oval copper alloy dish that had been silvered, and fragments of a disc that was a Roman calendar (Maxe-Werly 1871). The case is similar for the jug-handle from a well in at Jupille-sur-Meuse, Belgium (Tassinari 1973: 136). These examples all appear to be valuable items and are unlikely to have been merely thrown away, suggesting special deposition. A detached foot-handle was found in fill 6436 of well 5735 in Silchester (Clarke and Fulford 2011: 43). Further special deposits came from the same fill: a bucket handle, a maple writing-tablet, and a dog's scapula (Clarke and Fulford 2011: 313-314). Crummy interprets this jug-handle as a votive deposit (Crummy 2011: 114), which is likely, since animal bones in wells are indicative of structured deposition (Merrifield 1987: 32) and dog bones are of particular significance (Morris 2008:

9). While it is possible that complete jugs found in wells were used for drawing water and dropped in accidentally, the assemblages found with the foot-handled jugs in wells point to ritual deposition, either as a marker for a stage in a well's biography (van Driel-Murray 2011a: 337; van Haasteren and Groot 2013: 25), or as part of a votive process (van Driel-Murray 1999: 136).

Rivers and water-logged ground have also yielded foot-handled jugs. This corpus contains examples taken from the river Saône, near Chalon-sur-Saône, Lux, Boyer, and Beauregard-Jassens (Joconde 2021). Three of these were isolated finds, and were possibly dropped while collecting water. However, the examples from Lux and Chalon-sur-Saône were found near river crossings (Dumont 2002: 58) and might be foundation offerings (Eckardt 2021: 21–22) or *ex votos* for a safe river crossing (Dumont 2002: 66). Foot-handled jugs from the Waal near Nijmegen (den Boesterd 1956: 81), the Danube at Budafok-Háros, Hungary (Szabó 1981: 52), and one from Schallemmersdorf, Austria (Sedlmayer 1999: 18), were also isolated finds. Szabó (1981: 63) suggests such jugs were vessels used to store water for ritual purposes from *in vivo flumine* rather than for domestic water collection, and that the nature of the sites is related to the rites of sacrifice.

In other riverine deposits foot-handled jugs form part of assemblages. The Boyer jug was accompanied by other vessels including a copper alloy pan (Bonnamour 1977: 21). One foot-handled jug from the Waal near Nijmegen was found with another type of jug, a pot with a lid, a large vessel, and a *patera* (Rijksmuseum van Oudheden 2021). This resembles the sets of flagons and *paterae* often carved on the sides of Roman altars (Henig 1984: 131: Mustață 2017: 48–53), so there could be an element of sacrifice in these deposits. One jug was found filled with Hadrianic coins at Épagnette in a peat bog near the river Somme (Tassinari 1973: 136), possibly a votive watery setting. This coin hoard would have increased the value of the offering.

It is debateable whether we should class the jug from Hauxton as a watery find. Hurrell (1904: 496) reports that it was found above Hauxton Mill 'between the mill stream and the rivulet which carries off the water when the mill is not working', and rivers change course over time, so it could conform to the pattern. However, both Liversidge (1958: 11) and Eggers (1966: 99) suggest that the accompanying finds of two further copper alloy jugs, four glass vessels, an iron lamp, and ceramics, including a barbotine cup, may indicate a burial similar to those in Belgic 'tumuli', and therefore high-status. Nevertheless, many of the Roman foot-handled jugs from watery contexts seem to have been deposited for ritual purposes, as votives, as markers of a stage in the biography of a well, or as symbols of sacrificial rites.

It is quite common to find foot-handled jugs in hoards with other bronzes or with Roman coins, some of which have already been discussed. A group of three copper alloy jugs found by a detectorist near Nunnington, North Yorkshire, includes two with foot-handles (PAS YORYM-68EAC1). A jug found between Chaumont and Langres, France, was filled with Roman coins (Tassinari 1973: 136). The jug from Nida-Heddernheim, Germany, was found with other bronzes (Szabó 1981: 64), as was a handle from Enns-Lauriacum, Austria (Sedlmayer 1999: 18 and fig. 25). As well as a foot-handled jug, the 'Vieille Bruyère' sand quarry at Givry, France, yielded an assemblage of two cauldrons, a balance rod, a second copper alloy jug, four copper alloy bowls, three tinned dishes, some greenish pottery and some glass vials (Moisin 1954: 181). The Weißenburg hoard, which includes a foot-handled jug, comprises 114 objects, including 18 copper alloy statuettes, 10 other figurative bronzes, 11 silver votive sheets, three copper alloy face masks, an iron helmet, 20 copper alloy vessels, 18 copper alloy fittings, and 33 iron implements (Donderer 2004: 235). It was thought this hoard may have been left by plunderers (Donderer 2004: 236) but Donderer argues that the hoard was carefully deposited, which does not fit with looters (2004: 238). It may have been a temple treasure, based on the cult statues in the hoard, but Donderer suggests that the assemblage is too heterogeneous (2004: 236) and should be regarded as having been left by a metal goods trader (2004: 242).

Two of the hoards featuring foot-handled jugs come from beyond the Limes in Romania. The hoard from Mălăieștii de Jos contained 74 coins dating from Vespasian to Valerian I, five bracelets, a pendant, a fibula, and two silver ingots (Spânu *et al.* 2016: 237). The hoard was not buried in a funerary setting or in a house (Spânu *et al.* 2016: 237). Indeed, Spânu *et al.* argue that, since the hoard comprises a jug and coins from the Roman Empire together with jewellery that 'reflected the preferences of the *Barbaricum* elites', it is 'a significant cultural landmark for the crossroads of the Principate in its nadir phase with the earliest migrations taking wing in the Lower Danube region in the last decades of the third century' (Spânu *et al.* 2016: 255). The Muncelu de Sus jug contained 667 coins, ranging from the late republic to Marcus Aurelius (Sanie *et al.* 1980: 249). This hoard is, therefore, much earlier than that from Mălăieștii de Jos. Three further coin-hoards of a similar date and seven silver vessels were discovered at the same site (Sanie *et al.* 1980: 249). Sanie *et al.* (1980: 266) suggest that, due to the value of these deposits, Muncelu de Sus may have been the residence of an important Dacian leader and the coins were *stipendia* received by one of the Costoboc kings which were buried as a result of Roman action in East Carpathia beginning with Marcus Aurelius (Sanie *et al.* 1980: 266). In these two cases, the hoards containing foot-handled jugs appear to have been markers of status.

Hoards containing foot-handled jugs may have had a variety of different and overlapping significances (Millett 1994: 100), which were possibly not the same as within the Roman Empire. Religious symbols are common on objects found in hoards (Millett 1994: 100). The feet on the handles may represent deities, so this could be why these vessels were considered appropriate containers for, and components of, valuable hoards. Some hoards may be collections of valuable metal for recycling. Others may be markers of power and status. The foot symbolised domination (Dio Cassius 50.24.3 and 52.34.8; SHA. *Max*.28; SHA.*Prob*.20), so the inclusion of foot-handled jugs seems appropriate. The hoards could also be votive deposits (Millett 1994: 103; Gerrard 2009: 179).

This section has explored the social significance of 82 foot-handled jugs or detached handles, which were found across the northern areas of the Roman Empire as an example of Roman foot-shaped artefacts. Foot-handled jugs may have been more valuable compared with other types due to their relative rarity (Szabó 1981: 63), hence their appropriateness as markers of status. Many foot-handled jugs appear to have been of ritual significance, being used in funerary and sanctuary settings, and as votive deposits, possibly because the depiction of feet on the handles represents deities (Croom 2010: 74).

5.3 Knife or razor handles in the shape of feet

A peculiarly Romano-British example of representations of feet and footwear is that of handles in the form of legs finishing in feet. This study has catalogued 37 such handles, all but eight of them from Britain (Figure 5.15). Two bone or ivory handles which represent just a foot were found in Ostia and one in Chartres. Two further bone or ivory handles which are similar in style to the British copper alloy handles came from Italy, a third one from Ostia (inventory number 4305), and one found in Alba Fucens (*Artefacts* 2021 CNF-4078). A further example was found in Las Ermitas en Espejo, Spain. The other exceptions were found in Schwirzheim (Menzel 1966: 80) and Cologne, Germany (Franken 1996: 126–127) and are both copper alloy (Figure 5.14). The example from Cologne is the only one to include a depiction of hobnailing, possibly because it depicts a closed boot, rather than a sandal.

The foot length of these handles varies between 10 and 24.3 millimetres, with an average of 18.7 millimetres. The leg-length is less representative, as they appear to have broken off at different points (see Figure 5.16).

The function of the handles is unclear (Worrell 2005: 453; Allason-Jones 2009: 442). Henig suggests votive feet for healing shrines (2015). Lloyd-Morgan favours an attachment for delicate furnishings, such as a furniture foot

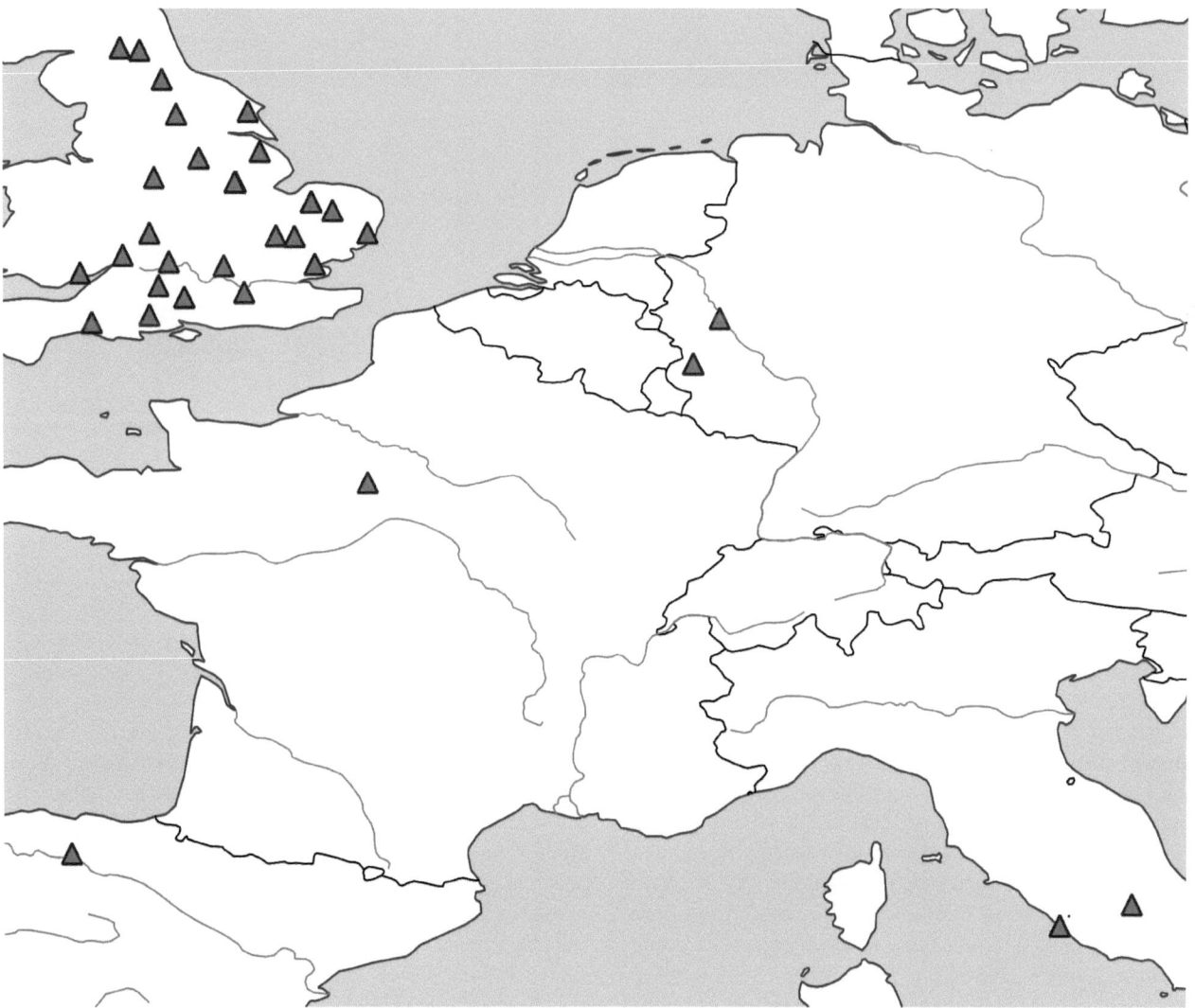

Figure 5.14: Map to show the geographical distribution of Roman knife/razor handles in the form of feet.

Roman Feet and Shoes

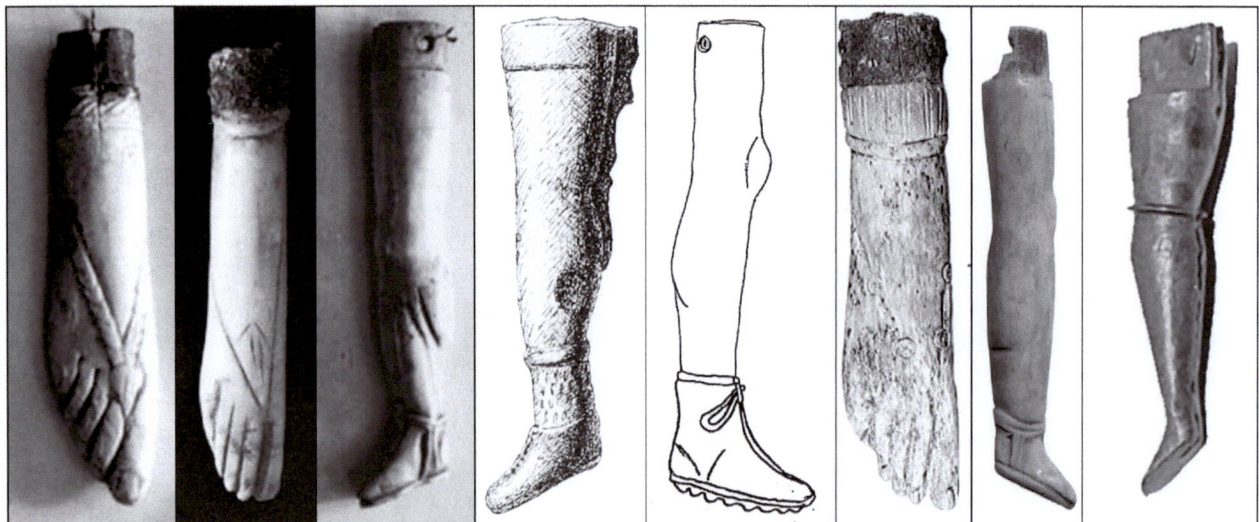

Figure 5.15: Knife/razor handles from: Ostia (Museo Ostiense 4304, unknown, and 4305); Schwirzheim (Dehn et al. 1937: fig.2); Cologne (Author's drawing); Alba Fucens, Chartres, and Espejo (Artefacts CNF-4078 Bianchi; CNF-4087 Canny; CNF-4036_4 Feugère).

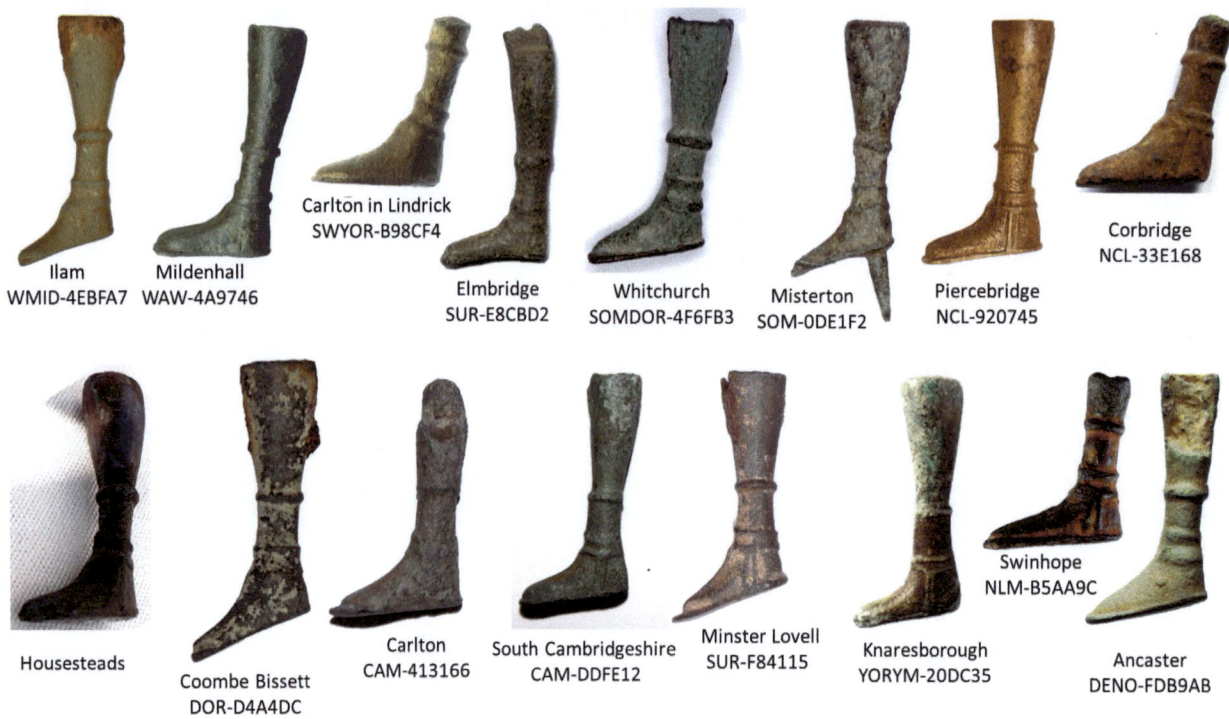

Figure 5.16: Roman knife/razor handles showing socks with sandals (Portable Antiquities Scheme).

(1994: 181; 2000: 368). Allason-Jones proposes a support for small candelabra or dishes (2009: 442) and possibly boxes (2008: D11.33). Some have been misidentified as part of a figurine (PAS NLM-DB6484). However, Menzel calls them handles for folding knives (1966: 80) and Feugère *et al.* call them clasp-knives (2021). Feugère and Božič have also suggested that small, folding Roman knives are pen-knives, part of Roman writing equipment (Božič 2001: 29; Feugère 2003: 10; Božič and Feugère 2004: 37-39). Worrell thinks they are likely to have been knife handles (2005: 453) and Köstner argues for knife or razor handles (2016: 22). There are 21 such handles in the Portable Antiquities Scheme database, 19 of which are identified as knife or razor handles, and three of which have evidence of iron corrosion from a blade (SOM-0DE1F2; DOR-D4A4DC; SUR-F84115). This, therefore, seems the most probable function of these handles.

Because they were found by detectorists, 20 of the handles have no precise archaeological context, making definitive dating difficult. However, since 25 of the 35 handles in this study's corpus are wearing the same style of sandal over socks (Figure 5.16), and footwear can be used as dating evidence (van Driel-Murray 2001a), it has been suggested that the sandals' design indicates a date of the late third and early fourth centuries. The footwear is reminiscent of wide soled men's *soleae* (PAS SOM-0DE1F2 and SOMDOR-4F6FB3; Köstner 2016: 22) that were fashionable then (van Driel-Murray 2001a: 194–195). Two handles from Housesteads fort come from contexts securely dated to the late third and early fourth centuries (Rushworth 2009: 91 and 188). A handle from Heybridge also fits this date range (Henig 2015).

Lloyd-Morgan compares a foot-handle from Alcester to a similar third-century item (1994: 181). The Caerleon foot-handle was found in the yard of building 12 in a context (1226/SG125 (1157)) whose date does not extend beyond the middle of the fourth century (Evans 2000: 122). The strong similarity between 22 of the copper alloy knife or razor handles (Figure 5.16) and the dating evidence, points to a date of late third to early fourth century for this style of handle. The Ostia handles, which are different, may be earlier, although the handle from Chartres, which is similar to the Ostia foot, does date to the third century.

The lack of data for archaeological context impacts on the analysis of the site type distribution of the handles (Figure 5.17). Four come from military sites: two from the north-east corner of Housesteads fort, one from Caerleon, and one from Piercebridge Roman fort. The knife/razor handles do not seem to be particularly associated with the army, however, as nine come from general, urban locations. Among these are a bone or ivory knife handle from Ostia (inventory number 4304), which portrays a right foot wearing the kind of sandal associated with statues of goddesses (Goldman 2001: 107), so this might be a religious symbol. Only two are known to have been found on villa/rural sites, although 20 whose data come from PAS are likely to have been from rural sites. Information on find settings is also scarce due to the data sources. Only the following two knife/razor handles have a known find setting.

The Heybridge handle (SF5806) is classed by Henig as a religious object (2015) and was found near a well, in pit 10910, with other artefacts including a jet pin (SF5768), bone pins (SF5772, SF5776), a spindle-whorl (SF5771), and box fittings (SF5769) (Atkinson and Preston 2015).

Henig suggests that the handle is connected to the cult of Mercury, patron of travellers (2015), but also Psychopomp (Crummy 2007: 227). A second handle from Piercebridge was found in the River Tees (PAS NCL-920745). Walton, who recorded the find, comments that the material from the Tees at Piercebridge represents a rich and important votive deposit (2008: 293). She also notes that, as an object associated with the body, it may have been imbued with some form of ritual significance, particularly in this watery setting (2021: 81).

It should be noted that Roman knife handles have been found in the shape of gladiators (for example, PAS NCL-393023 and LON-88EF5E) hunting scenes (for example, PAS SUR-817DAD and DEV-8DA53D) and erotica (for example, PAS GLO-481969 and WAW-0A2FF7), so Roman knife or razor handles in the form of lower legs with feet may just be novelty forms (Figure 5.18). Roman knife or razor handles occur in the form of other body parts. Augusta Raurica has a group of 14 in the shape of a hand (Kaufmann-Heinimann 1998: 33), five of which are holding round objects. Such hands are thought to have acted as powerful apotropaic charms (Eckardt 2014: 176). Handles in the form of human heads are sometimes found, such as four from Augusta Raurica (Kaufmann-Heinimann 1998: 33-34; 109) and two on the PAS database (YORYM-4482B0 and BUC-410F94). Heads were also thought to be powerful (Croxford 2003: 88–9; Eckardt 2014: 168) and the residence of the spirit or soul (Clarke 1996: 75). There are some knife or razor handles that depict deities: Venus is known (PAS ESS-7F7F06; NMS-14DDF6; WAW-378661), as is a hunter-god from Yorkshire (Crummy and Holmes 2003: 9), which may support an argument for religious symbolism. Handles in the form of busts of Minerva are also known (for example, PAS KENT-AE9C22 and LANCUM-B19766). These are described as razor or spatula handles on the PAS database. Minerva handles represent the goddess of wisdom (Eckardt 2014: 188) and are evidence for literacy (Eckardt 2014: 191). Small knives may also be part of Roman writing equipment (Božič and Feugère 2004: 37-39). The foot-handles are,

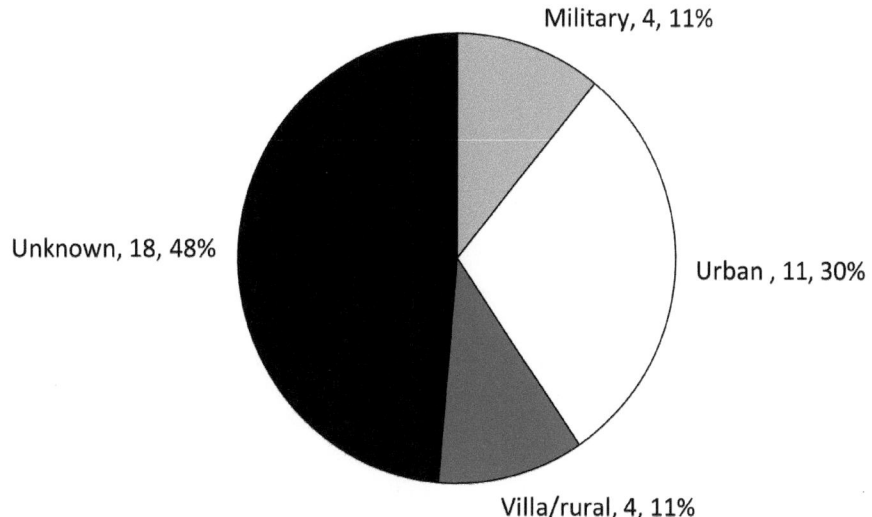

Figure 5.17: Chart to show the site type of 37 foot-shaped Roman knife/razor handles.

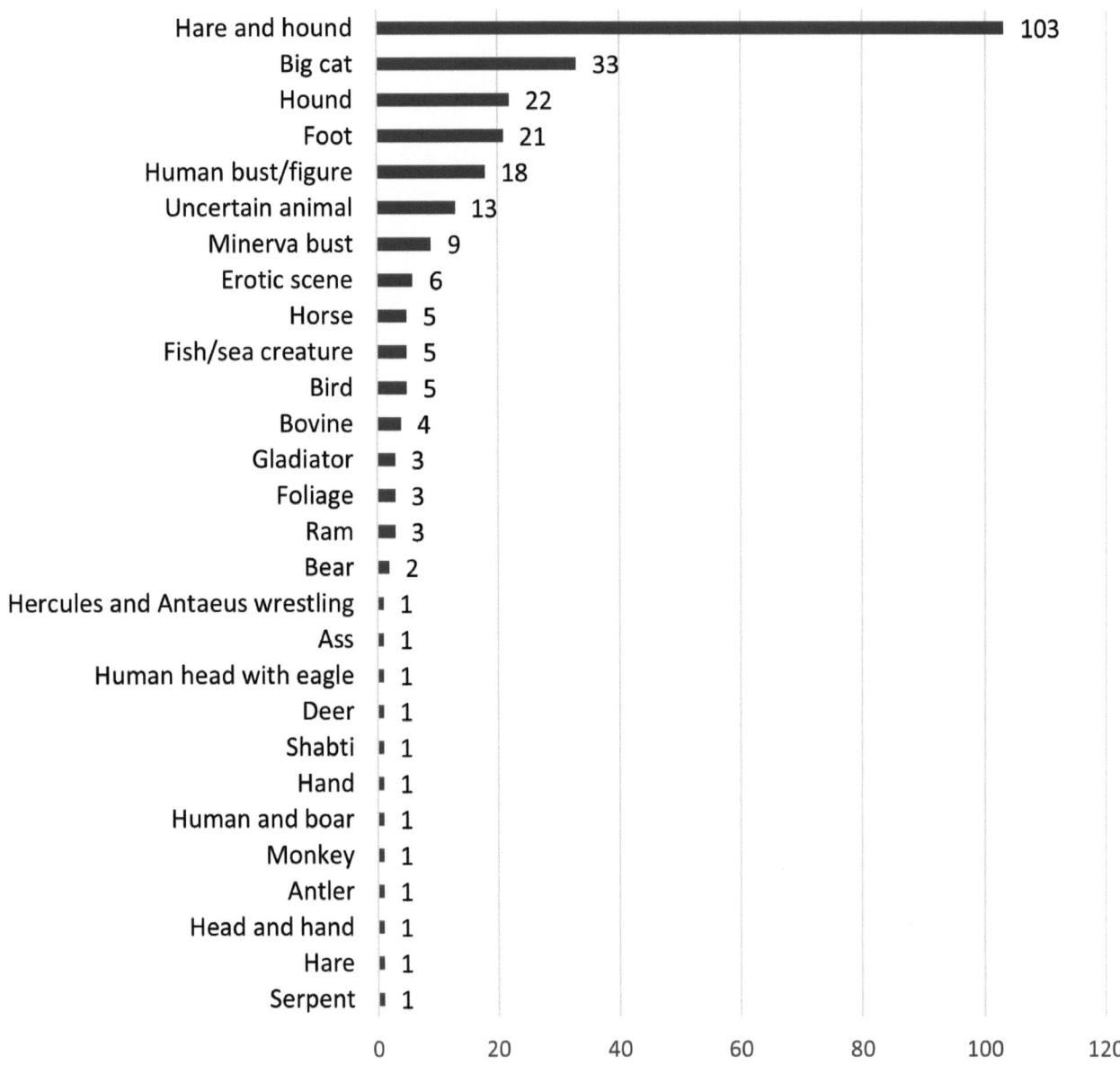

Figure 5.18: Chart to show the proportions of ornamentation type in 258 Roman knife/razor handles with representative designs in the PAS database.

therefore, polysemous, ranging in significance from a representation of fashionable footwear to being used as votive objects in religious settings. They may also have played an apotropaic role.

5.4 Furniture feet

This section considers the various significances of Roman furniture attachments in the shape of human feet. It will examine their chronological, spatial and find setting distribution, and discuss their range of symbolism. This study has catalogued 54 sets of furniture feet.[1] Originally the feet would have been in groups, usually of three or four, depending on the type of furniture, but some sets have lost components over time. Of the 54 sets, 28 are single feet, 14 left, 13 right, and one indeterminate because there is

no photograph and the British Museum does not mention its chirality (no. 1824,0498.39). There are 13 pairs and 13 sets of multiple feet, which comprise anything from three to six (Figure 5.19).

The geographical distribution of the corpus ranges from western Spain eastwards to Turkey, with a concentration in the north-western provinces (Figure 5.20). Three sets in the corpus were found in Britain, in antiquarian finds from Wroxeter (British Museum no. SLAntiq.33), and the Bartlow Hills (Liversidge 1955: 29–31) and Lexden tumuli (Laver 1927: 248–249). Given their wide distribution, it is clear that such feet correspond to a type of decoration particularly appreciated in the provinces (Dieudonné-Glad et al. 2013: 140). They frequently come from a light, folding seat, made up of four bars connected at half height with a leather seat (Dieudonné-Glad et al. 2013: 140). Examples of these were found in the Great Barrow of the Bartlow Hills (Figure 5.21a), which still had the leather

---

[1] Franken (1996: 60–61) lists others. Details of some proved impossible to obtain.

The ubiquity of Roman foot- and shoe-shaped artefacts

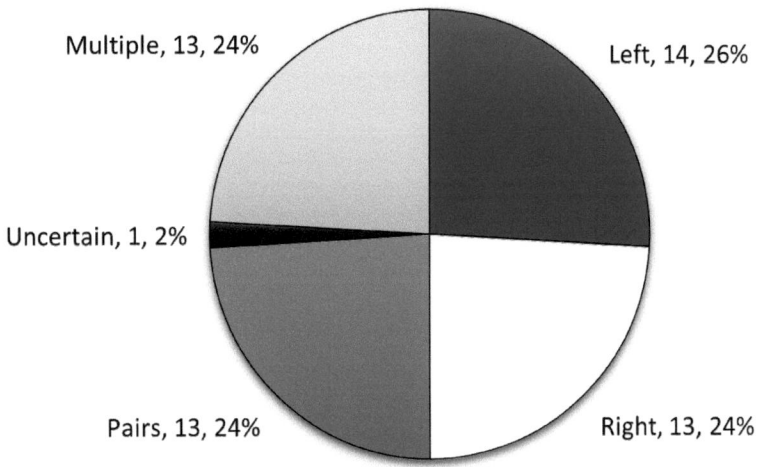

Figure 5.19: Chart to show the chirality of 54 sets of Roman furniture 'feet'.

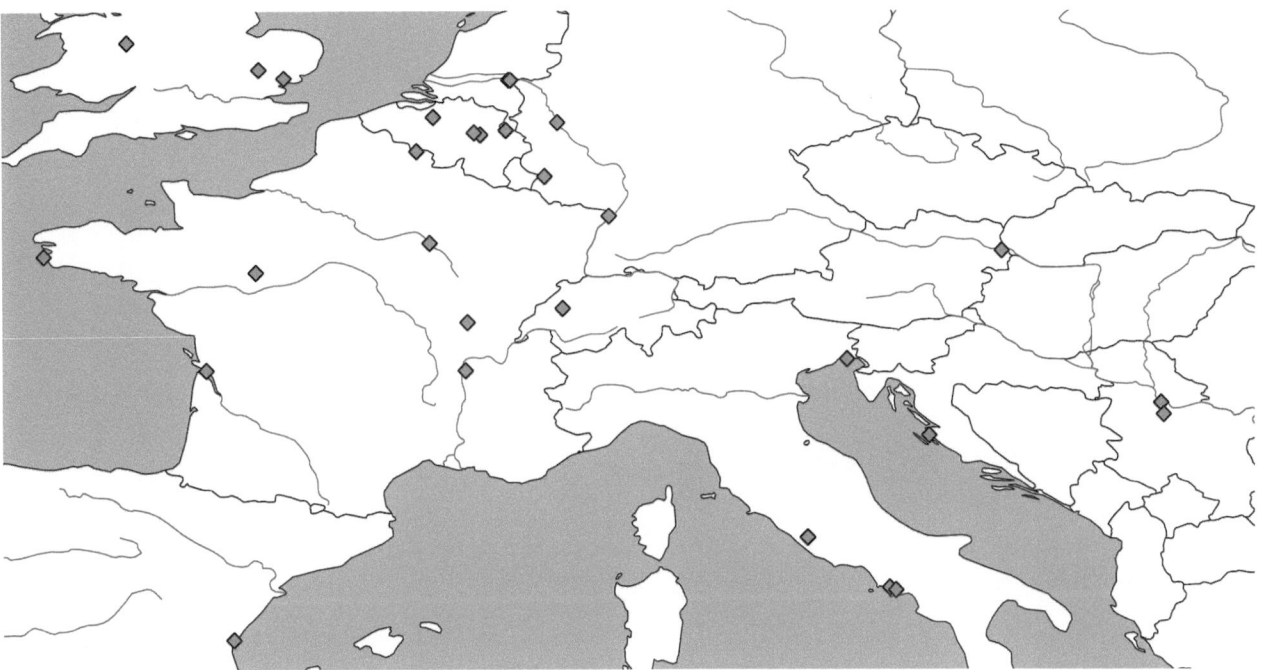

Figure 5.20: Map to show the distribution of Roman furniture 'feet'.

attached (Liversidge 1955: 30), and at the Roman villa in, Schophem, Belgium (Figure 5.21b; Liversidge 1955: 31). The frame of a different type of folding seat with human 'feet' (Figure 5.21c) was found at Nijmegen (Liversidge 1955: 33–34; Collectie Gelderland 2020b). It has a curved frame and can be called a '*sella curulis*' (Mols 1994a: 293). Two of the feet from this chair were preserved, while the other two were restored (Mols 1994a: 293). This stool, although rare, is not unique: a very similar specimen was found in the river Scheldt, Belgium (Mols 1994a: 293). Virtually identical feet were also found in Volubilis, Morocco[2] and in the Lexden tumulus near Colchester (Mols 1994a: 293). A third type, which had only three legs, also existed (Franken 1996: 59–60).

The Latin word for foot, *pes*, was also used for furniture attachments (Lewis and Short 1979), and they may be an example of a witty novelty because of the pun. Roman furniture feet in the shape of animals' paws also exist, providing further evidence of this interpretation. However, there may be a deeper symbolism involved in these furniture feet. One suggestion is that, because the attachments are often associated with folding seats (Franken 1996: 60; Hoss 2020: 58), they could come from *sellae curules* (Franken 1996: 60; Pozo-Rodríguez 2004: 444), the Roman magistrate's seat. The folding stools also bear a resemblance to the *sella castrensis*, or campaigning chair. Roman coins sometimes depict emperors seated on such furniture, for example , a sestertius of Trajan (Figure 5.22a; Roman Imperial Coinage (RIC) II Trajan 666) with Dacians literally at his feet. This illustrates the Roman idea of the foot as a symbol of power.

---

[2] Unfortunately, literature relating to the Belgian and Moroccan examples was unobtainable at the time of writing.

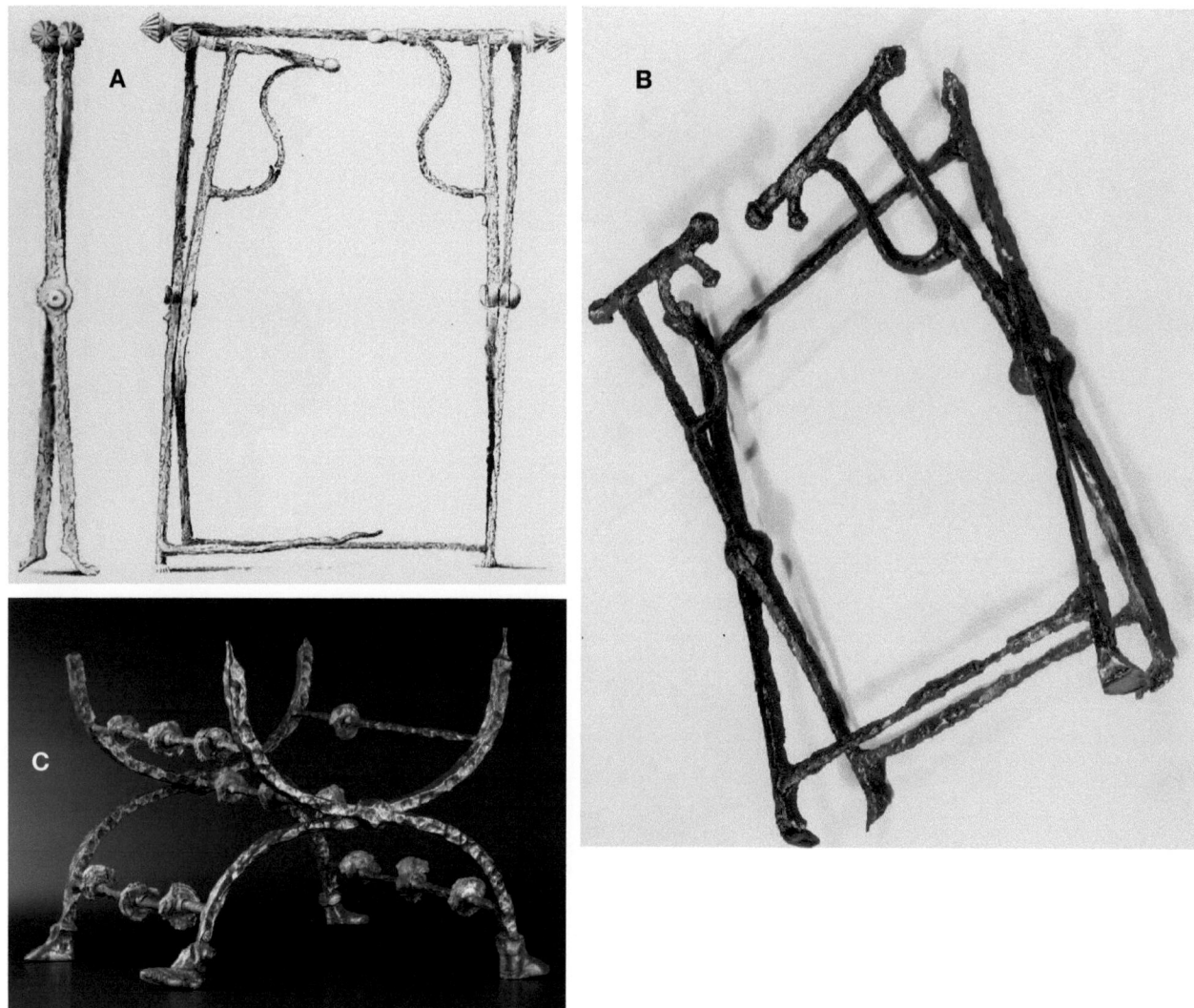

Figure 5.21: Roman folding stools with human feet: a) Bartlow Hills burial (Gage 1836: pl.32.2); b) Schophem Roman villa (KIK-IRPA B170629); c) Hunnerberg necropolis, Nijmegen (Het Valkhof Inv. no. CC.279).

The metaphor of trampling underfoot as a sign of domination occurs in Dio Cassius' accounts of Cleopatra (50.24.3) and how Augustus should handle the law (52.34.8). This idea persists in reports of later emperors, for example, kissing feet as a sign of obeisance (*SHA. Max.*8.7). Nine princes of different tribes are said to have prostrated themselves at Probus' feet (*SHA.Prob.*14) and he 'put down all barbarian nations under his feet' (*SHA. Prob.*20). Iconography expressing this idea can be seen in Panzer statues of emperors, for example Hadrian with non-Romans at his feet, such as that from the theatre at Hierapytna, Crete (Figure 5.22b). Furniture feet could, therefore, be symbols of power. However, only five sets of furniture feet in this study are known to come from military sites, whereas 26 were found in urban locations (Figure 5.23), and probably have more to do with displaying power in terms of wealth and status than in a military sense.

Furniture 'feet' have been found in rural burials (Figure 5.24). Frames of folding seats ending in human feet were found in the Bartlow Hills (Liversidge 1955: 29–31), and the *tumulus* at Avernas-le-Bauduin, Belgium (Liversidge 1955: 31), which also produced three pairs of copper alloy furniture feet (Faider-Feytmans 1979: 132). The Bartlow Hills cremation burial was accompanied by a wooden chest containing two strigils, several glass and copper alloy vessels including a *patera*, and a copper alloy lamp (Gage 1836: 302–305). A furniture foot found in the Lexden tumulus, which dates to about 15 BCE, is thought to have come from a folding seat (Mols 1994a: 293). The tomb also included a Roman copper alloy table, a figurine of Cupid holding a goose, a silver medallion modelled on a Roman coin of Augustus, and at least 17 Mediterranean wine amphorae (Historic England 2021).

The inclusion of Roman wares in a later Iron Age tomb is remarkable and indicates a powerful, wealthy person (Historic England 2021). These Roman barrow burials display high status (Eckardt *et al.* 2009: 80), and the inclusion of folding chairs in élite burials elsewhere is not unknown: 42 have been found in richly furnished graves, which date from the first to third centuries, in the European border provinces, from Britain to Thrace (Mráv 2013: 106).

The ubiquity of Roman foot- and shoe-shaped artefacts

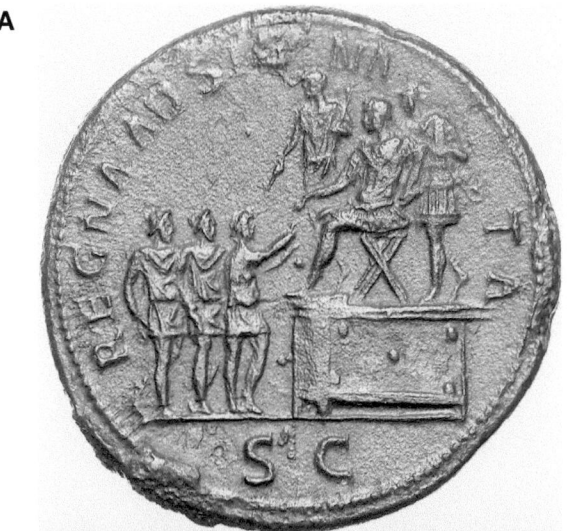

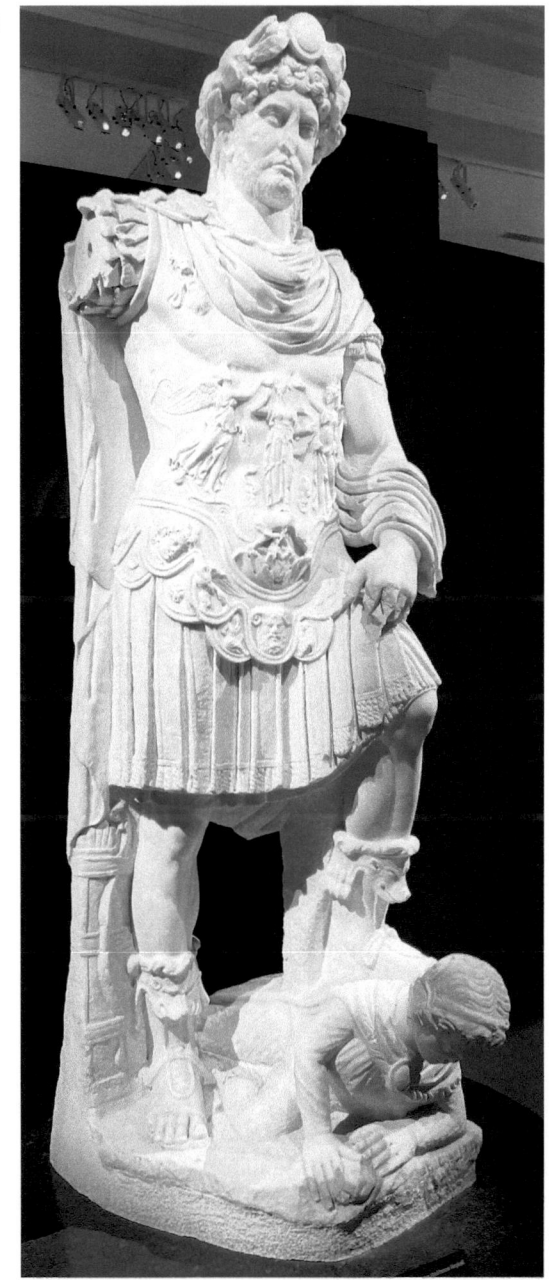

Figure 5.22: a) Sestertius RIC II Trajan 666 (Münzkabinett der Staatlichen Museen Berlin): b) Panzer statue of Hadrian from the theatre at Hierapytna, Crete. (Photo: Raddato).

Three further burials contained furniture feet. A set of four feet and an iron link came from a grave in Kesseldorf, Alsace, for which there are few details. A pair of bare feet came from grave 197, Luxemburger Straße, Cologne (Franken 1996: 61), along the route of the *Via Agrippa*. The frame of an elaborate iron and copper alloy folding chair (Figure 5.21c) was found in grave 49 of the Hunnerberg necropolis, Nijmegen, with a lot of pottery vessels and lamps (Vermeulen 1932: Pl. XV). These are also fairly high-status burials.

Further evidence for the use of furniture with feet in association with burials can be seen on some grave-markers, such as several in the Grosvenor Museum, Chester, where there is a funerary banquet that includes a three-legged table with 'feet' (RIB 497; 523; 558; 562; 563; 567; 568; 3162). The deposition of furniture with human feet in graves is also appropriate because of the apotropaic role of the foot, especially when shod, and the association of footwear with protection on the journey to the Underworld (van Driel-Murray 1999a: 131–132).

Mráv (2013) suggests that folding stools may be associated with bathing. He provides much iconographical evidence of chairs being used in baths (2013: 111–113) and at toilet (2013: 113–116). The Bartlow Hills burial included two strigils and a patera, which were used for personal cleansing. Mráv discusses archaeological finds, including a folding frame from a chariot burial at Érd, Hungary (2013: 117–119) that also contained two strigils and a copper alloy flask. Hoss considers a furniture foot from the baths at Heerlen that probably belonged to a folding stool (2020: 58). It demonstrates considerable luxury (Hoss 2020: 26). Indeed, Roman bathing was associated with comfort and luxury (Dunbabin 1990: 101; Fagan 1999: 176). Burial with such luxury goods would, therefore, have displayed wealth and status. As well as being fun, furniture attachments in the form of human feet can signify power, wealth and status. They were also deemed appropriate grave furniture, and may also symbolize the luxury of bathing (Dunbabin 1990:101).

5.5 Flasks in the form of feet

Bathing and luxury are evident in another type of foot-shaped Roman artefact: the oil flask, *unguentarium*, or *balsamarium*, which this section will consider. Foot-shaped containers for oils and perfumes were not unique to Roman culture. There are many examples of ancient Greek *aryballoi* in the form of sandalled human feet (for example, Smith 2018: 207–211). The oils contained in them could have been used in bathing, sympotic, erotic, or funerary settings (Smith 2018: 195). A large proportion of left-footed *aryballoi* were found in graves (Smith 2018: 203). Shoe-vessels were also known in other areas of Europe in the Iron Age (Forrer 1942: 50; Kohle 2013: 53). Many of these came from funerary settings too (Forrer 1942: 44), particularly cremation burials (Kohle 2013: 55).

Roman vessels in the shape of feet are the successors to

Roman Feet and Shoes

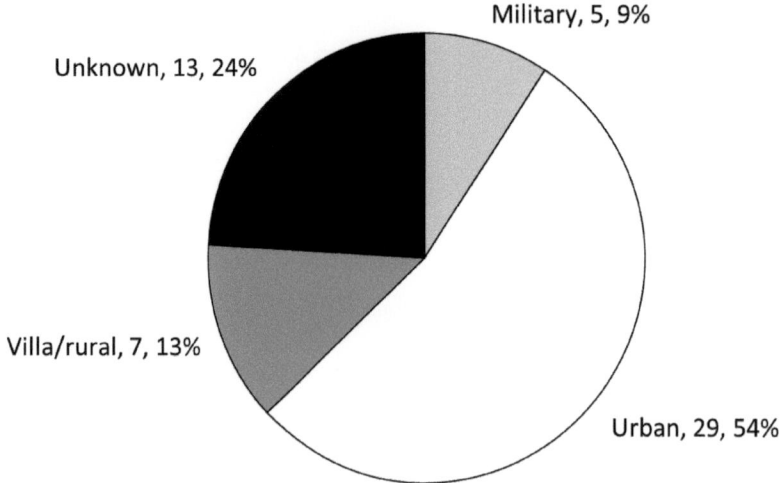

Figure 5.23: Chart to show the site type of 54 sets of Roman furniture 'feet'.

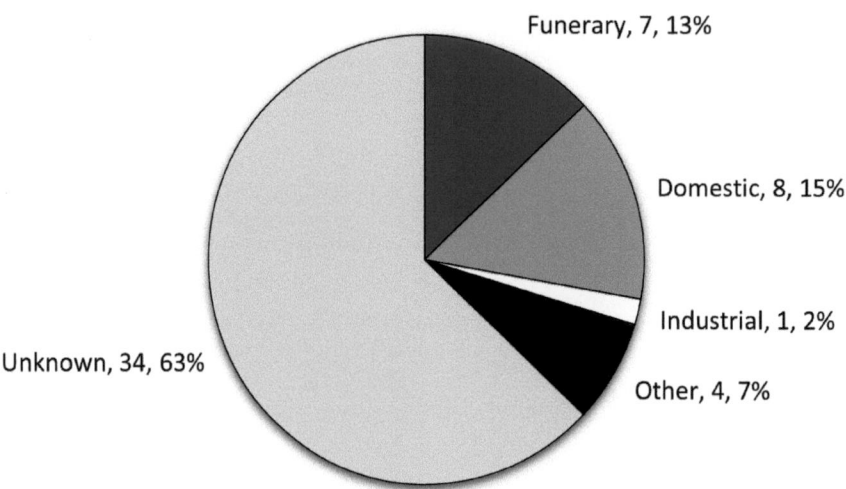

Figure 5.24: Chart to show the find setting of 54 sets of Roman furniture 'feet'.

these traditions. Coombe suggests they were used as grave goods, bathing equipment, and for ritual perfuming, such as foot washing (2006: 8). While there are many Ancient Greek examples (see Figure 6.6), the Roman equivalent is quite rare (Coombe 2006: 12), and this study could only catalogue 23. This may be because the metal flasks were melted down and recycled, or because there are more in private collections. Indeed, in this study, seven examples were found on auction websites and are now in private hands. A further four, now in museums, came from private collections. Only 15 come from a known country (Figure 5.25), just nine have a recorded site type, and a mere six come from a known find setting. Their rarity may have made them more special.

The majority of these foot-shaped *balsamaria* date to the second and third centuries (Figure 5.26). Thirteen depict a very similar shoe style, the 'Ramshaw' (see Figure 6.21), which began in the late second century (van Driel-Murray 2001a: 190) and remained popular for over 150 years (van Driel-Murray 2011a: 366). This could mean that three Ramshaw-style flasks known from auctions may be earlier than the estimated date ranges of fourth to sixth century

(Royal Athena Galleries 2016: 54; 2017: 34; Gorny and Mosch 2016: 64–65). It could also help to date Coombe's 'uncertain' example (2006: 15–16).

Although usually interpreted as containers for perfumed oil (Vierneisel 1979: 181; Harden 1987: 138; Coombe 2006: 23), the contents of these foot-shaped vessels may have varied. The terracotta vessel found in the *domus del chirurgo*, Rimini, is thought to have been a therapeutic device which held hot water into which the patient would have inserted their foot (Ortalli and Maioli 2021). A boot-shaped copper alloy container found in Reims may have held perfumed oil (Forrer 1942: 85; van Driel-Murray 2001b: 3) but may also have been an ink-well (MAN 75452). Not all copper alloy flasks appear suitable for liquids, as the sole was simply attached and therefore not always water-tight (Creemers 2006: 34–8).

Because many of the examples in the corpus are from private, antiquarian collections, there is a lack of adequate recording of their find sites and settings. Where the site type is known (Figure 5.27), six are urban: three of them unspecified, one from the foot of the Palatine in Rome, one

The ubiquity of Roman foot- and shoe-shaped artefacts

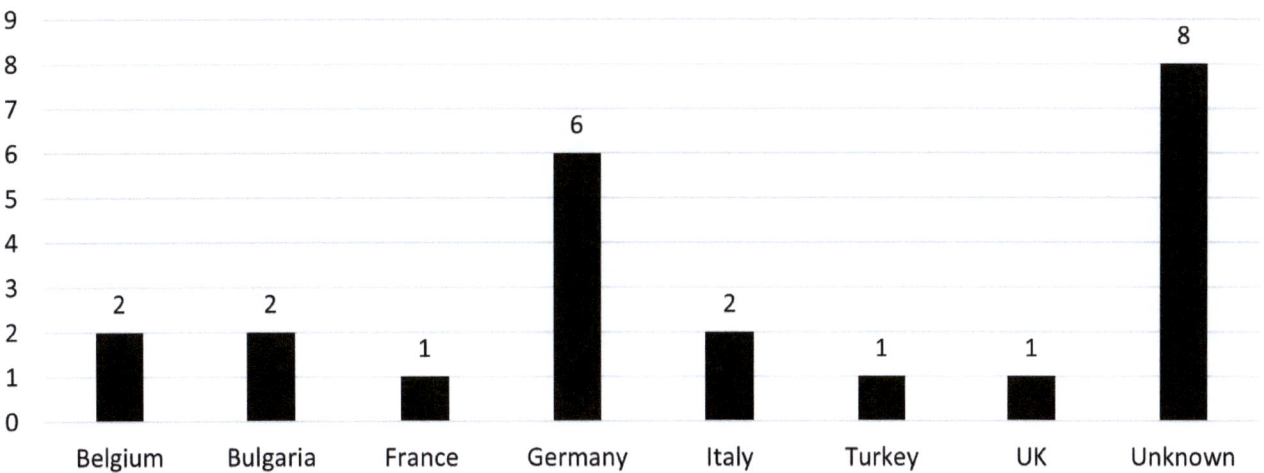

Figure 5.25: Chart to show the modern find country of 23 Roman oil flasks in the shape of feet.

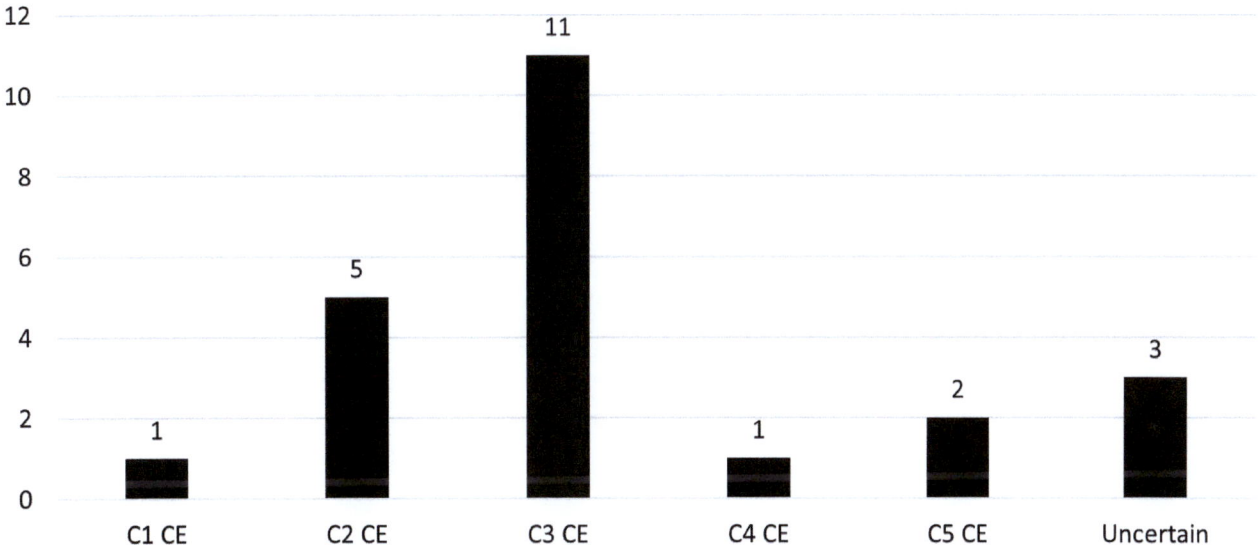

Figure 5.26: Chart to show the date range of 23 Roman oil flasks in the shape of feet.

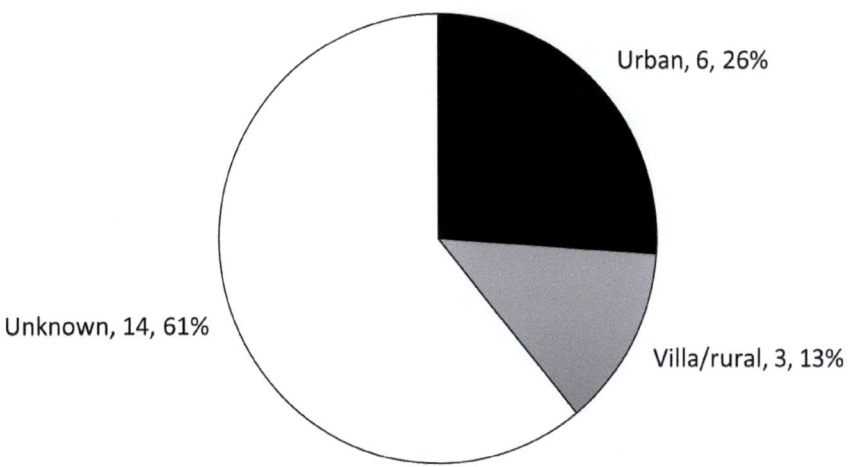

Figure 5.27: Chart to show the site type of 23 Roman flasks in the shape of feet.

from Reims, and one from Speyer. The other urban finds are from the domus del chirurgo, Rimini, and the pair of flasks from Cologne. Only three are known to have come from rural sites. The Hoeselt flask and the Hardwick boot are discussed in detail below. A copper alloy flask was found in the foundations of a villa at Willemeau, Belgium (Faider-Feytmans 1979: 126). It might have been hidden, or was possibly a foundation offering.

Three of the flasks were found in burials (Figure 5.28). Two form a pair of glass oil-flasks fashioned in the shape of *soleae* with imitations of hobnails on the underside (Figure 5.29). These came from a woman's grave found at 129 Severinstraße, Cologne, which included an ornate bone spindle and an *as* of Augustus (RIC 360) (Harden 1987: 138). The burial is thought to date to the third century due to the style of the glass decorations (Harden 1987: 138).

The interpretation of this unusual deposit is multi-layered. Wilmott (2018) suggests that the flasks may have been 'just a bit of fun'. They may also represent the luxury of Roman bathing (Dunbabin 1990: 101; Fagan 1999: 176), or the Roman custom of perfuming feet (see Pliny *NH*13.4). The footwear style could have been chosen to show the femininity of the deceased, as this style of sandal was worn by women (Goldman 2001: 107). The assemblage of grave goods is reminiscent of Plutarch's Gaia Caecilia, whose sandals and spindle were 'tokens of her love of home and of her industry respectively' (*Moralia* 271e). This deposit is, therefore, polysemous.

A copper alloy *balsamarium* was found in a grave in Hoeselt, Belgium (Figure 5.30). The Gallo-Romeins Museum in Tongeren describes it as a spice container, as it was not water-tight. Shoes as appropriate grave goods have been discussed extensively elsewhere. Perfumed oils and spices were linked to rituals of anointing the dead (Anderson-Stojanović 1987: 121).

A terracotta perfume bottle in the British Museum (1875,0309.22) is thought to have been found in Knidos, Turkey. It is dated to the first or second centuries, which is plausible from the style of the boot. Its sole is decorated with hobnails which depict the Greek letters alpha and omega, and a swastika, or cross (Figure 5.31). A swastika depicted in hobnails is thought to have been an apotropaic symbol (van Driel-Murray 1999a: 132). It is possible that these are very early Christian symbols. The phrase 'I am the Alpha and the Omega' occurs three times in the New Testament (Revelation 1:8; 21:6; 22:13). The swastika, or *crux gammata*, is found on many early Christian tombs

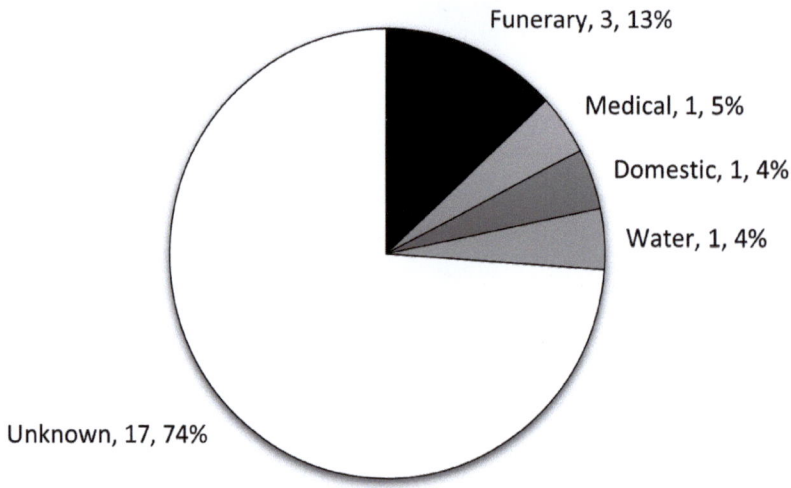

Figure 5.28: Chart to show the find setting of 23 Roman flasks in the shape of feet.

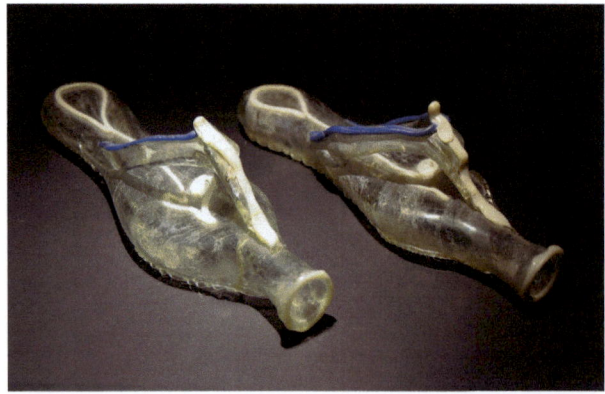

Figure 5.29: Two sandal-shaped glass flasks from a Roman burial in Cologne (Photo: Raddato).

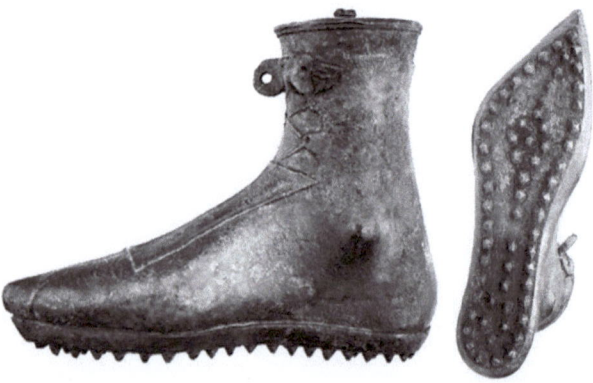

Figure 5.30: Balsamarium from a grave in Hoeselt. (Photo: Gallo-Roman Museum Tongeren).

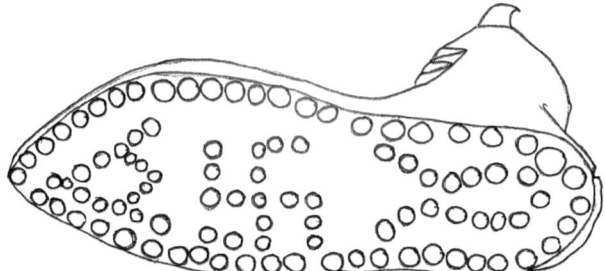

Figure 5.31: Roman perfume bottle from Knidos showing hobnailing. (Author's drawing).

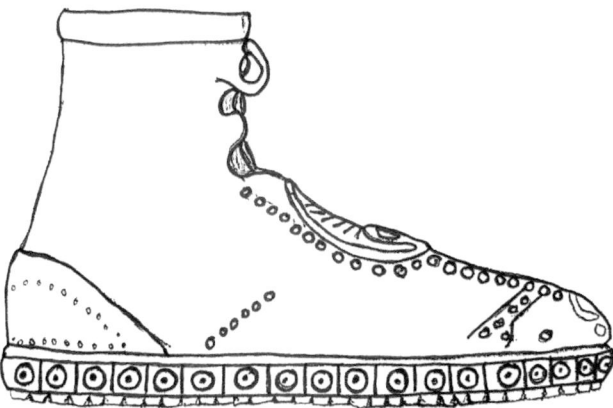

Figure 5.32: The Hardwick Boot (Author's drawing).

as a veiled symbol of the cross (Encyclopaedia Britannica 2020).

Perhaps the most closely studied copper alloy foot-flask is known as the 'Hardwick Boot' (Figure 5.32), and is the only one known to have been found in Britain. This isolated discovery was made in 1999 on land owned by Brasenose College, Oxford, in a gravel pit on the edge of the Upper Thames (Coombe 2006: 1). Coombe compares the footwear style to a Ramshaw boot (see Figure 6.21), but says that the way the footwear is depicted in the Hardwick Boot is inaccurate (Coombe 2006: 7). Van Driel-Murray, who also studied the flask, suggests that it is a copy made in Late Antiquity, based on the unusual hobnails and the inaccuracies in the shoe-style (2001b: 2). She argues that it was possibly a Coptic or Byzantine import (2001b: 2). Coombe proposes a second century date of manufacture, due to the shoe style (2006: 7). Since the style did not become really popular until around 200 CE (van Driel-Murray 2011a: 366), a slightly later date may be more accurate.

The purpose of the flask is also unclear. Coombe discusses its proximity to nine cremations and three inhumations, and to a possible temple or shrine (2006: 6). She also speculates about an as-yet-undiscovered bathhouse (2006: 25) and even that the flask could be an ancient joke (2006: 23). Van Driel-Murray argues that, considering the role of footwear in preparedness for spiritual journeys, the flask may have played a liturgical role (2001b: 2). One might also justify an interpretation of a water offering, given that the flask was found in a gravel pit in a river valley.

Balsamaria in the form of feet, then, appear to have been special, whether as valuable items that demonstrate wealth and status, or as ritual objects. Like many foot-shaped artefacts, a single flask may embody a multiplicity of meanings.

5.6 Conclusions

This chapter has presented a series of case studies of a variety of Roman small finds representing feet and footwear, exploring their social significance. The discussions are based on a corpus of 216 foot-shaped artefacts of seven different types. Although not all types of object were found in all areas, in general they were found across the Roman Empire, with a concentration in the north-western provinces (Figure 5.33.)

Only 131 items in this study's corpus have a known date of manufacture (Figure 5.34). The range extends from the late first century BCE to the fifth century CE, with the majority falling in the second to third centuries. This is in line with the date ranges of Roman footlamps and sandal *fibulae*, the research into which is discussed in the case studies in the following chapters.

Most of the feet are single, with some pairs and, in the case of furniture feet, sets of three or more (Figure 5.35). Of the 155 single feet, 89 (44%) are right, which is to be expected, given Roman beliefs about good luck associated with the right. However, 63 (31%) represent left feet, which is harder to explain. This may be linked to the persistence of local beliefs, as seen in the Iron Age amulets, or to some form of resistance. It could also indicate the contractual use of left and right shoes proposed by van Driel-Murray (1999a: 136). It is also possible that, as in Ancient Greece, the left side symbolised movement, or reflected the feminine, as found in the Hippocratic treatises, bringing healing and restorative qualities (Lloyd 1973: 172; Smith 2018: 206). The shoe symbolism may have been apotropaic enough, without the effect of chirality (Eckardt 2013: 231).

Where it is known, the site type of these artefacts (Figure 5.36) shows that many of them came from an urban context, where there would have been ready access to manufacturers and markets. Sixteen objects are from military sites, and their spread may be partly due to the army (Sedlmayer 1999: 19). Only three come from villa or rural locations, perhaps emphasizing the popularity of foot-shaped artefacts in towns. The 'other' category includes two objects from industrial sites, the medical foot, a jug found in a sand quarry, and the Mălăieștii de Jos hoard, whose interpretation is uncertain.

In many cases (125 or 60%), the find settings of this selection of foot-shaped artefacts are unknown (Figure 5.37), which does skew the data and makes analysis more difficult. Of the remaining 84, 10 come from domestic

Roman Feet and Shoes

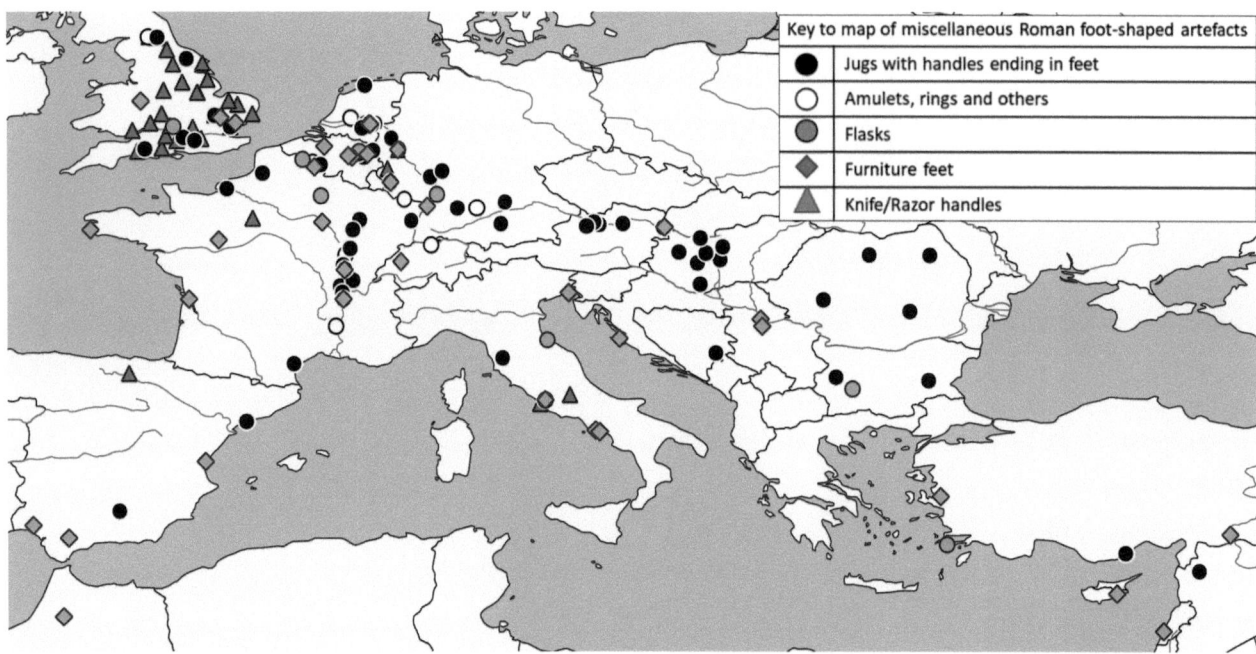

Figure 5.33: Map to show the distribution of 217 selected Roman foot-shaped artefacts.

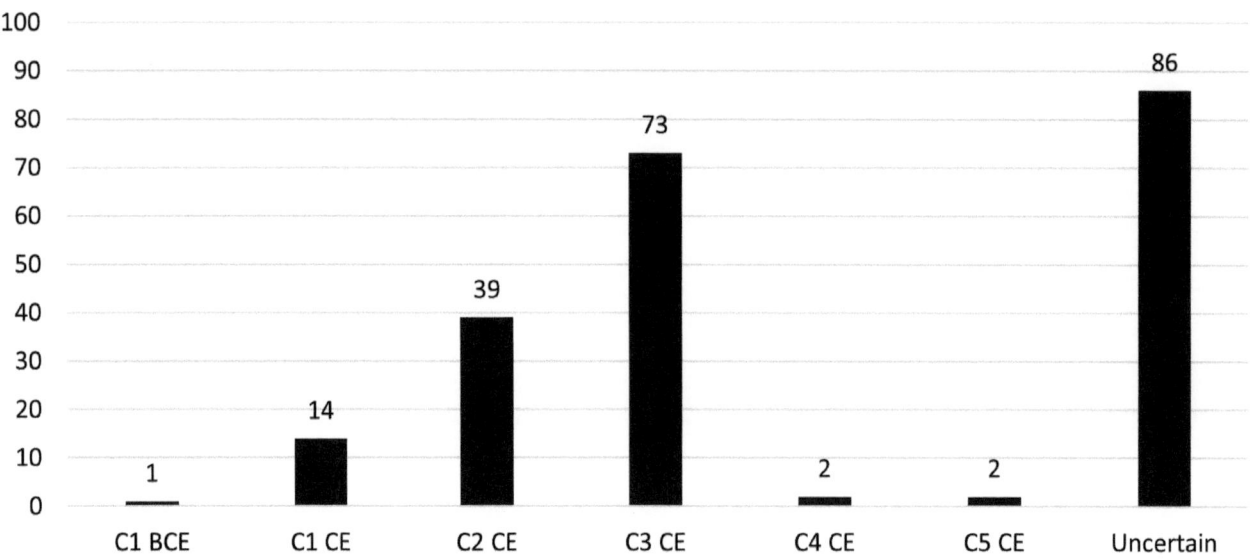

Figure 5.34: Chart to show the date range of 217 sets of selected Roman foot-shaped artefacts.

settings and 25 from find settings labelled 'other'. These artefacts are mostly from unspecified areas of military sites, but five are classified as part of hoards, one is medical, and one came from the *macellum-forum* of Aubigné-Racan. A further 48 examples come from graves, temples or shrines, and watery settings. This is 23% of all find settings in this selection and 57% of all known find settings. Objects in this study's complete corpus which come from a ritual setting comprise 44% of those with a known find setting, and 26% of all foot-shaped items in this sample. One could, therefore, say that the ritual use of foot- and shoe-shaped artefacts was reasonably common.

The symbolism of this miscellaneous selection of Roman artefacts in the form of feet and footwear is varied and multi-layered. It is unnecessary to consider 'deposition in the ground or in wet places as either sacred or profane', since these actions were probably 'invested with significance in both spheres' (Millett 1994: 104). While some of the objects may be mere novelties, many of them were chosen to display power, wealth and status. Some were religious offerings or added to the preparedness of the dead for the journey to the Underworld. Amulets and other objects were regarded as having apotropaic properties. The depiction of hobnailing on many of the artefacts in this sample is realistic in some instances and fanciful in others, but always sends a message about the owner. It also strengthens the talismanic qualities of the foot-shaped item.

This chapter has, therefore, helped to demonstrate the themes which run through this study. The variety of artefacts, and their geographical distribution, has shown how ubiquitous, polysemous, and important representations of feet were in Roman life.

The ubiquity of Roman foot- and shoe-shaped artefacts

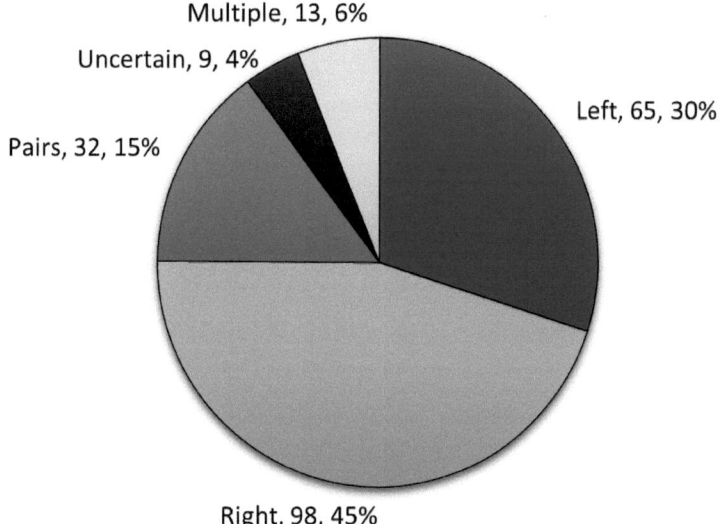

Figure 5.35: Chart to show the chirality of 217 sets of selected Roman foot-shaped artefacts.

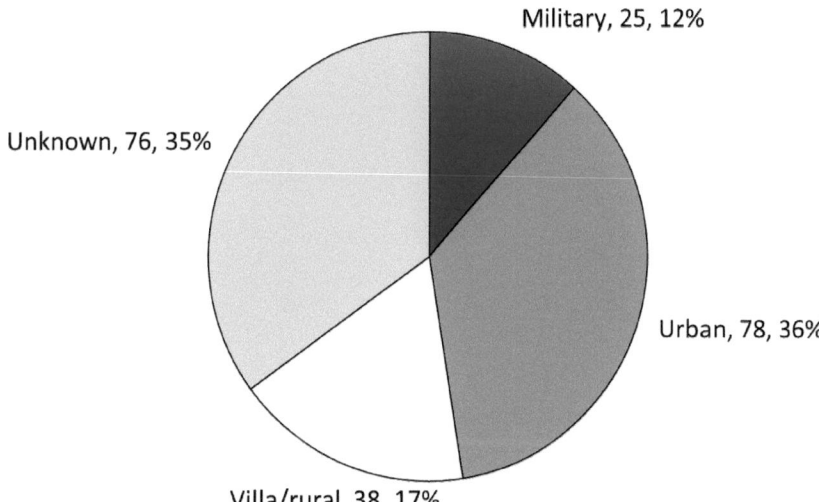

Figure 5.36: Chart to show the site type of 217 sets of selected Roman foot-shaped items.

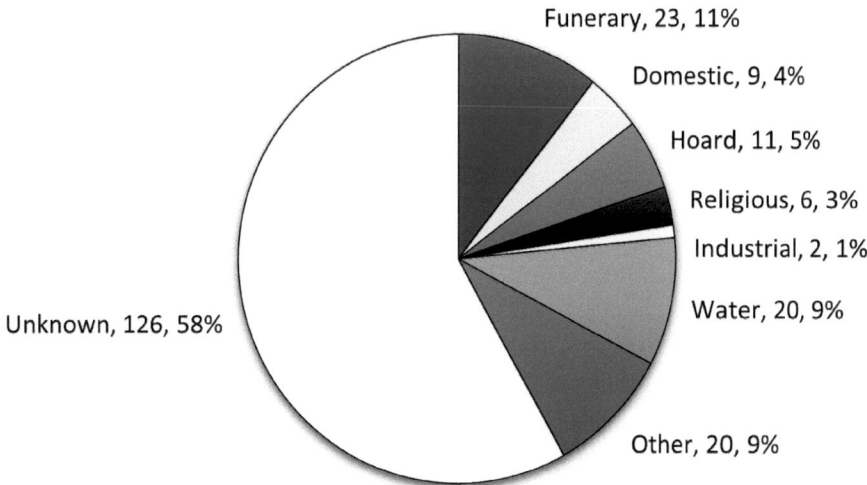

Figure 5.37: Chart to show the find setting of 217 sets of selected Roman foot-shaped artefacts.

6

Roman footlamps: a case study

This chapter comprises a case study of Roman lamps in the shape of feet, most of which are shod. While Roman lamps in general have been studied widely, lamps in the shape of feet have previously only been treated in works on other lamps, or as individual curiosities. So far there has been little work on Roman footlamps as a discreet type of artefact (Eckardt 2013: 229). In part, this chapter is intended to rectify this. Its main aim is to illustrate how multi-faceted the possible significances of this particular representation of feet and footwear are. Footlamps are a good subject for a case study because they have been found across the Roman Empire (Figure 6.1), especially in the north-western provinces (Figure 6.2). They bring several insights into why representations of feet and footwear may have been chosen as suitable iconographic subjects for decorative artefacts.

It has been suggested that some Roman foot-shaped artefacts were mere novelties. This could be true for some footlamps. Their novelty value may have made footlamps objects of desire, an attitude shared by those who collected original footlamps on their Grand Tours, or bought reproductions for their cabinets of curiosity. A footlamp in the British Museum (inv. no. 2011,5016.10) is a nineteenth-century replica of a Roman footlamp found in Pompeii (Figure 6.3). Interest in these artefacts certainly dates back as far as the seventeenth century. The earliest reference this study found to a footlamp is from 1652, in Liceti's *De lucernis antiquorum reconditis* (Figure 6.4). However, the significance of these unusual lamps runs a lot deeper than mere amusement.

Footlamps were the most common type of Roman plastic lamp (Loeschcke 1919: 161; Hill 1946: 70; Grandjouan 1961: 33; Weitzman 1979: 337). Nevertheless, Roman plastic lamps, which were made in the form of animals, objects and people, are rare in the empire (Eckardt 2002: 213) for example, of the more than 4,000 Roman lamps in the Römisch-Germanisches Museum, Cologne, only 74 are plastic lamps (Möhring 1989). In comparison with more ordinary lamps, footlamps are very scarce, for example, only one out of 550 Roman lamps in the Museum of London is a footlamp, and the British Museum has only 12 footlamps in a collection of 4,388 lamps. While 46 of the footlamps in this study's database are known to have been found in Germany, and 45 in Italy, only two are known to have been found in Britain, one from Southwark and one from Corsham, Wiltshire, although one may have been found in Carlisle.

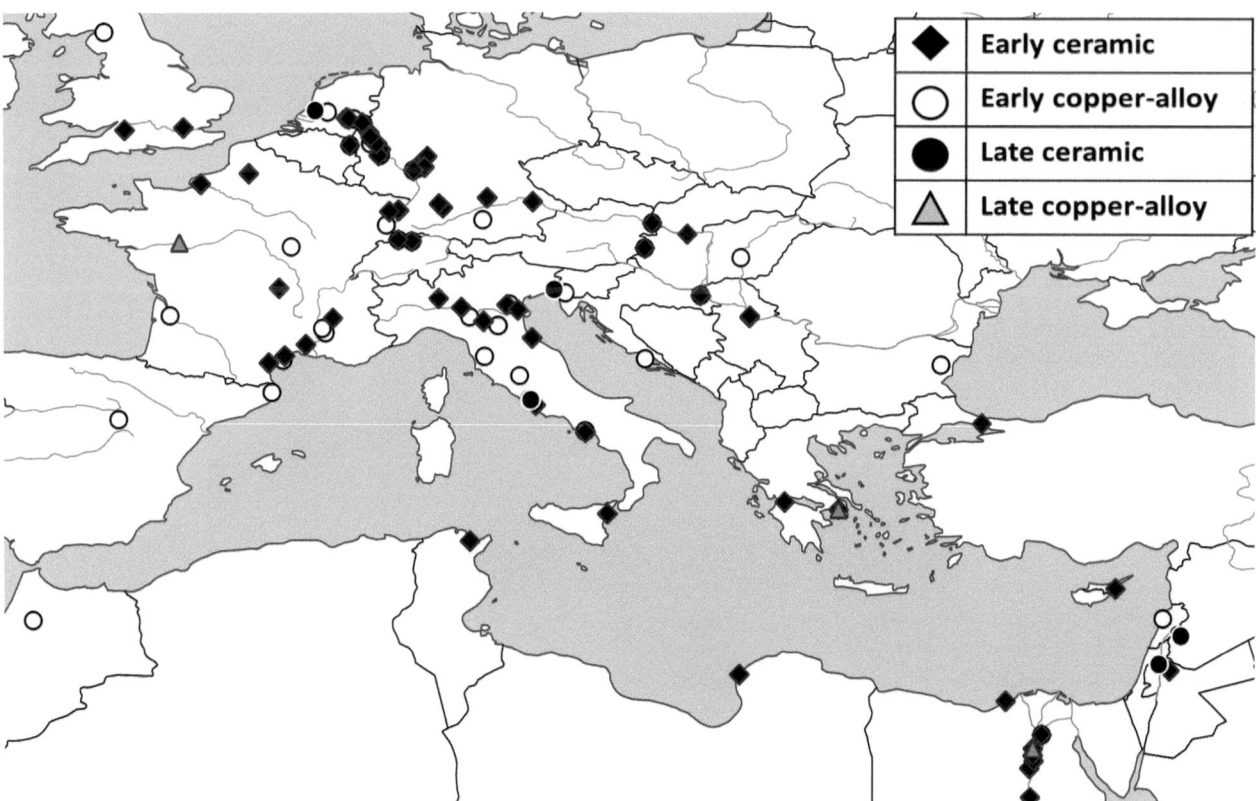

Figure 6.1: Map to show the known geographical distribution of 178 footlamps across the Roman Empire.

Roman Feet and Shoes

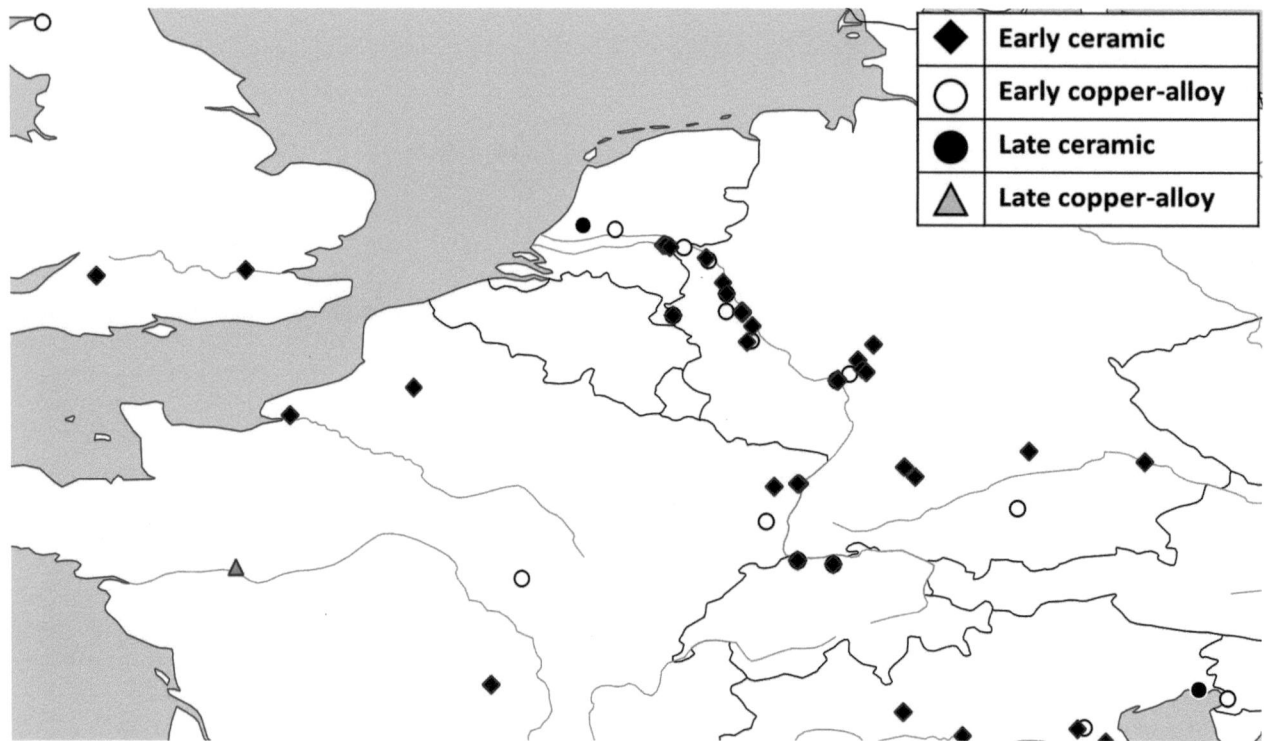

Figure 6.2: Map to show the known geographical distribution of Roman footlamps across the north-western provinces.

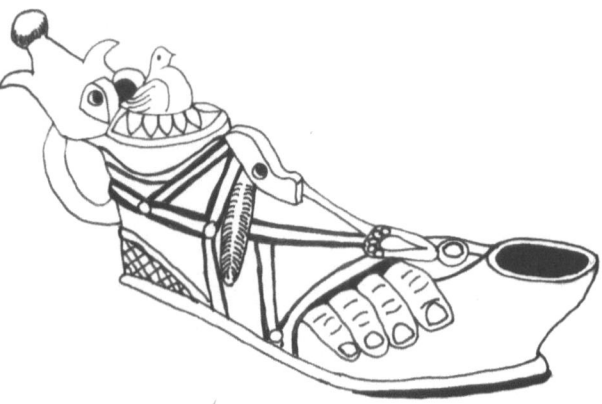

Figure 6.3: Footlamp in a 'crepida' with a bird on the lid from Pompeii.

This could indicate that footlamps were manufactured for a specific purpose. It may be because Roman footlamps are eminently collectable and many have ended up in private hands: 33 in the corpus are known to be privately owned after being auctioned. Their rarity value may have rendered them more desirable. Additionally, some copper alloy footlamps may have been melted down and recycled.

This chapter will discuss methodology, the construction of a footlamp database, and some of the findings from the data analysis. It will consider what these may show about the different social significances of Roman lamps in the shape of feet. The prestige accorded to fashionability will be discussed, along with socio-economic status demonstrated by footlamps and military influence on the popularity of footlamps. This chapter will explore the ornamentation

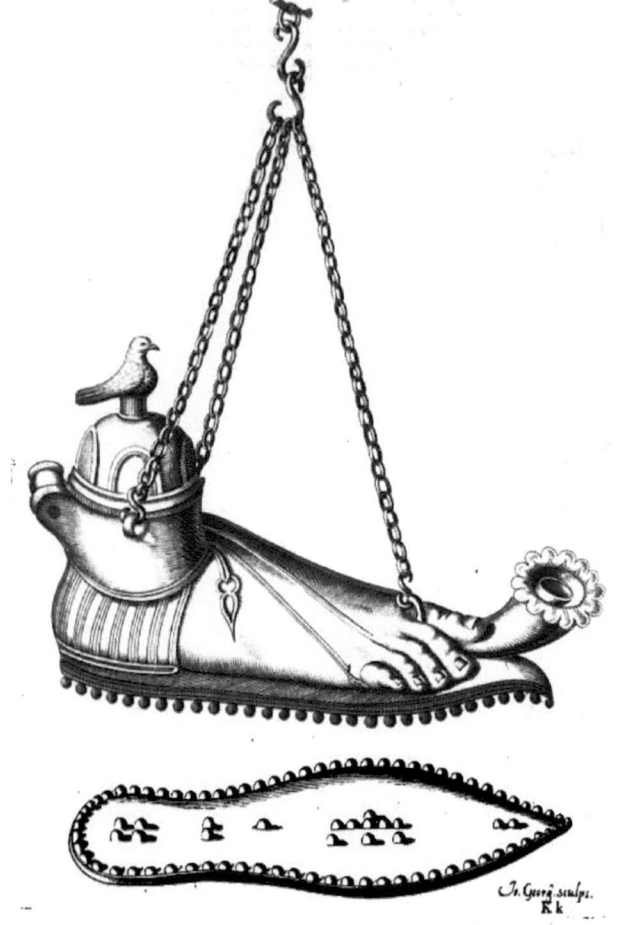

Figure 6.4: Footlamp from Licetus 1652: 770.

found on footlamps and suggest how the motifs could be interpreted as religious symbolism linked to specific cults, such as Christianity, Serapis, Isis and Bacchus. It will examine the apotropaic qualities of footlamps and investigate why they were appropriate as grave goods. The argument will be that footlamps embodied a range of meanings, which would have been different for each individual owner, user or beholder.

6.1 Methodology

In order to conduct this case study, data on footlamps were collected from books, papers, museum catalogues, and online auction websites. The resulting database catalogues 245 footlamps from across the Roman Empire. There are probably further, unpublished footlamps in museums and in private ownership. The information recorded in the database includes the footlamps' dates, find locations and, if possible, find settings. Pictures were also useful, where available, to help assess the lamps' chirality, ornamentation and the possible significance thereof. The database also logs size, chirality, materials, ornamentation, shoe-style and hobnailing, where the lamps were made, and where they are now. Unfortunately, it was not possible to collect a complete dataset for every lamp, as the information is not always available, especially for footlamps found in the antiquarian era. The various papers on Roman footlamps come in a range of languages, and some footlamps are only mentioned as footnotes in other literature. Other scholars have commented on the lack of publication of some Roman lamps (Galavaris 2006: 43; Harris 1980: 127).

The majority of the footlamps were excavated over a century ago and were in private collections before being donated to museum collections. This means that little is known about their precise find locations, site types and settings. Only 180 (73.5%) of the 245 catalogued lamps have a known find location. This situation is worsened because most of the information about the footlamps in the corpus comes from museum catalogues or studies of lamps in general, and very little is from excavation reports. Just 112 (46%) have a known site type, and even fewer (81 or 33%) have a known find setting. In fact, only six of the footlamps have a recorded archaeological context that includes the other artefacts found in the assemblage. The paucity of recording means some of the data are inevitably skewed. The problem of bias is further exacerbated by the types of site excavated, in that there may be a concentration on military or funerary settings. Nevertheless, analysis can still be carried out on the material, as long as these biases are taken into account.

Combinations of the data were examined and analysed for emerging patterns because identifying these trends can help to interpret the social significance of Roman footlamps. In addition, analogies were sought with the ornamentation and find settings of other Roman lamps, and with actual Roman shoes. This helped when considering the themes of the lamps' decoration, and whether the footwear depicted was realistic.

6.2 Background data

One of the first sets of data considered was the dating of Roman footlamps. There are a few Roman footlamps from the republican era and the form may have developed from Greek foot-shaped vessels such as *gutti* (Figure 6.5) and perfume bottles (Figure 6.6). There are also some early, votive footlamps (Figure 6.7). The vast majority of Roman footlamps come from the first and second centuries CE (Figure 6.8). This is in line with the production of other types of Roman plastic lamp (Möhring 1989: 806). There is a big dip in the third century, and then they become more popular in the fourth and fifth centuries. This later rise in popularity has been attributed to footlamps being adopted into Christian symbolism, which will be discussed later. There may also be an element of reviving a past style, a reworking of old material culture in a new social and symbolic context (Eckardt 2004: 46).

The form and placement of the nozzle and wick hole have been linked to the approximate date of the manufacture of footlamps. Loeschcke's influential typology of Roman footlamps has four categories:

a. the foot rests on an oil reservoir which is visible around the foot and which supports the nozzle;
b. the nozzle juts out from under the foot;
c. a small nozzle protrudes at the front of the foot;
d. the wick hole is carved out of the big toe where the nail would be.

Loeschcke (1919: 45) suggests that the first two types date firmly to the first century, the third to the late first and early second centuries, while the last type is second century.

In 1989 Möhring claimed Loeschcke's typology was still valid, as was his dating for lamps with a wick hole in the big toe (Möhring 1989: 834). However, several lamps from a definite first century context have such a wick hole, for example the footlamp from Southwark, which was found in a pre-Boudican level (Drummond-Murray *et*

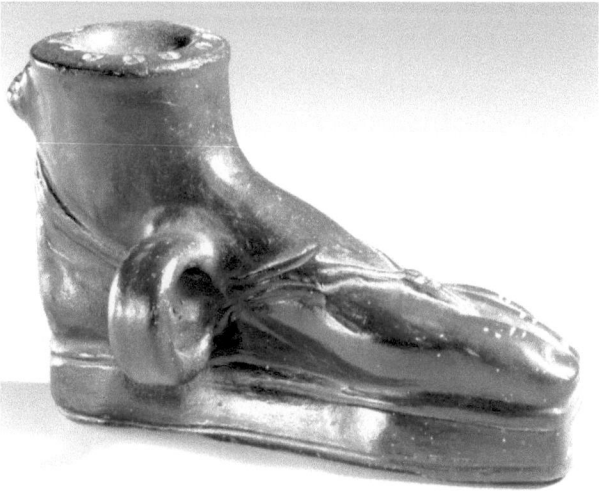

Figure 6.5: Ancient Greek foot-shaped guttus. (Metropolitan Museum of Art no. 06.1021.263).

Roman Feet and Shoes

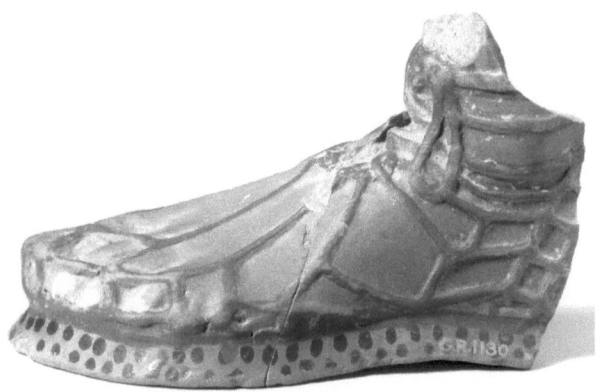

Figure 6.6: Ancient Greek Foot-shaped perfume bottle. (Metropolitan Museum of Art no.98.8.5).

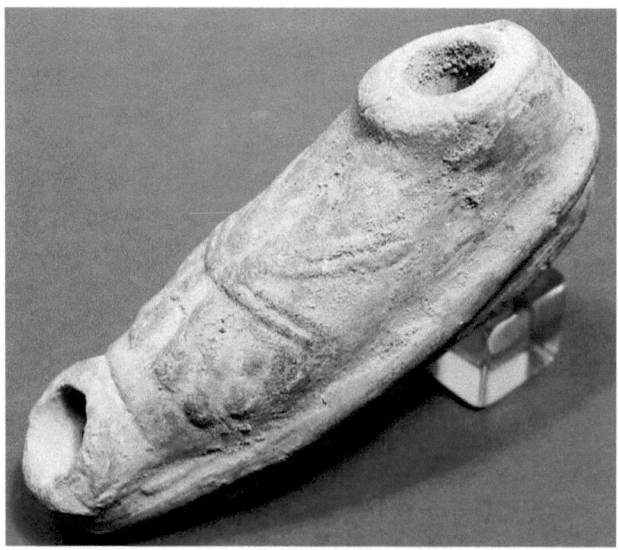

Figure 6.7: 2nd century BCE votive footlamp. (Photo: eBay)

al. 2002: 31). Perhaps the dating aspect of Loeschcke's typology should be reconsidered because this discrepancy may mean that some of the dates are insecure, depending on how the dating was determined.

There is a slight correlation between date and material: earlier footlamps tend to be ceramic and later ones copper alloy, but there is no hard and fast rule. There is a similar link between size and material: copper alloy lamps tend to be larger, but there are exceptions, as can be seen from Figure 6.9. Sadly, the length of footlamps is not always published, not even by Loeschcke: dimensions are readily available for only 168 of the footlamps in the corpus.

Footlamps vary in length, with the majority in the 101–150-millimetre range. The smallest in the corpus is 48mm long, came from a first-century tomb in Egypt, and is now in the archaeological museum in Krakow (Figure 6.10). The longest measures 280mm (Figure 6.11). It was auctioned online and is now in the hands of a private collector. Based on archaeological finds in forts, the smallest Roman babies' shoes start at 110mm long (Driel-Murray 1995: 4) and 77 footlamps in the corpus are shorter than this. Roman adult shoe sizes begin at 190mm (Driel-Murray 1995: 18), with some men's shoes as large as 290mm (UK size 12 or European size 45), so only six footlamps could be classed as adult-sized.

Knowing the type of site and setting in which the footlamps were found can provide an indication of their social significance. Unfortunately, this is another aspect of footlamp data that is not always recorded (see Figure 6.12 and 6.13). This is often true of footlamps found and collected on a 'grand tour' as part of a cabinet of curiosities. Of the twelve footlamps in the British Museum's collection, none has a recorded find setting, and only one has a definite find location: Benghazi, Libya (inv.

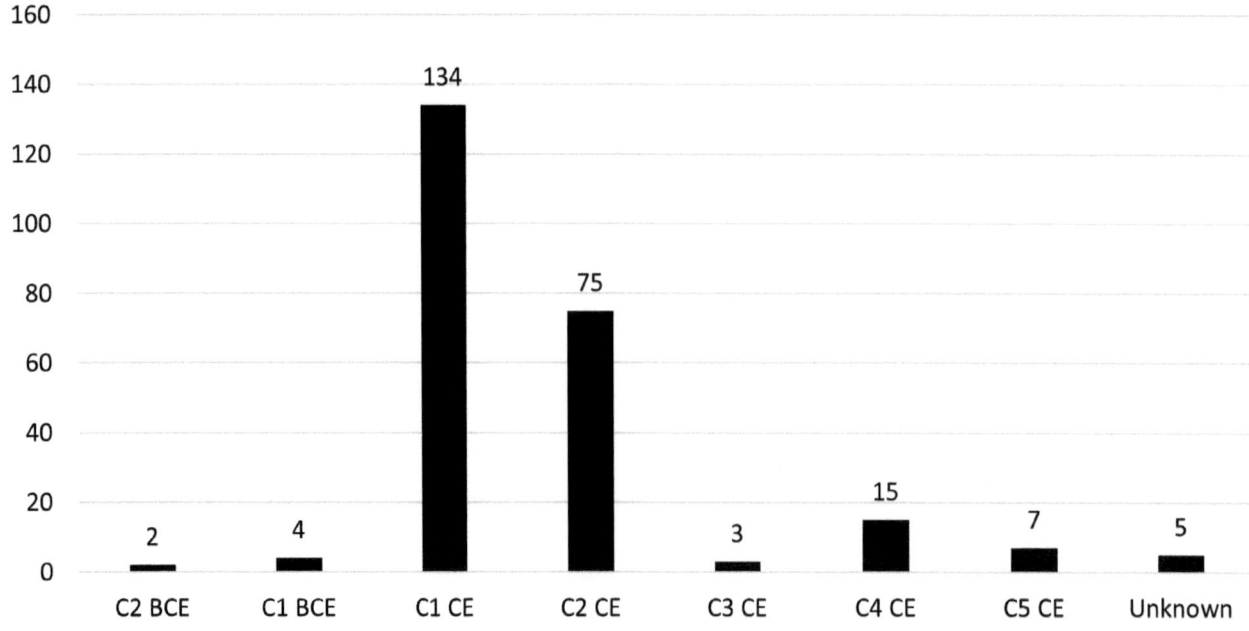

Figure 6.8: Chart to show the date of manufacture for 245 Roman footlamps.

Roman footlamps: a case study

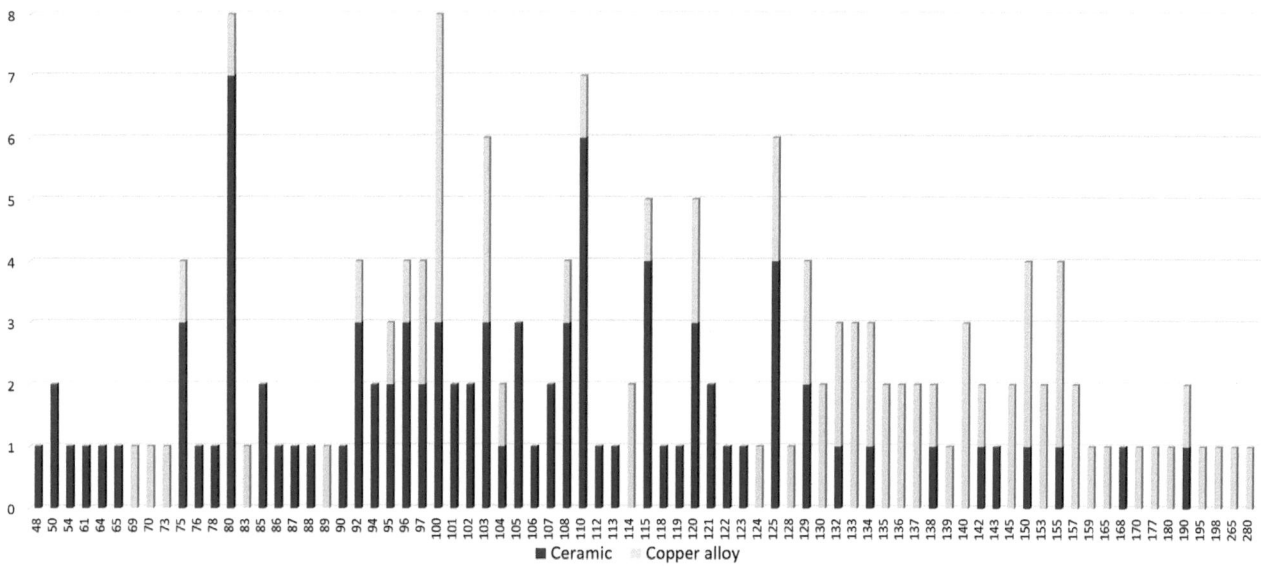

Figure 6.9: Chart to show the length in millimetres, and the materials, of 170 Roman footlamps.

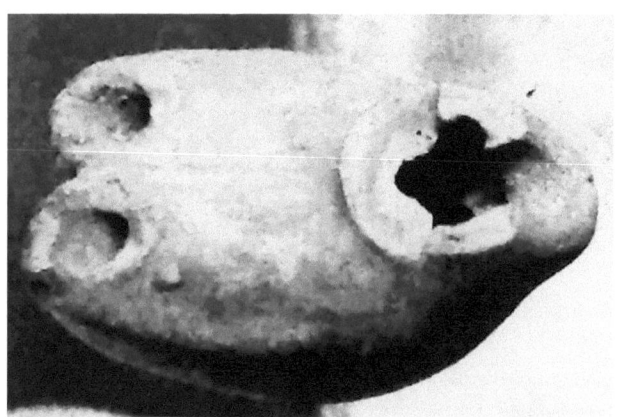

Figure 6.10: Lamp from a Roman-Egyptian tomb: Muzeum Archeologiczne, Krakow. (Photo: Author's own).

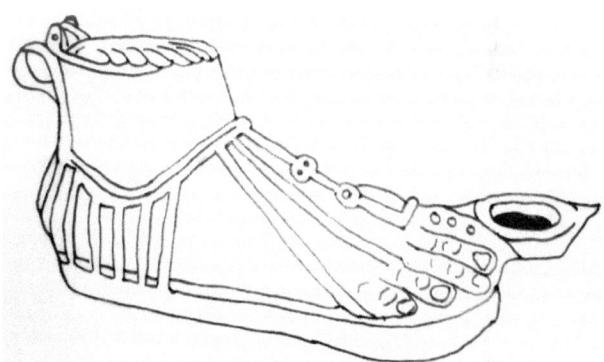

Figure 6.11: Life-size footlamp in private ownership.

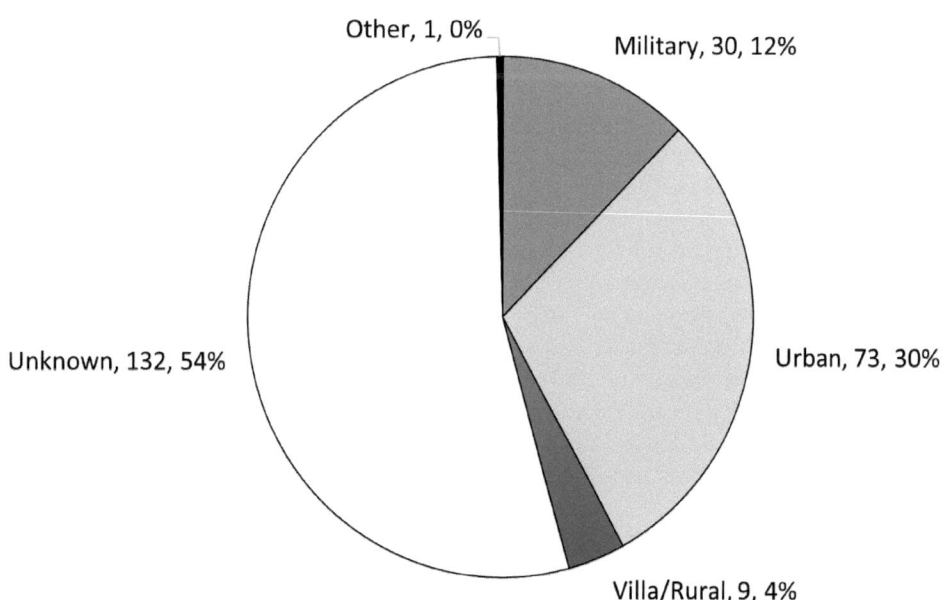

Figure 6.12: Chart to show the site type of 245 Roman foot-shaped lamps.

Roman Feet and Shoes

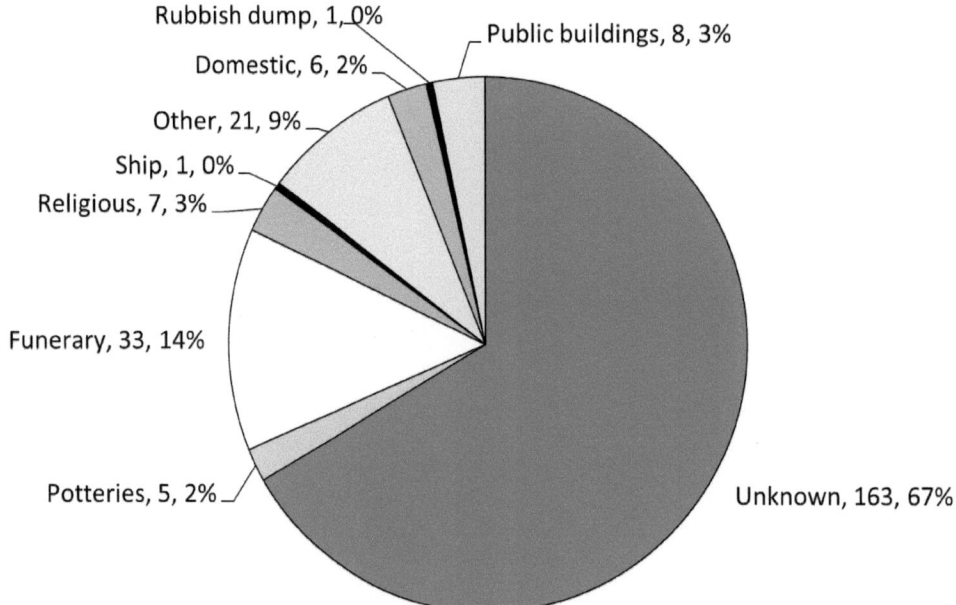

Figure 6.13: Chart to show the find settings for 245 Roman footlamps.

no. 1856,1001.31). More recent discoveries of footlamps tend to record site types and find settings as a matter of course. Nevertheless, this information is lacking for over half of the 245 footlamps.

The site type is recorded for 110 (46%) of the footlamps in this study's corpus. In line with general findings, 70 come from urban locations, and 30 from military sites, while only nine were found in villas or other rural sites. The single footlamp from an 'other' site type was found in a shipwreck off Agde, France (Musée de l'Éphèbe 2022).

Of the footlamps whose find setting is known, the largest group is 33 from funerary settings. This quantity may be due to their ritual use in burials, or could simply be that artefacts are more likely to survive in funerary contexts. Most of the funerary footlamps are from urban sites, three are villa/rural, and five are from military sites. Military sites also account for two lamps from the baths at Heerlen. Six of the footlamps were found in the potteries in which they were made. Seven footlamps come from religious settings, four from temples, and three with definite associations with lararia. Among the footlamps from urban sites are three from theatres, two from the Athens Agora and one, the Southwark lamp, was found in a rubbish dump. This footlamp is one of the few where the precise archaeological context is recorded. It was found during the building of the London Bridge underground station ticket office, in a pre-Boudiccan layer between two later buildings, on the edge of a rubbish deposit (Drummond-Murray et al. 2002: 31). The footlamp was found with the copper alloy handle of a vessel, possibly a skillet or colander (Drummond-Murray et al. 2002: 214 and 218).

As discussed in Chapter 2, chirality is an important quality of Roman footwear. Because of the significance of right and left in Roman culture, this aspect of Roman footlamps was included in the database (Figure 6.14). 165 of the footlamps in the study depict right feet (see Figure 6.3), but 47 represent left feet and 30 portray pairs of feet, such as those in the Getty Museum L.A. (Figure 6.15 and Figure 6.16). It is, therefore, clearly not true that footlamps are invariably right feet, as some scholars claim (for example, Driel-Murray 1999a: 136; Manzoni 1976: 82).

There are, in addition, two matching pairs of footlamps, one from Lillebonne in France (Figure 6.17) and one from Greece, now in the Loeb collection in Munich (Figure 6.18). It is impossible to tell whether footlamps were generally made in pairs, but some evidently were.

6.3 Fashion and footwear style

The footlamps were sorted into seven categories according to footwear style: boot, *solea*, strappy (sandals with thin straps, like the lamp in Figure 6.15), *crepida*, *caliga*, bare, and sandal (those not covered by any of the other categories). This enabled the study of how realistic the portrayal of footwear on the lamps is. It also allowed an investigation into whether some types of ornamentation were peculiar to certain shoe styles.

Roman shoe-making technologies brought an improvement in footwear, which led to fashions that spread across the Roman Empire (Driel-Murray 2011a: 342). It is therefore possible that one of the inspirations for the production and consumption of footlamps was Roman shoe fashion. Buyers may have valued the products as a means to show off their modishness, thus gaining social prestige and exhibiting status.

Some of the footwear styles represented on the footlamps are seen in actual Roman shoes. Examples of *soleae* as worn by the footlamp in Figure 6.19a are also known

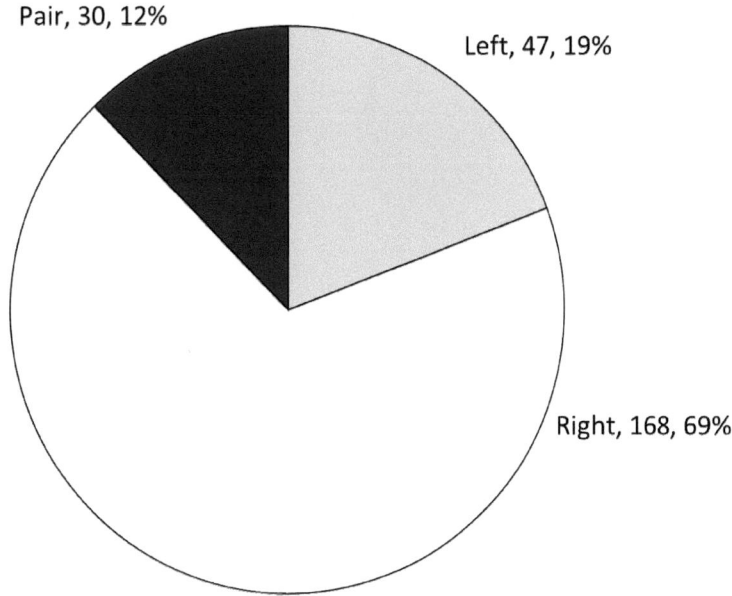

Figure 6.14: Chart to show the proportions of chirality in 245 Roman footlamps.

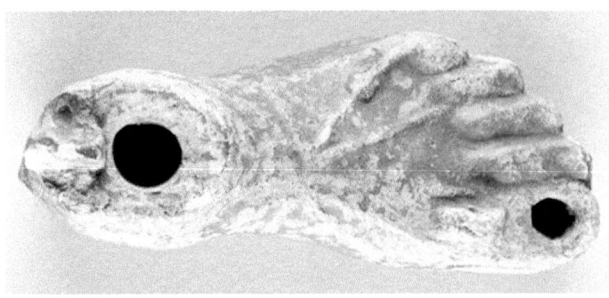

Figure 6.15: Left-footed lamp (Photo: J. Paul Getty Museum inv. no. 83.AQ.377.502).

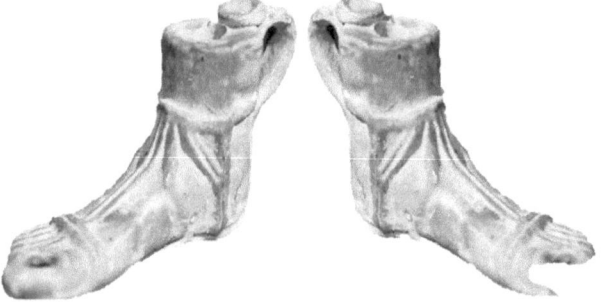

Figure 6.17: Pair of footlamps from Lillebonne, France. (Photo: Author's own).

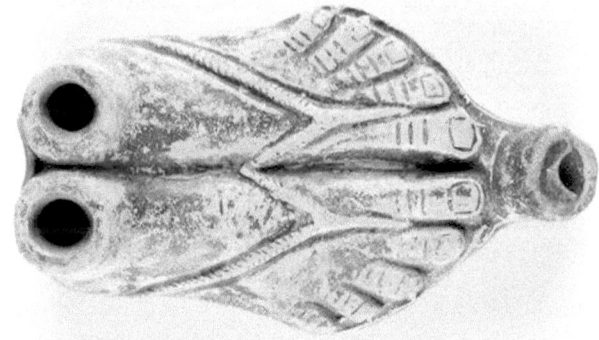

Figure 6.16: Two-footed lamp. (Photo: Photo: J. Paul Getty Museum inv. no. 83.AQ.377.501).

archaeologically, for example, Figure 6.19b, an Augustan-age sandal from Comacchio, Italy. Although these footlamps demonstrate footwear fashion, they also show the kinds of shoe depicted on early imperial statues. The *solea* is seen on many sculptures of women, especially goddesses (Goldman 2002: 107). The real strappy sandal in Figure 6.19c is a low *caliga* from Mainz (see also Göpfrich 1986: 19). The sandal on the footlamp from Southwark (Figure 6.19d) bears a close resemblance to this contemporary style of shoe. Such shoes also appear

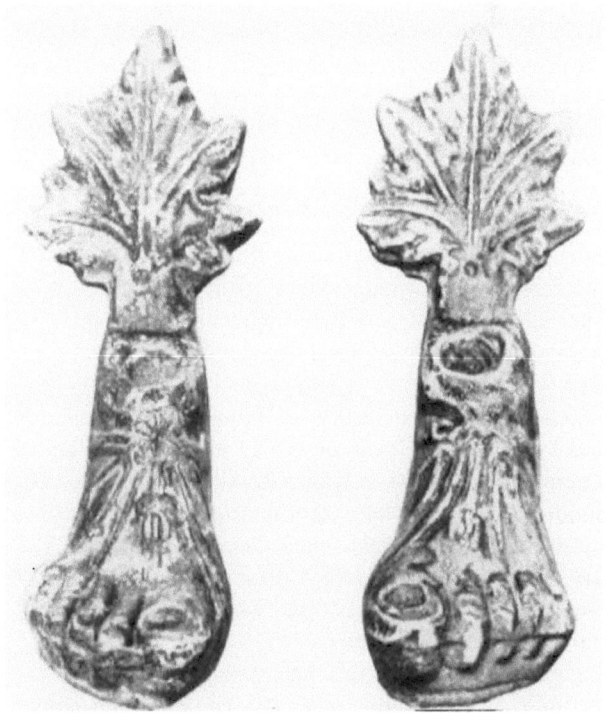

Figure 6.18: Pair of footlamps, Loeb collection, Munich. (Photo: Sieveking 1930: Tafel 25).

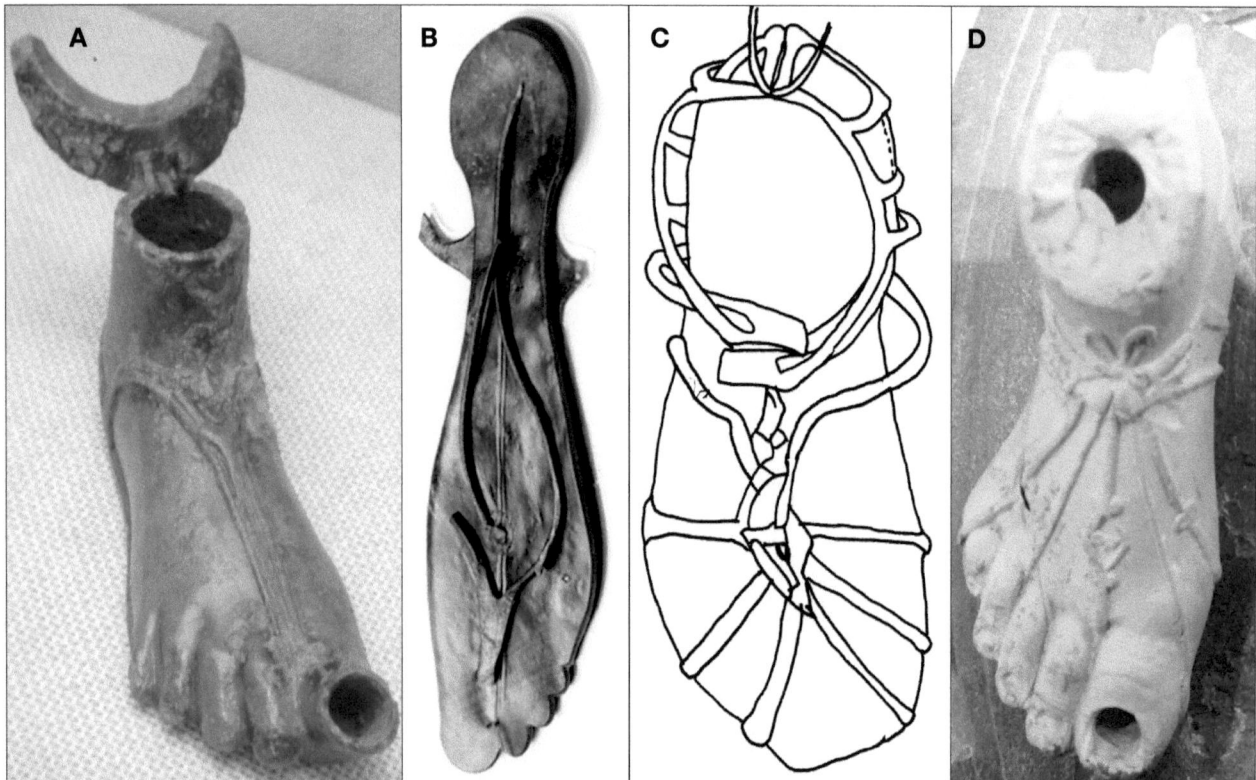

Figure 6.19: a) Footlamp in a solea. Xanten LVR-Römermuseum 33775; b) solea from the Comacchio shipwreck; c) Low caliga 16 from Mainz; d) Southwark footlamp in strappy sandal. (Photos: Author's own).

on first-century military monuments, such as the Arch of Titus in Rome, and tombstones, for example, that of Caecilius Avitus (RIB 492).

Recent research has shown that footwear tends to be portrayed more accurately in later Roman art (Shaw 2017: 50). An unusual third-century footlamp (Driel-Murray 2011a: 367; see also Figure 6.20 below) shows a contemporary type of boot known as the Ramshaw (Figure 6.21), which has been found across the Roman Empire (Driel-Murray 2011a: 367). Nevertheless, much of the footwear depicted on lamps has not been found archaeologically, yet seems to resemble that portrayed on statues of a similar period, where it was used as a code for the identity of the wearer (Shaw 2017: 48). The *crepida*, a sandal associated with philosophers and healers, is an example (see Figure 6.22 and Chapter 2).

Inaccuracy in the depiction of footwear styles can be found in those footlamps described by some scholars as wearing *caligae* (for example, Xanthopoulou 2010: 20: Houben 1839: 53). There is, of course, no guarantee that the Romans would have called this style '*caligae*'. The boots on these lamps do not resemble the real *caligae* excavated in such places as Mainz and Castleford (compare Figure 6.23 and 6.24). This may be because 15 of the 22 footlamps of this type were made in the fourth and fifth centuries, long after 100 CE when the *caliga* disappears from the archaeological record (Driel-Murray 2011a: 345). There may be a continuation of this style of

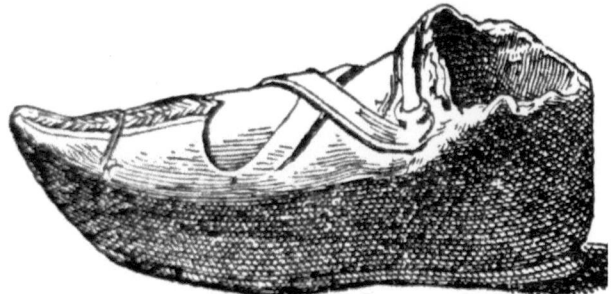

Figure 6.20: Footlamp (or flask) in the Louvre. (Forrer 1942: 86 Fig. 22).

footlamp linked to military identity. The *caliga* continued to be represented in art until the early third century, for example, on the Arch of Septimius Severus, which was dedicated in 203 CE. The later '*caliga*' lamps could be based on earlier examples, of which there are three in the corpus. It may therefore be an instance of the reworking of old material culture (Eckardt 2004: 46) to embody a new ideology, in this case Christianity; later lamps of this kind feature Christian iconography.

Thus, we see that, while some footlamps do depict shoe fashion, most of them seem to be wearing styles in keeping with the footwear seen on Roman sculpture. As such, they are associated with an aspect of the wearer's identity. Therefore, care is needed when using footlamps as evidence for actual Roman footwear.

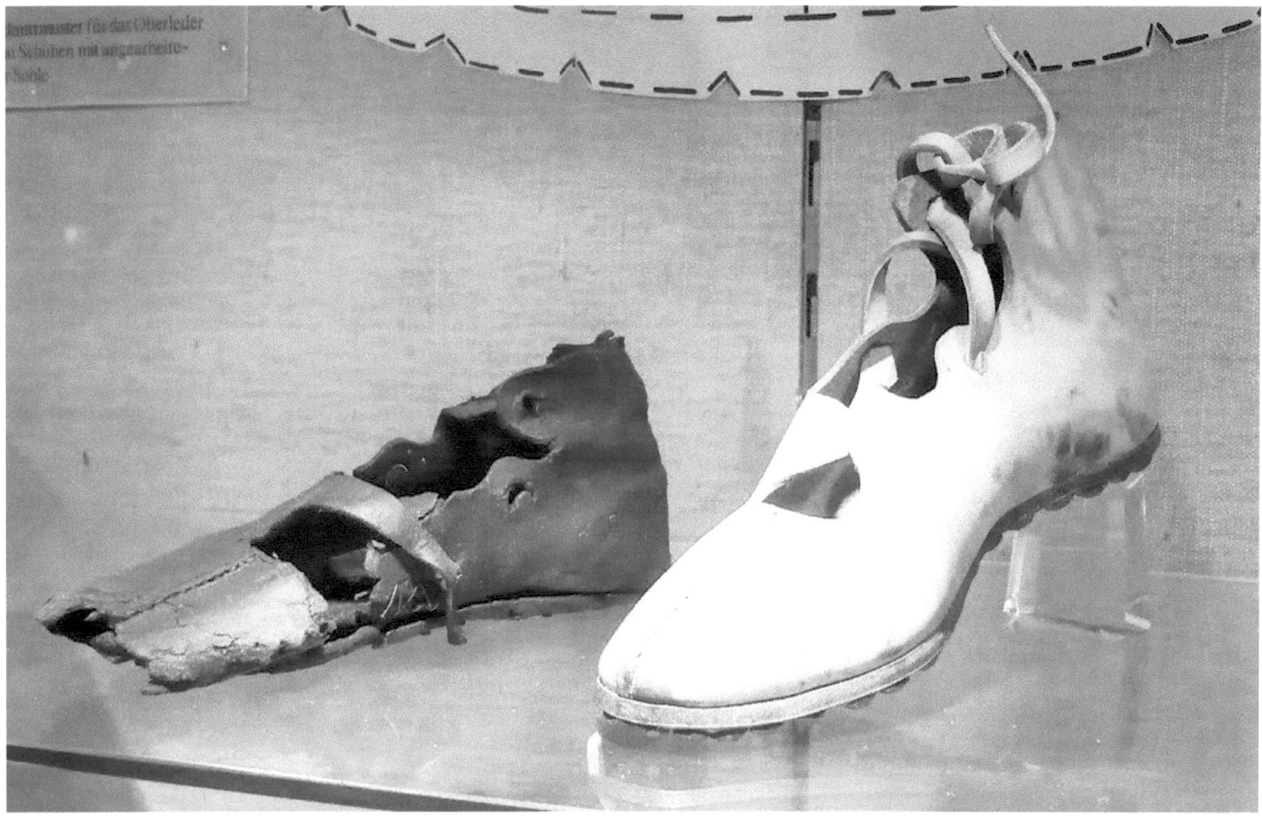

Figure 6.21: 'Ramshaw' boot and reconstruction, Saalburg. (Photo: Roberto Pastrana).

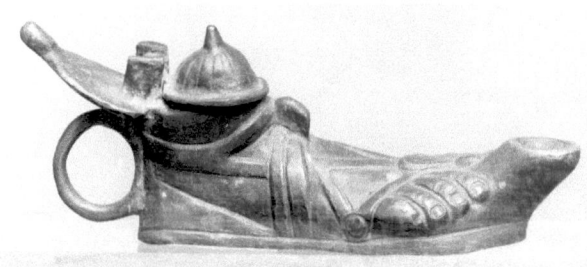

Figure 6.22: Example of a crepida on a footlamp. (Photo: Staatliche Museen zu Berlin 30260).

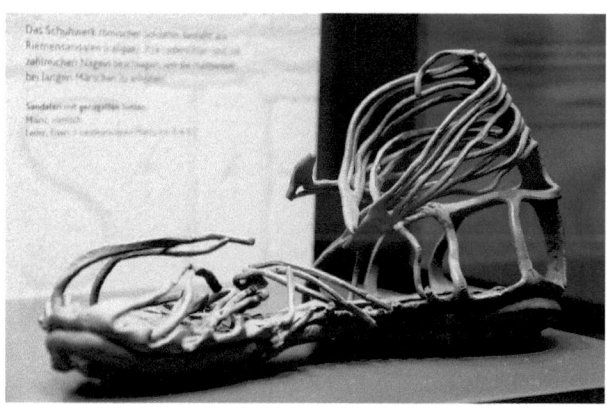

Figure 6.24: Mainz caliga 9. (Photo: Raddato).

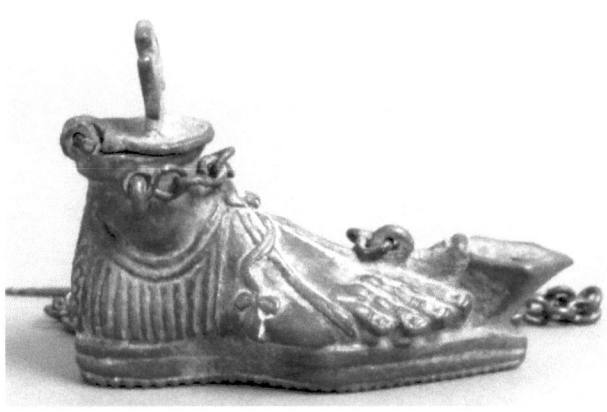

Figure 6.23: Footlamp wearing a 'caliga'. (Photo: Metropolitan Museum of Art, New York; inv. no. 62.10.2).

6.4 Hobnailing on Roman footlamps

As we saw in Chapter 3, Roman hobnailing also followed trends and 92 (38%) of the 245 catalogued footlamps are known to include representations of hobnailing. Some of the lamps depict nailing patterns like those seen on actual footwear (Figure 6.25–6.30). Other hobnailing patterns spell makers' names, such as 'Vitalis' (Figure 6.31), a Hadrianic potter from Mainz (Möhring 1989: 841). Hobnailing can also depict symbols, such as a cross (Figure 6.32: see also Xanthopoulou 2010: 20). As the soles of numerous footlamps rested on a surface, the hobnailing was not always visible during use. Hobnailing must, therefore, have been an important feature of footlamps. It is probable that the hobnailing on footlamps shared some

Roman Feet and Shoes

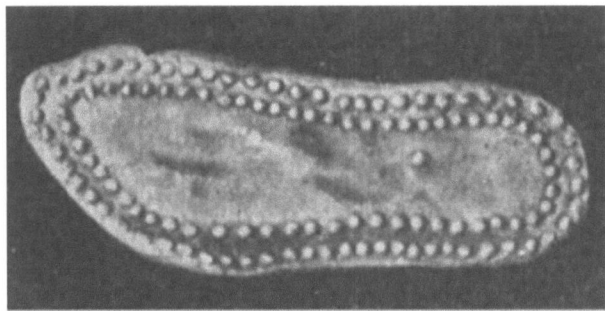

Figure 6.25: Hobnailing on a footlamp from Cologne. (Fremersdorf 1926: 46, Figure 2c).

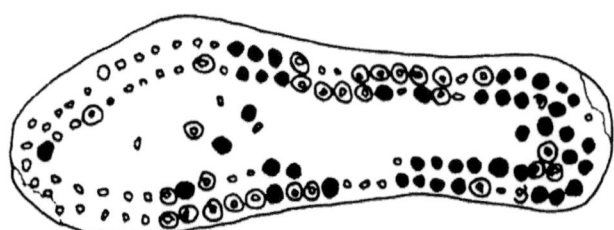

Figure 6.26: Hobnailing on a shoe from Carlisle. (Photo: Padley 1991: 238, Figure 211).

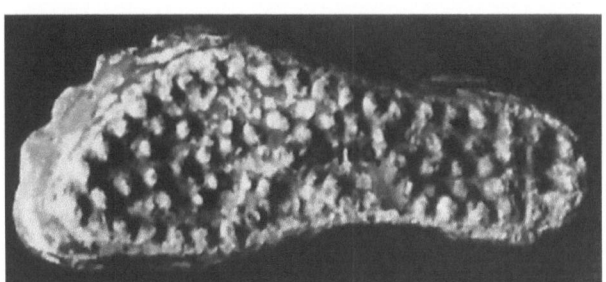

Figure 6.27: Hobnailing on a footlamp from Cologne. (Fremersdorf 1926: 46, Figure 2b).

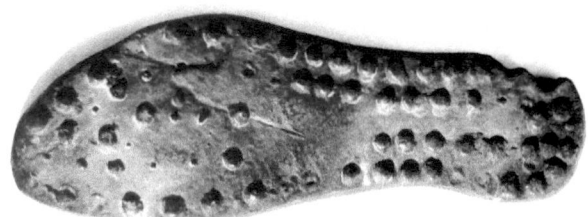

Figure 6.28: Hobnailing on a caliga. (Forrer 1942 Tafel 33).

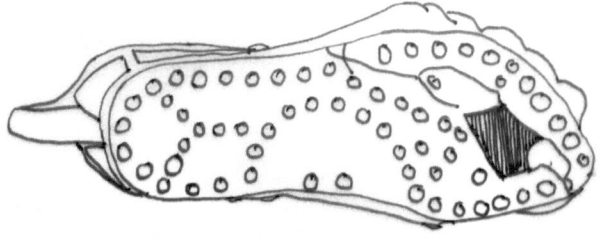

Figure 6.29: Hobnailing on the footlamp from Southwark. (Author's drawing).

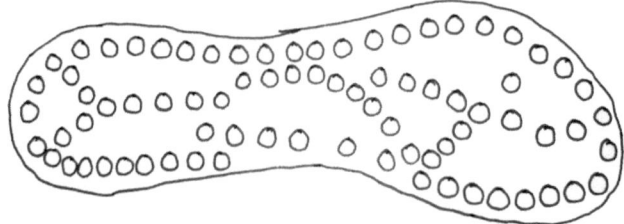

Figure 6.30: Hobnailing on a shoe from Valkenburg. (Author's drawing).

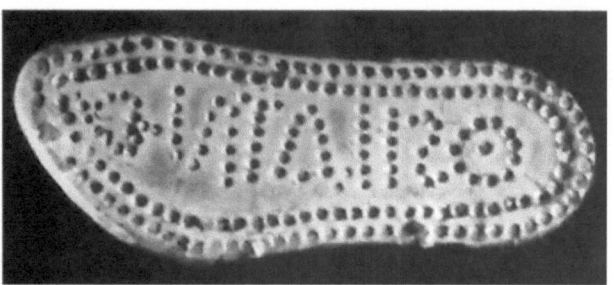

Figure 6.31: Hobnailing as a potter's mark on a footlamp from Cologne. (Photo: Fremersdorf 1926: 46, fig. 2a).

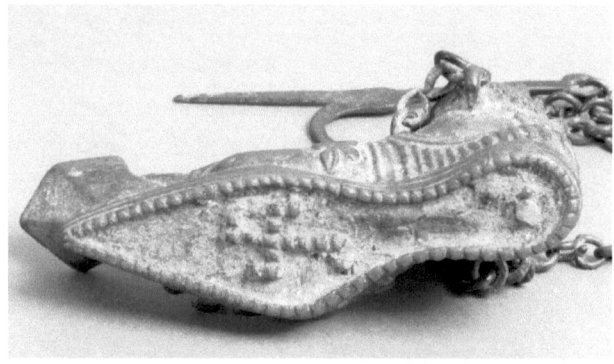

Figure 6.32: Footlamp with a cross depicted in hobnailing. (Photo: Metropolitan Museum of Art, New York).

of the functions of hobnailing on real shoes, as a statement of identity, group membership, and an apotropaic device (Driel-Murray 1999a: 132).

It seems likely that, influenced by the popularity of attractive hobnailing patterns, footlamp makers mimicked the hobnailing to attract customers and to demonstrate their skills as craftspeople. This display of fashion and skill may have elicited a higher price, and thus may be a marker of status. Clearly, then, hobnailing was a significant, multivalent component of Roman footlamps.

6.5 Patterns in ornamentation

An analysis of the decoration found on footlamps reveals common patterns in motifs. Sixteen of the footlamps are quite plain, the only decoration being simple straps with, perhaps, some hobnailing (Figure 6.33). There is some correlation between ornamentation and shoe style. Four lamps depicting pairs of feet in *soleae* have crescent moon handles (Figure 6.34). Nine copper alloy lamps

Roman footlamps: a case study

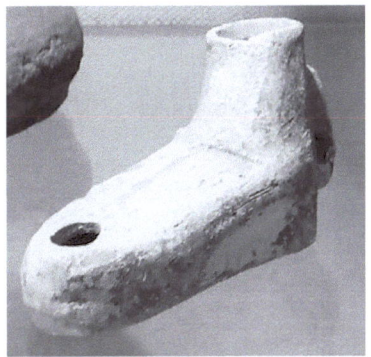

Figure 6.33: Fairly plain footlamp, Saalburg. (Photo: Roberto Pastrana).

wearing *crepidae* feature birds on their lids (see Figure 6.3). There is a group of twelve footlamps with similar straps and vine-leaf handles (see Figure 6.18). There are a further 21 footlamps with this strap design, but whose handles have broken off, as is often the case (27% of the study's footlamps have missing handles). Because of their similarity to complete lamps, it is likely that these also had vine-leaf handles (Bailey 1988: 457; Drummond-Murray *et al.* 2002: 218; Koutoussaki 2007: 22). The possible significance of these recurring themes in decoration is discussed below. That there are such commonalities in ornamentation may show how popular footlamps were across the north-western provinces.

Some of the ornamentation on footlamps is extraordinary. Two of the lamps in the database feature oversized eagles, one from Augst (Figure 6.35) and one in the Bally Shoe Museum (Figure 6.36). The eagles could be symbols of Jupiter, or of Serapis (Steiger 1980: 67; Santoro l'Hoir 1983: 232). Thanks to syncretism, the eagle may represent both deities at once (Steiger 1980: 67). In addition, the eagle was also the symbol of the Roman army (Steiger 1980: 67; Nicgorski 2014: 160), giving the lamps a possible military significance and linking them to the Imperial cult.

Two copper alloy footlamps sport flying gryphons as handles (Figure 6.37). They both date to the fourth century and were made in Italy. Gryphons may be symbols of Apollo or, as on other copper alloy lamps, Christ (Radovanović 2018: 226–227; Popović *et al.* 1969: 48).

A further two footlamps have heads on top of the shoes, one whose provenience is unknown (Figure 6.38) and one from a pottery in Cologne (Figure 6.39). The heads include what one scholar describes as 'phallic topknots' (Möhring 1989: 842). These unusual footlamps may have been mere novelties, or have had a ritual or apotropaic function. A footlamp in the British Museum, which was made in Italy and found in Libya, has a sphinx handle (inv. no. 1856,1001.31). The sphinx was a guardian spirit

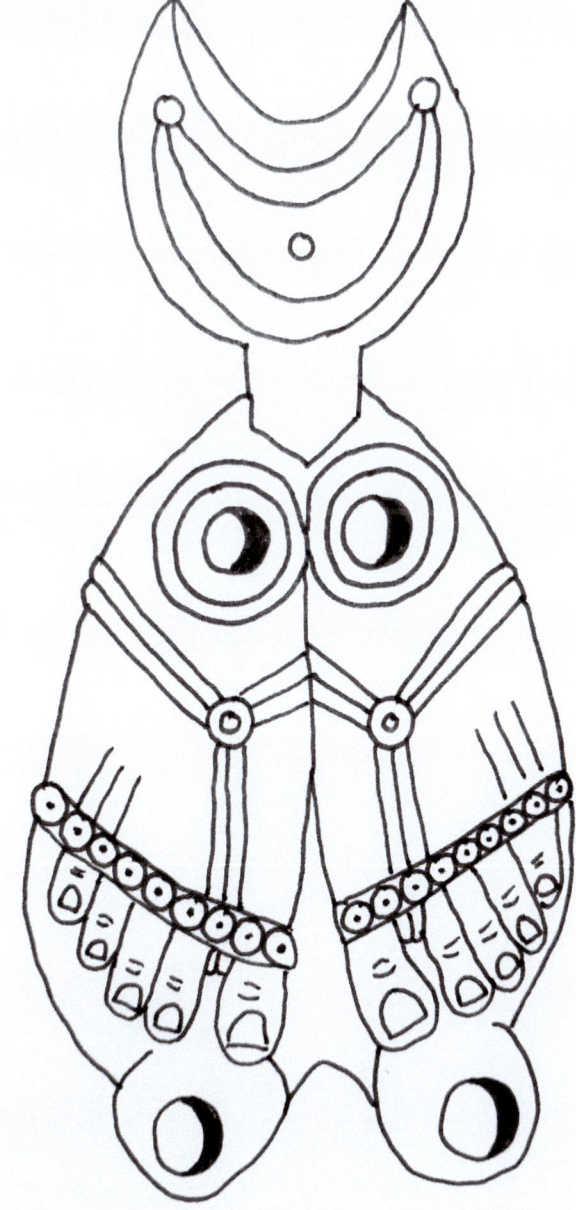

Figure 6.34: Double footlamp with crescent moon handle. (Author's drawing).

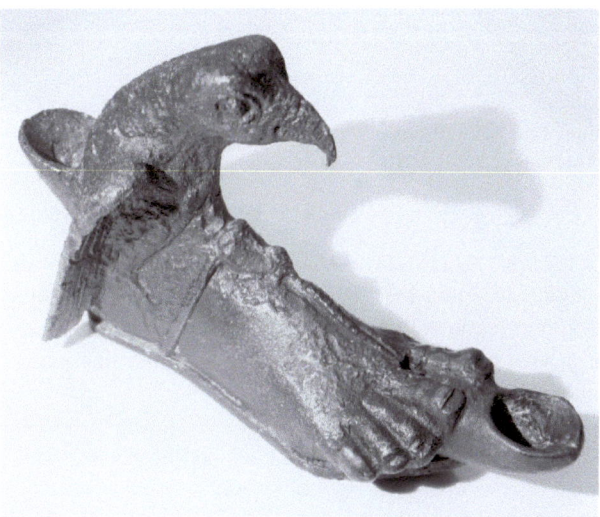

Figure 6.35: Eagle footlamp found in Augst. (Photo: KIM BL).

Roman Feet and Shoes

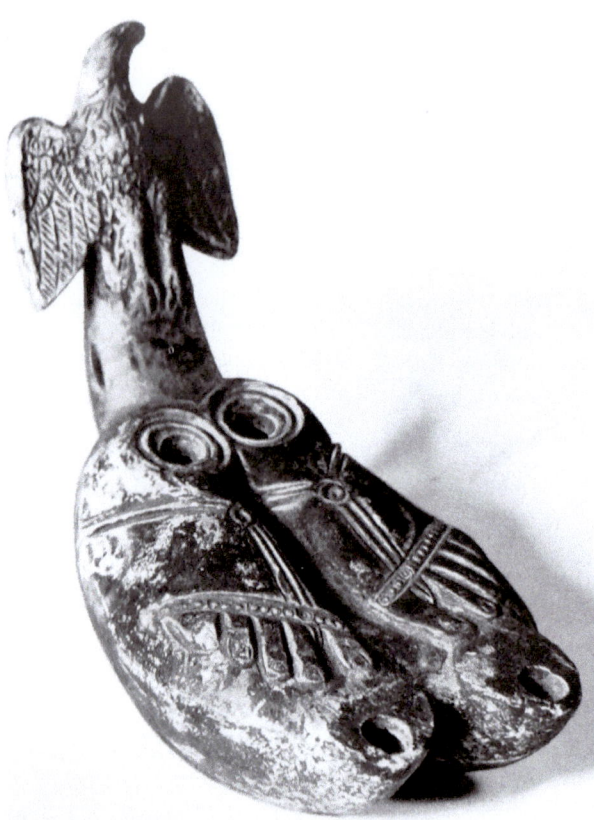

Figure 6.36: Bally Schuhmuseum eagle footlamp. (Photo: Forrer 1942: 88).

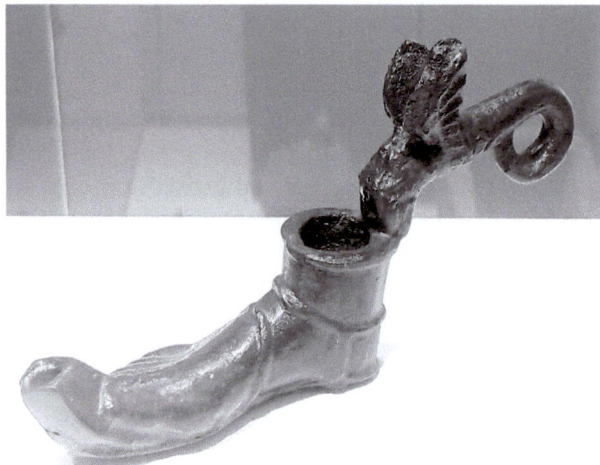

Figure 6.37: Footlamp with Gryphon, Allard Pierson Museum. (Photo: Author's own).

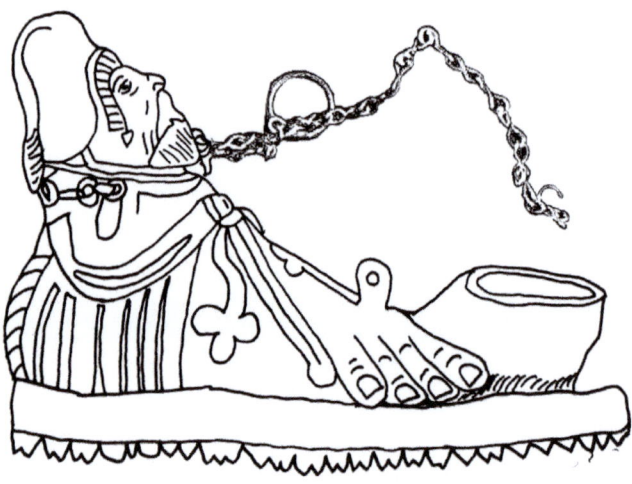

Figure 6.38: Footlamp with head.

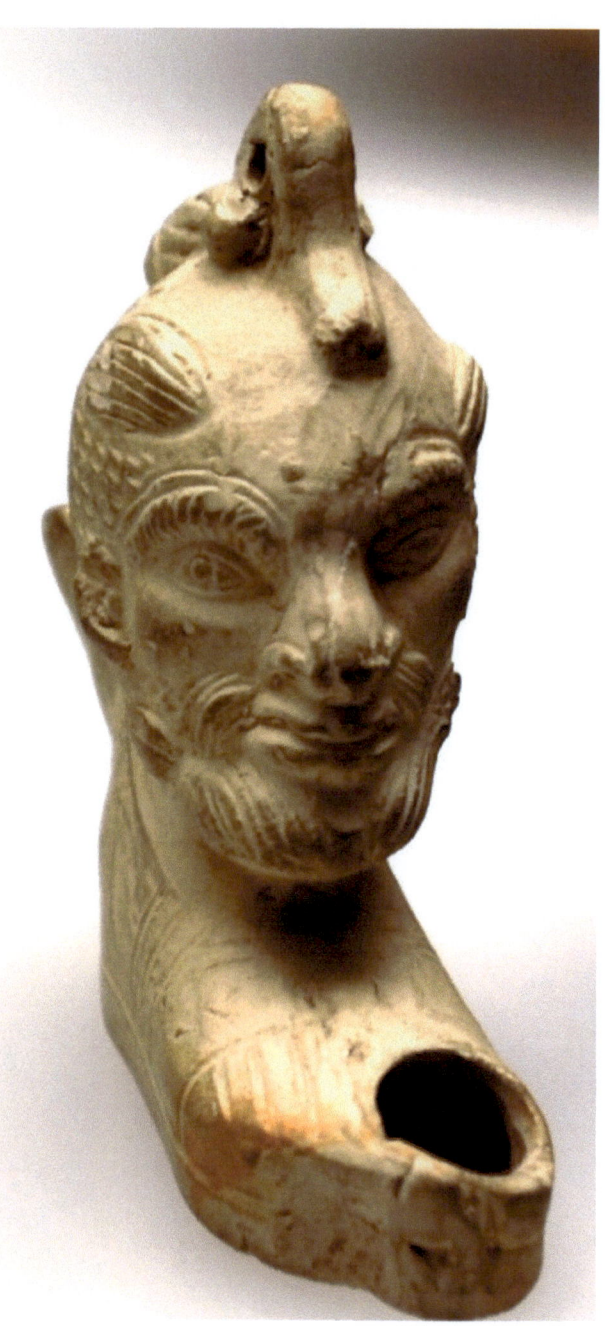

Figure 6.39: Footlamp with Satyr's head from Cologne. (Photo: Rien Bongers).

(Schachter 2012) and was common in Roman funerary art (Davies 2012) so it is, perhaps, surprising that only one footlamp features this motif. Such exceptional footlamps may have been specially commissioned rather than mass-produced.

6.6 Footlamp distribution and socio-economic status

Roman footlamps displayed status not only through their modishness, but also because of their economic implications. Regular Roman oil-lamps were inexpensive;

according to CIL 4.5380, ordinary lamps in Pompeii may have cost as little as one *as*. Thanks to inflation, the price rose to four denarii under Diocletian's Maximum price edict (15.79). Because of their relatively unusual designs and rarity value, footlamps may have cost more. Transporting these lamps to their destinations would have added to their price (Harris 1980: 134), as would the cost of olive oil for fuel, especially in areas where it had to be imported, such as Britain, representing a significant level of status and wealth (Eckardt 2000: 8–9).

The value of Roman footlamps might be demonstrated by how far they were transported from their area of manufacture. Although the details for both locations are only available for 80 out of the 245 footlamps, this is about a third of the dataset and an analysis may give some insight into their social significance. Sixteen footlamps are known to have been manufactured in Egypt, fifteen of which have recorded find locations. Two of these Egyptian lamps were found in Germany, one in Weißenburg and one in the Saalburg, both of them in military settings. Fifty-one footlamps are known to have been made in Italy. Of the forty-two with recorded find locations, most remained in Italy, twelve of them in Rome itself. However, seven were found elsewhere: one in Rouen, one in Hungary, one in the Netherlands, one in Germany, two in Switzerland and one in Benghazi, Libya. Those found in Switzerland were in private houses, while the German one came from a military setting. Six footlamps were made in the Netherlands, of which only one, a pottery mould, was found there. Two came from funerary settings in Cologne, one from a temple in Hungary, one from a fort in Switzerland and one from a rubbish deposit in Southwark.

It appears, then, that many of the footlamps with a known area of manufacture remained in that place. Local lamp-makers may have copied or adapted the design from footlamps they had seen, and the repetition of designs would tend to suggest this. There are certainly signs that some pottery footlamps were produced in numbers. Moulds have been found in potteries in Mannheim, Germany (Stupperich 2016: 15), Berg en Dal in the Netherlands (Rijksmuseum van Oudheden Inv. No. e 1944/1.81), and Szombathely, Hungary (Fitz 1998: 112). Two footlamps were also found in potteries, one in Cologne (Möhring 1989: 842), and one in Lezoux, France (Bémont and Chew 2007: 15). Two very similar footlamps made by the potter Vitalis, based in Mainz, are known from the name in their hobnailing designs (Figure 6.31) (Bonner Jahrbuch 88: 108; Fremersdorf 1926: 46; Möhring 1989: 839-840).

A trio of virtually identical footlamps may illustrate that they could be produced in numbers and still display wealth and status. The three lamps were found in Southwark (see Figure 6.19d), Vindonissa, Switzerland, and Savaria (Szombathely), Hungary. The Southwark footlamp was made in the Netherlands (Drummond-Murray et al. 2002: 218) and it is likely that the others were too. They probably all once sported a vine-leaf handle, which has since broken off (Drummond-Murray et al. 2002: 218). The Hungarian lamp was excavated in a temple to Isis, and the Vindonissa lamp came from a military setting (Wiedemer 1962: 43). The Southwark lamp is a bit of an oddity, given that it was found in a rubbish deposit (Drummond-Murray et al. 2002: 31). It may, and this is purely speculative, have been buried by its owner to protect it, and the copper alloy vessel found with it, from the effects of the Boudiccan revolt. It may simply have been broken and thrown away—the vine-leaf handle is missing and the upper and sole are cracked—but would still have been high status when in use. Many factors, therefore, may have contributed to the distribution of footlamps, among them trade and fashion.

6.7 The role of the army in footlamp distribution

Military postings may have played a role in the diffusion of Roman footlamps (Radišič 2008: 370). Forty-six percent of the 110 footlamps from known site types came from military sites. A map of known find locations shows a clear line of footlamps following the Limes along the Rhine and the Danube (Figure 6.40). This is in line with other scholars' findings on the distribution of footlamps. Drummond-Murray et al. comment that many ceramic footlamps were found in military areas of the north-western provinces (2002: 31). Harris suggests that the distribution of some lamps must be due to legionary soldiers (1980: 139). Of the footlamps known to have travelled from where they were made, four were found in military settings. Some footlamps from unknown settings may also be military, coming from sites along the *Limes* such as Xanten, Mainz and Nijmegen. It is thought that the Southwark footlamp might have been made in an army workshop in the Netherlands (Drummond-Murray et al. 2002: 218), and the similar lamps from Vindonissa and Savaria probably were too. The Vindonissa lamp was found in an officer's quarters in the fort (Wiedemer 1962: 34). Rather than costing extra to transport, it is possible that the footlamps were bought by soldiers posted to the Netherlands, who took them to their final destinations.

Apart from the attractive qualities of footlamps, there are other reasons why the Roman army may have been involved in their distribution. It is widely thought that some footlamps were associated with eastern religions, such as the cult of Serapis (see below), which were popular with soldiers. As a deity of resurrection, Serapis could have been comforting to men who faced death as an occupational hazard. The popularity of the cult of Serapis with emperors may have recommended it to the army, which was under imperial command. Hadrian had his own Serapeum at Tivoli. Vespasian visited the Serapeum at Alexandria just after being declared emperor by the Egyptian garrison (Tac.*Hist*.4.81.1–3; Suet.*Vesp*.7.2.).

Many emperors from the first to the late fourth centuries featured Serapis on their coinage (for example: Domitian, RIC IIa 812; Commodus, RIC III 246; Caracalla, RIC IV 289; Gallienus, RIC V 19; Constantius I, RIC VI 96; Julian, RIC VIII 494). The army became a vehicle for spreading the cult of Serapis (Stoll 2007: 468). For instance, dedicatory

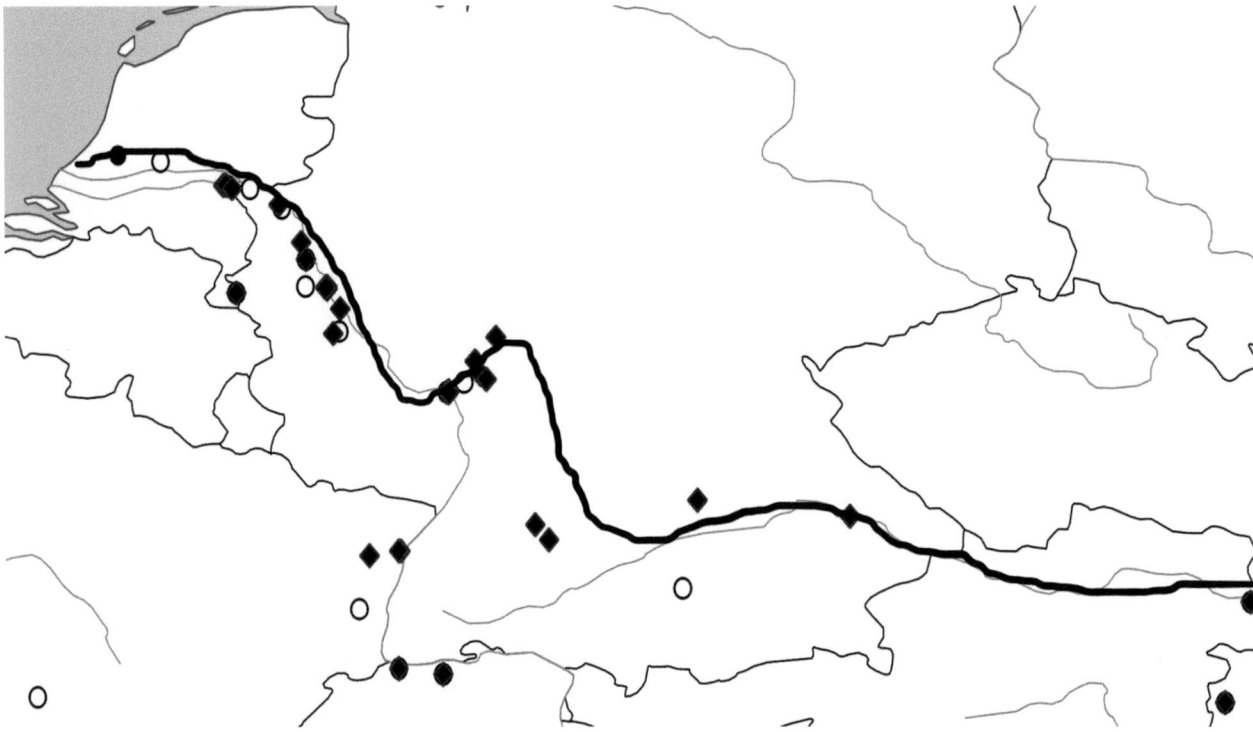

Figure 6.40: Map showing the spread of Roman footlamps along the Limes.

inscriptions to Serapis connected to the army have been found at York (CIL 7.240) and Stockstadt, Bavaria (CIL 13.6638). By the same token, the army may have played a role, however incidental, in the distribution of footlamps, and the data show some evidence of this.

6.8 Footlamps and religion

According to the Theodosian Code (XVI.10.12), lamps were lit for the gods. Footlamps played a role in Roman religious activity, not least because the representation of a foot has been interpreted as a symbol of divine power (Puccio 2010: 138) or divine presence (Dunbabin 1990: 86). Four of the footlamps in the database are from temples in Windisch, Switzerland (Loeschcke 1919: 161), Padua (Padova Cultura 2019) and Modena, Italy (Aemilia online 2019), and Szombathely, Hungary (Fitz 1998: 112). Two footlamps from town houses in Augst (Kaufmann-Heinimann 1998: 102 and 109), one from Mèze, France (Rouquette 1969: 239) and one from Pompeii (Niccolini 1890: 95) were found with *lararia*. The Pompeii footlamp (see Figure 6.3) is one of the few with a precise find setting. It was found in a *lararium* niche in the south wall of the atrium in the House of Caprasius Felix (IX.vii.20) with a pair of copper alloy *lares* (Niccolini 1890: 95), the bases of which are inlaid with silver, and a seated statuette of Fortuna holding a cornucopia (Boyce 1937: 88). The lamp depicts a right foot wearing a *crepida*; there is a bird on the lid and the sandal straps are ornate. The quality of the statuettes and the footlamp indicates a wealthy household.

It is possible that a further six lamps from domestic settings were also connected with private worship. Three additional footlamps are from theatres at Volterra, Augst and Beit She'an, and may have been associated with the temples or shrines there (Hanson 1959: 59). Footlamps therefore seem to have been valued as religious equipment.

6.9 Footlamps and Christianity

Footlamps may carry ornamentation that is emblematic of a particular religious affiliation or deity. Of the 22 Late Roman footlamps in the corpus, ten are copper alloy with Christian iconography in the form of crosses, many of them on the sole; two of these also feature doves. One of the lamps with a cross comes from Damascus and is almost identical to a lamp in the Metropolitan Museum of Art. The latter bears no overtly Christian symbols, but the museum claims it is Christian.

It is also possible that the foot itself was adopted as a Christian symbol by the early Church. Some early Christian catacombs are decorated with a pair of sandals, which have been interpreted as a symbol of mission (Arnold 1997: 232). Although it bears no obviously Christian motifs, a further footlamp, found in Saint-Pierre-du-Lac, has been interpreted as Christian (Delestre 1979: 175) due to its link with Psalm 119, verse 105, 'The word is a light unto my feet and a light unto my path'. Many scholars suggest this link (Deonna 1927: 262; Hill 1946: 71; Grandjouan 1961: 33; Ostoia 1969: 49; Delestre 1979: 175; Reynolds-Brown 1979: 338). This is a possibility, since psalms were used in the early church (Ephesians 5.18b–19a; Colossians 3.16; Tert.*Apol*.39.18; Jer.*Ep*.52.10). On the other hand, it may be an assumption based on early twentieth-century ideas, and there is no further evidence to support this connection (Galavaris 2006: 45). Nevertheless, there are a number of references to feet and sandals in the New Testament, for example, Christ washing the feet of his disciples at the Last Supper (John 13), and John the Baptist describing Jesus as one whose sandals he was not worthy to untie (Matthew 3.1; Mark 1.7; Luke 3.15; John 1.27; Acts 13:25). The symbolism on these footlamps may not necessarily demonstrate that their owners had Christian beliefs as, in the late empire, hanging bronze lamps were status symbols (Ellis 1995: 70). There is, however, no reason why these footlamps could not have signified both Christianity and high status simultaneously. Whatever the truth, there are footlamps with explicitly Christian symbols.

6.10 Footlamps and Graeco-Roman deities

Like Christ, some Graeco-Roman deities are associated with death, resurrection and life after death. For example, one copper alloy footlamp has a figurine of Diana on the lid (Figure 6.41). This does not seem to be unusual, since Möhring (1989: 805) writes about lamps with statuettes as carrying handles, citing one in the form of Artemis. A further nine footlamps have crescent moons for handles, some of which may also represent Diana. Diana presided over transitions and liminal situations, especially rites of passage (Sourvinou-Inwood 2012). One of Diana's roles was as a goddess of the Underworld, or at least of ushering people between life and death (Green 2007:133).

Feet are associated with Mercury (Galavaris 2006: 44). Crummy notes that, since Mercury is the patron of travellers, footwear is one of his defining characteristics (2007: 226). A footlamp from Padua features a wing at the ankle, which might symbolise Mercury. One of Mercury's roles was to guide the dead to the underworld. Thus, we see another chthonic deity linked with feet.

Some scholars have argued that footlamps are peculiar to the cult of Serapis, especially those that feature an *uraeus* (Deonna 1927: 246; Santoro-l'Hoir 1983: 226; Bailey 1996: 12). Serapis certainly figures in the decoration on other oil lamps (for example, British Museum inv. nos. 1814,0704.824; 1824,0478.3; 1987,0402.27). Foot iconography, such as giant sculpted feet and images on coins (Dow and Upson 1944: 58), is linked to the cult of Serapis, a deity of fertility, healing, power and death (Nicgorski 2014: 154). It might, therefore, seem reasonable to connect footlamps with Serapis.

On the other hand, the argument that all footlamps are associated with the cult of Serapis (Hill 1946: 71) is not convincing. Many large 'feet of Serapis' are unshod (see Dow and Upson 1944: 73 figure 10; Parkin 2018: 183 figure 7.3). This is not unusual in Roman iconography depicting deities (Croom 2010: 74) and, while some of the catalogued footlamps do portray bare feet, there is no additional evidence to link them to Serapis. Serapis is also sometimes depicted wearing *crepidae* (for example, Fitzwilliam Museum 2022) appropriate footwear for his role as a healer. Undoubtedly, some of the footlamps do sport *crepidae*, and may well refer to Serapis. However, the footlamps that some scholars argue are connected with

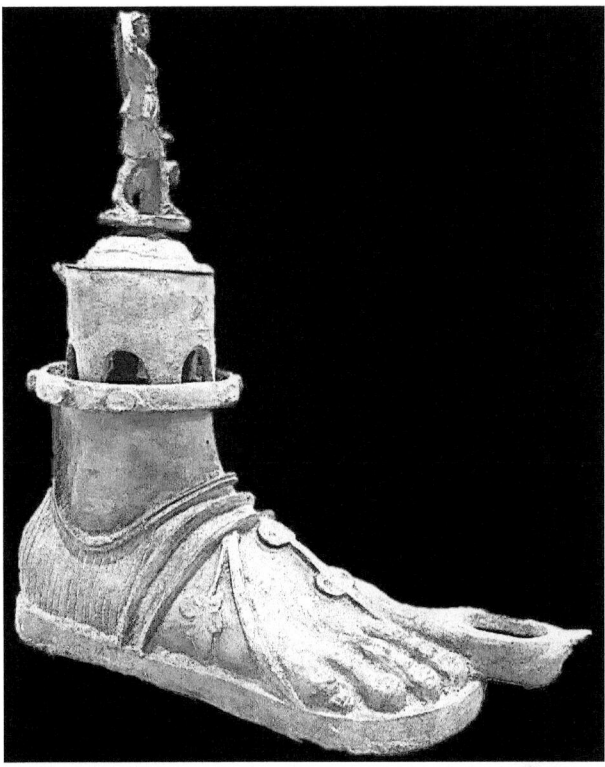

Figure 6.41: Footlamp with Diana statuette. (Photo: eBay).

Serapis, are wearing *soleae* (Figure 6.42 and 6.43), the type of sandal seen on Roman depictions of women, especially female deities and nymphs (Goldman 2002: 107). There are certainly a number of Roman statues of Isis wearing such *soleae* (for example, Capitoline Museums inv. no. MC0744). The *uraeus* is also one of her symbols. It could therefore be suggested that footlamps which combine this iconography and shoe-style are more likely to represent the cult of Isis. Indeed, one of the footlamps recorded as being found in a temple came from the Iseum in Szombathely.

Sphinxes are linked to Isis, for example, a painting from Herculaneum of an Iseum with sphinxes flanking the door (Museo Archeologico Nazionale, Naples, inv. no. 8924), so the footlamp with a sphinx handle (British Museum no. 1856,1001.31) might represent Isis. The moon was also a symbol associated with Isis, so the crescents found on footlamps may refer to her, rather than to Diana. Moons could also symbolise both goddesses simultaneously, since there was an element of syncretism between Isis and Diana (Apul.*Met.*11.5).

Iconography associated with Bacchus is evident on some of the footlamps in the database. Twelve have vine leaves, one of his symbols, for handles, and 21 others of a similar type might once have had such handles, but they have broken off. On six of these footlamps, the vine leaf is coupled with a scallop shell. This is another emblem associated with Bacchus (Eckardt 2002: 124). The Mildenhall Bacchic dish (British Museum no. 1946,1007.1) contains a ring of scallop shells among other Bacchic images, and a lead sarcophagus found in Snodland, Kent (Figure 6.44),

Roman Feet and Shoes

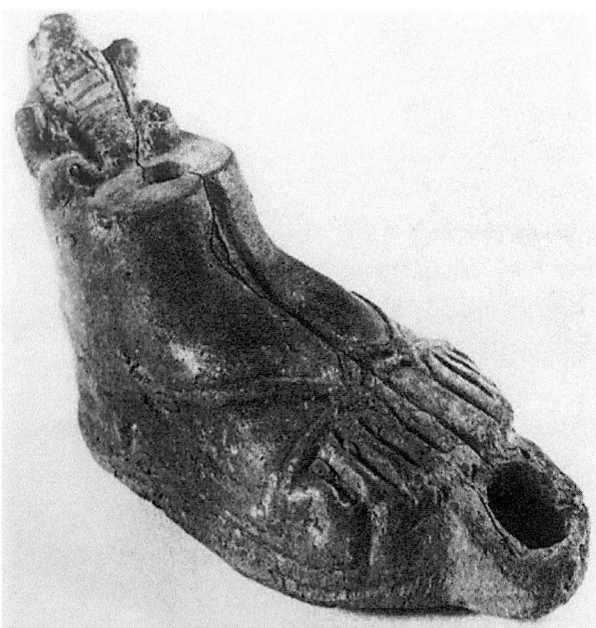

Figure 6.42: Double footlamp with soleae and Uraeus. (Photo: Detroit Institute of Arts Inv. no. 72.425).

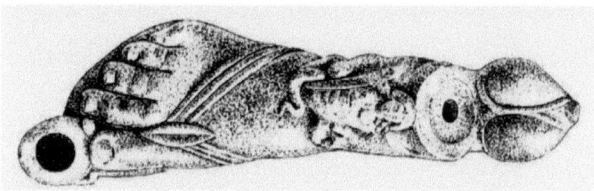

Figure 6.43: Right-footed lamp with solea and Uraeus. (Photo: Paul Perdrizet 1921: pl 15).

has a decoration of scallop shells together with a maenad and a satyr (Jessup 1954: 36). An ornate copper alloy footlamp in the National Archaeological Institute in Sofia combines a vine-leaf handle and a theatre mask, which is, again, attributable to Bacchus (Figure 6.45). It seems likely, therefore, that some of the footlamps are connected to the worship of Bacchus. As with Diana and Isis, there was syncretism between Bacchus and Serapis (Hdt.II.42 and 123), so vine leaves could stand for both. In addition, like Diana, Mercury, Isis and Serapis, Bacchus was god of, among other things, reincarnation and the afterlife (Henrichs 2012).

6.11 Magic footlamps?

Apotropaic objects were ubiquitous in Roman daily life (Dasen 2018; 129). They were thought to afford protection against the evil eye or conduct the dead safely to the underworld (Parker and McKie 2018: 5). Roman superstitions regarding the lucky nature of right feet are well documented and 67% of the footlamps in the database depict right feet. Footlamps usually feature some kind of footwear and the metaphorical protection provided by shoes was discussed above, so the form alone may have sufficed as an amulet (Galavaris 2006: 44). Iron Age amuletic jewellery in the shape of feet (see Chapter 5.1) has been discovered across Europe, some of it in tombs,

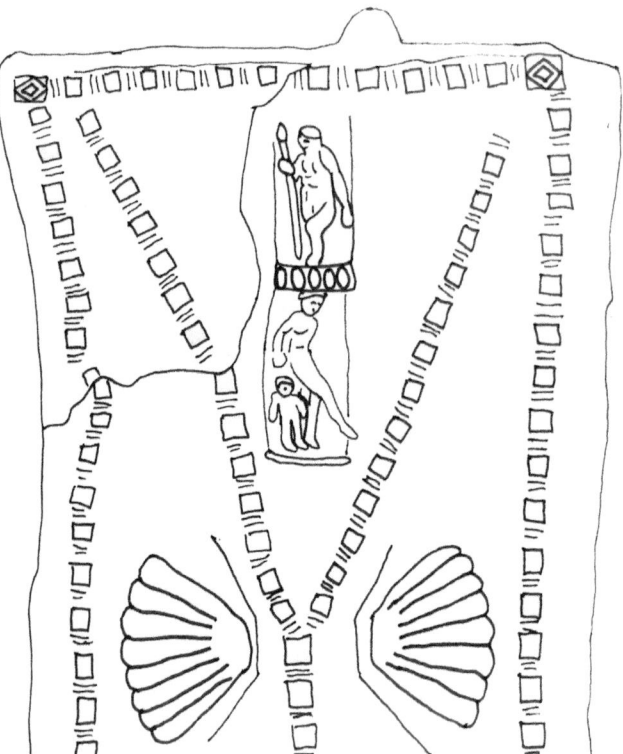

Figure 6.44: Bacchic figures on the Holborough sarcophagus. (Author's drawing).

(Feugère 1998: 23), so we may be seeing a continuation of this idea in Roman era feet. The light from lamps was also thought to ward off evil (Deonna 1927: 238), so footlamps might have been considered very effective. As far as apotropaic qualities in graves are concerned, it appears that the mere symbol of light was enough to protect the deceased (Santoro l'Hoir 1983: 229), so the small size of some footlamps did not diminish their amuletic effect.

Some of the symbolism in the ornamentation may have provided additional apotropaic value to the footlamps. Effigies of deities have a protective virtue (Deonna 1927: 257) as, presumably, do their symbols. As discussed earlier, the footlamps with large heads feature phallic symbols, a well-known Roman talisman (Whitmore 2018: 17). Deonna suggests that the crescent moon, seen on several of the footlamps, was a powerful apotropaic charm (1927: 258). The use of the *lunula* as an amulet seems to go back to ancient Egypt (Dasen 2018: 128). This also applies to shells (Dasen 2018: 128), which feature in the ornamentation on 17 of the footlamps. Henig suggests that shells may represent the womb and rebirth (1977: 200) or the soul's journey to the blessed isles (1977: 201), and therefore afford protection in funerary settings. Scallop-shell ornamentation can be seen on several lead sarcophagi in addition to Snodland: for example, from Lullingstone Villa, Spittalfields (Hall 1999:13) and Colchester (Crummy *et al.* 1993: 267). Lamps in the form of a pair of sandalled feet adorned with an *uraeus*, an apotropaic symbol according to Menzel (1952: 135), would have constituted a powerful amulet (Santoro l'Hoir 1983: 227). There are three such lamps in the dataset, together with

Roman footlamps: a case study

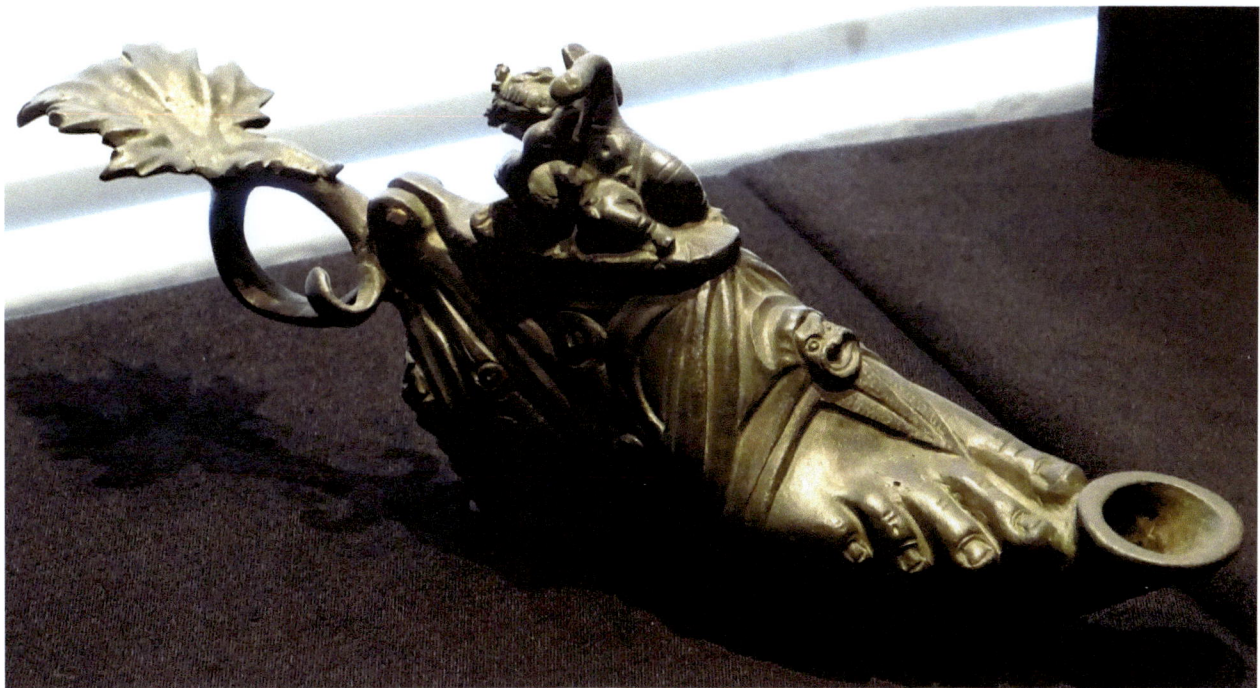

Figure 6.45: Ornate copper alloy footlamp. (Photo: Narodowe Muzeum Archeologiczne, Sofia).

three right-footed lamps with serpents. No doubt, they owe some of their talismanic virtues to the deities Isis and Serapis, whose symbol the *uraeus* is.

Another amuletic motif found on footlamps is the Medusa mask. The use of Gorgoneia as apotropaic symbols in funerary art was widespread in the Roman Empire (Santoro l'Hoir 1983: 230) because Medusa has associations with death and continuation (Parker 2016: 108). Their use on apotropaic jet pendants is also well known (Parker 2016: 110). Seven footlamps feature Medusa masks: four are pairs of feet with plane leaf handles (Figure 6.46); two are right feet with crescent moons (Figure 6.47), a quadruple charm.

A further footlamp has a mask that may be Medusa (Figure 6.48). Medusa heads are active symbols (Parker 2016: 108) which have the power to attract and hold evil influences, turning them away from the bearer of the amulet (Henig 1984, 179). As the aegis of Minerva, they may also have afforded the protection of that deity (Henig 1984, 179). It seems, then, that footlamps were valued for their apotropaic qualities, particularly when used in funerary settings.

6.12 Funerary footlamps

The religious affiliations discussed above share a common link with death and the afterlife. It appears that the association is appropriate for footlamps, as 33 in the corpus are from recognised funerary settings, that is 42% of footlamps with a known find setting. It seems likely that many of those from unknown settings may also be funerary (see Figure 6.13). Menzel argues that miniature forms of

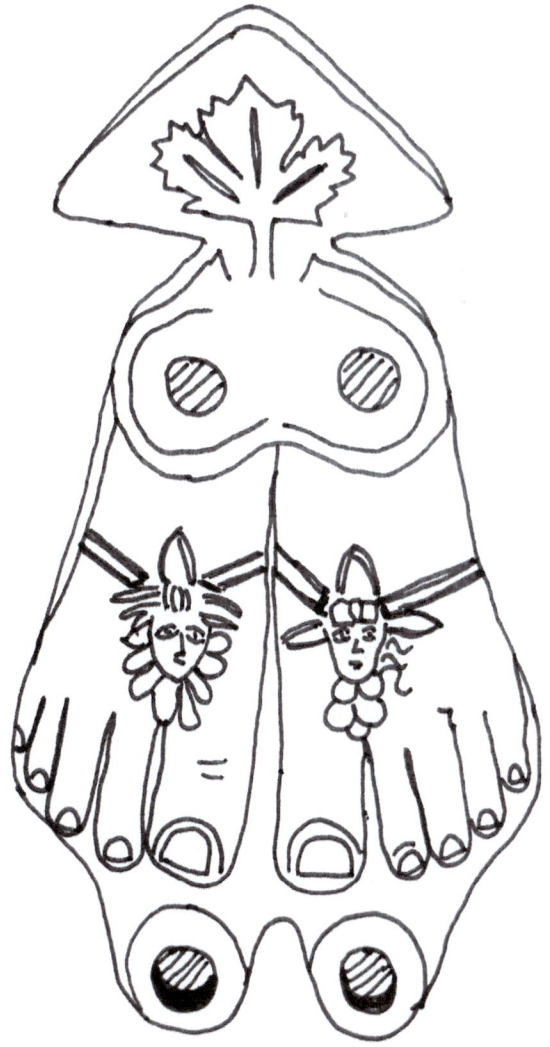

Figure 6.46: Double footlamp with Medusa masks.

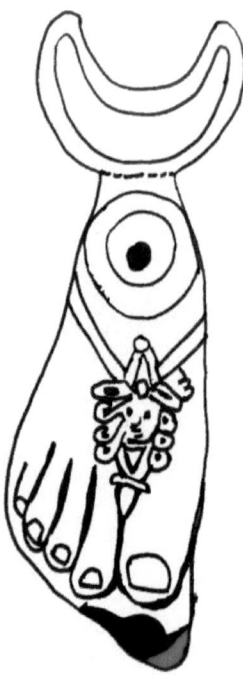

Figure 6.47: Right-footed lamp with Medusa mask and crescent.

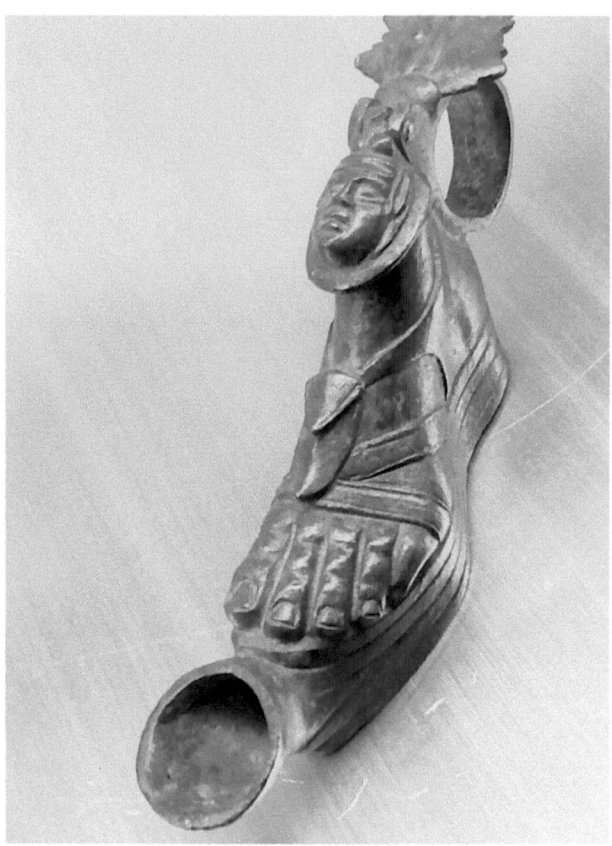

Figure 6.48: Possible Medusa mask, Museo Lázaro Galdiano, Madrid. (Photo: author's own).

lamp were made especially for burials (1952: 132). Some were so small that they could barely function as lights (Santoro l'Hoir 1983: 229). The average known length of footlamps in the dataset is 116 millimetres, while the average length of the footlamps known to have come from burials is 94 mm. Half of the footlamps from unknown find settings are shorter than the overall average for the corpus, of which 21 are shorter than the corpus average for footlamps in burials, so these may also have come from graves. One reason why the number of footlamps decreased may have been the decline in the use of lamps in inhumations (Philpott 1991: 192).

It should not be surprising that many footlamps come from funerary settings. The use of lamps in Roman burials is well attested (for example, Bailey 1963: 12; Eckardt 2000: 16; Philpott 1991: 192). Indeed, some cremation graves contained several lamps (Menzel 1952: 131; Philpott 1991: 192). Four of the six footlamps that have precise archaeological contexts with recorded assemblages were found in graves. A footlamp from Krefeld-Gellep was found in cremation grave 5211. The burial also contained two jugs, a dish, a round mirror, a rectangular mirror, and a plain, Loeschcke type X Firmalamp (Pirling *et al.* 2006: 69–70; 117; 140; 409; 420; 422). The pottery vessels are suggestive of provisions for feasting. The mirrors may indicate a female burial. They may also have been chosen to show socio-economic status.

A footlamp from Wehringen, Germany, came from cremation grave two. The cuboid grave was lined with tufa slabs and contained a glass urn with a metal lid that held only human remains (Walke 1962: 217). The lamp was in a niche above the grave and was apparently lit on memorial days, as there is soot around the wick-hole which indicates burning (Walke 1962: 217). No further grave furniture was recorded. This footlamp was, therefore, considered very special.

A double footlamp from Este is from cremation grave 67, which was found at a depth of two metres. The ashes were buried in half an amphora, above which were the footlamp, a greenish glass *balsamarium*, a simple clay lamp, a La Tène fibula, an iron ring with a chest and a *dupondius* of Augustus (Barnabei 1922: 22). This assemblage suggests an early imperial burial.

A footlamp from the Rue de Koenigshoffen, Strasbourg, is from a first-century cremation burial. It was only excavated in March 2019, but some details have been published online. The footlamp was found with five other disc lamps, a dish, a jug, a round mirror and a coin (Figure 6.49). This assemblage resembles that from Krefeld-Gellep. The lamp itself (Figure 6.50) is a left-footed version of the Southwark lamp (see Figure 6.19d).

Lamps tend to come from wealthier graves (Eckardt 2002: 115) and would, therefore, have been markers of identity and status. That footlamps were rarer may have increased the display of wealth. In addition, footlamps may have fulfilled a dual function. Shoes protect the feet, and actual shoes were deliberately placed in some Roman tombs (see Chapter 4), bringing metaphorical protection on the

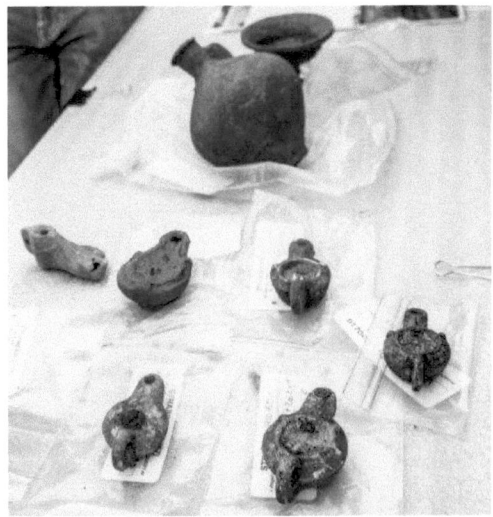

Figure 6.49: Footlamp in a funerary assemblage, Koenigshoeffen, Strasbourg. (Photo: Archéologie Alsace).

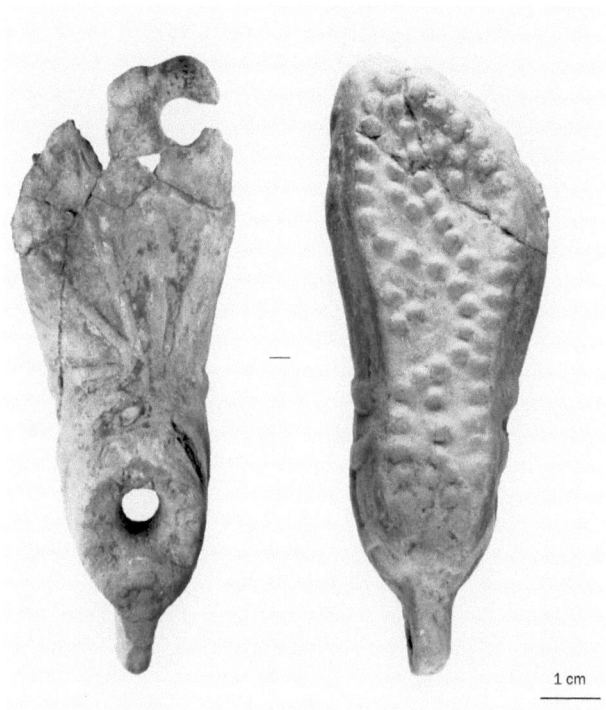

Figure 6.50: Detail of footlamp from rue de Koenigshoeffen, Strasbourg. (Photo: M. Higelin).

journey after death (Driel-Murray 1999a: 131). Shoe-shaped lamps may have shared this value (Pirling *et al.* 2006: 409).

Philpott suggests that, in the early Roman period, some people believed that the dead continued to live in the tomb and therefore needed footwear and lamps (1991: 193). Biddulph and Booth suggest that, in the context of graves, single shoes may have 'represented the living person in the realm of the dead, accompanying the deceased and connecting both worlds' (2006: 59). It may be that, because shoes connect humans to the earth, feet and footwear were seen as particularly appropriate offerings to chthonic forces (Driel-Murray 1999a: 137). A footlamp may therefore have fulfilled the functions of both lamps and shoes (Möhring 1989: 834). Perhaps an instance of this dual purpose can be seen in the footlamp from Krefeld-Gellep in Germany, which was not found with any actual footwear (Pirling *et al.* 2006: 409), although 101 of the graves there did contain shoes.

6.13 Conclusions

This chapter has highlighted various aspects of Roman lamps in the shape of feet. Roman footlamps were clearly socially significant on many levels across the Roman Empire and went far beyond mere amusement value, albeit in a limited range of contexts. Footlamps could be statements of fashion implying wealth and status. Their attractive qualities and comparative rarity would have enhanced their value, as would the maker's skill in producing fine detail, especially hobnailing (Eckardt 2013: 229). Footlamps seem to have been particularly valued by the Roman army, which helped to spread the designs across the empire. Footlamps served as religious objects in temples and lararia and symbolised many deities, sometimes more than one at a time. Deities with chthonic roles, Christianity, and eastern cults, especially that of Isis, were highly represented in the ornamentation on footlamps. As both lights and shoes, footlamps had an apotropaic value, possibly building on earlier ideas of feet as amulets. This talismanic significance was enhanced by some of the symbols added as decoration, such as Medusa masks and phallic symbols. Because of their apotropaic qualities and religious associations, Roman footlamps were often included in burials. They made particularly appropriate grave goods, representing both lights and shoes. Again, the funerary role of footlamps was protective. It was also a marker of identity and relative affluence.

Naturally, it would not be safe to assume that Roman footlamps held the same values for all people at all times across the Roman Empire. However, these artefacts enshrined all of the above values to a greater or lesser extent, depending on individual interpretations. As Miller says, consumers constantly give new meanings to products (Miller 1987: 169). Some footlamps may well have been just a bit of fun to their owners or buyers. Others may have simultaneously represented religious beliefs, apotropaic qualities, dual-function grave goods and a show of wealth and fashionability. This case study shows that there was considerable social significance in representations of feet and footwear, at least as far as Roman footlamps are concerned.

7

Roman sandal fibulae: a case study

Roman era brooches in the form of a shoe sole are found from South Shields in north-east England to as far south as Split, Croatia; from the Scilly Isles in the west to Olbia, Ukraine in the East (see Figure 7.1). Sandal *fibulae* are plate brooches of between 23 and 53 millimetres in length (Figure 7.2) and are usually enamelled in bright colours with representations of hobnailing. Apart from one silver example, they are made from copper alloy, so we are not dealing with elite jewellery. Although not popular outside the north-western provinces (Riha 1979: 11; Feugère 1985: 375), their wide distribution places this representation of Roman feet and footwear in the target research area, making sandal *fibulae* a good subject for a case study. Roman shoe brooches may not be as common as other types of *fibulae*, but they are the most common variety of skeuomorphic brooch (Johns 2012: 177; Croom 2018: 303), strengthening the case for their aptness as a subject for this study.

The aim of this chapter is to use this example of Roman representations of feet and footwear to illustrate further their multi-valent significances. Strands of significance seen in earlier chapters recur here: Roman shoe fashion, especially hobnailing, influencing the design of ornaments; the use of representations of Roman footwear in religious and funerary settings; and the apotropaic qualities of foot- and shoe-shaped artefacts. Sandal *fibulae* also provide an example of the synthesis of Roman and local ideas. The initial sections consider how the data were obtained and how the types of shoe brooch were classified. They analyse shoe brooch numbers and their geographical, chronological, and social distribution. The following parts examine how sandal *fibulae* were worn, the significance of their chirality, and their decoration, especially the representation of hobnailing. Lastly, the study discusses the apotropaic qualities of shoe brooches, their funerary use, and whether they shared the same symbolisms as actual shoes or lamps in graves, and their religious applications.

7.1 Data sources for shoe brooches

In order to gain a better insight into the symbolic significance of Roman sandal *fibulae*, this case study set out to catalogue as many as possible in detail in order to have a representative and robust sample. The total number in the database is 447.

While there are many studies of Roman brooches (for example Feugère 1985; Riha 1979 and 1994; Mackreth 2011), only two papers are dedicated to sandal *fibulae*: Eckardt (2013) and Croom (2018). This means that the data informing this study come from a variety of sources, some of which are discussed below. Of the 447 shoe brooches, 95 are antiquarian finds, 82 were found by detectorists, 34 were online sales and the provenance of 48 is unclear. This means that only 188, or 42%, come from more recent archaeological excavations, therefore not all of the information recorded was detailed, leading to gaps in the data.

The starting point for sandal *fibulae* from the United Kingdom was Eckardt's 'Shoe brooches in Roman Britain' (2013). She catalogues 63 (2013: 222–227) which were checked carefully for this study, for which Eckardt's bibliography proved invaluable. The sandal *fibula* from London's eastern cemetery (2013: 226, no. 45) has the same identity number in Barber and Bowsher (2000: 253) as a brooch in the Museum of London (2013: 227, no. 57), that is MSL87[1876]<684>. A sandal *fibula* in the Great North Museum, Newcastle, for which Eckardt has few details (2013: 224, no. 31), is the same brooch as that from Arbeia, South Shields (Eckardt 2013: 225, no. 42). This confusion probably arose because this sandal *fibula* was originally numbered as 1929.119.47 but was later assigned the number 1956.128.69.A. This shoe brooch is now referred to by its original number (Parkin 2019). Eckardt's catalogue therefore only includes 61 different Romano-British sandal *fibulae*. Nevertheless, the chapter

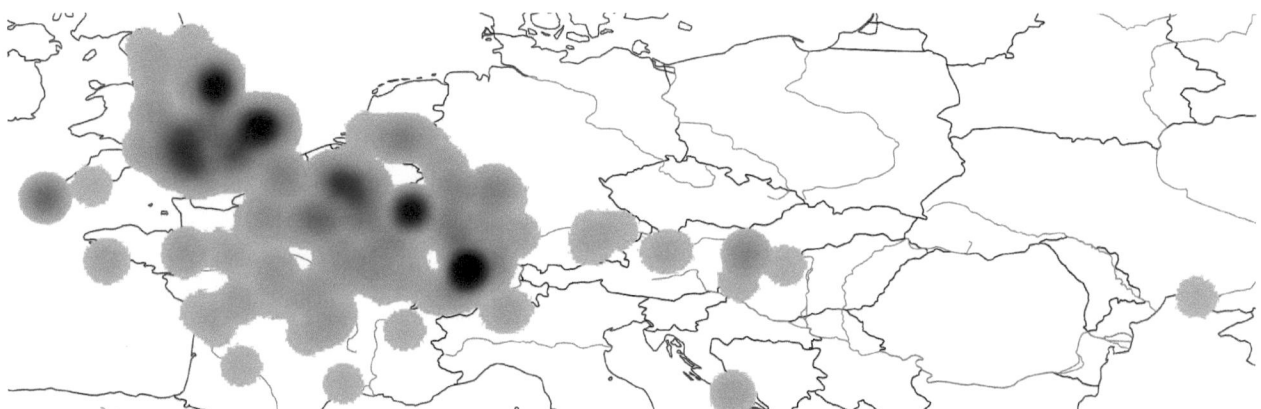

Figure 7.1: Heat map showing the geographical distribution of 363 Roman shoe brooches.

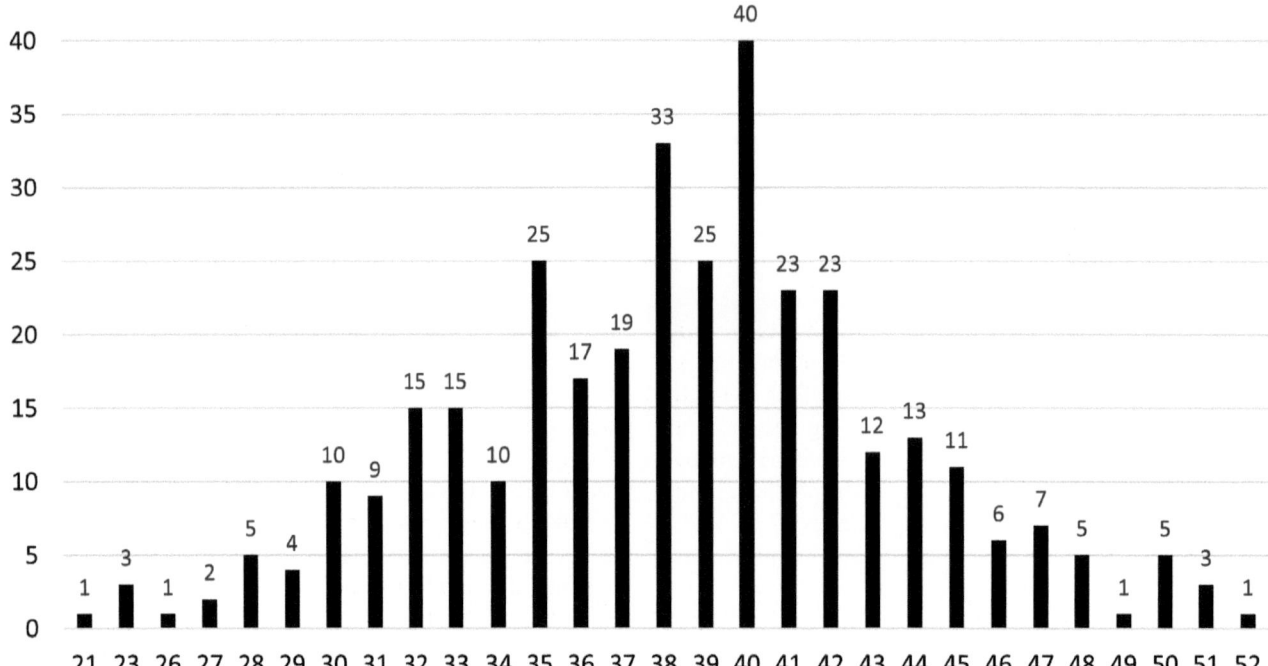

Figure 7.2: Chart to show the known length in millimetres of 344 Roman shoe brooches.

is a thorough consideration of many aspects of shoe brooches from Roman Britain.

The internet was helpful in obtaining some information. Data for 67 British shoe brooches come from the Portable Antiquities Scheme's online database. The main problems with this source are that no find setting is given, there is no picture for eight of the sandal *fibulae*, so their type and chirality cannot be judged, and the majority were returned to the finder, so there is no record of where these examples are. The online collections of the Museum of London, the British Museum, the Salisbury and South Wiltshire Museum, the Corinium Museum, and the Yorkshire Museum proved useful.

Feugère's *Les fibules en Gaule Méridionale* (1985) was the starting point for shoe brooches outside Roman Britain. This influential study categorises and catalogues all kinds of Roman brooches, including sandal *fibulae*, from Gaul and beyond, including Germany, Belgium, the Netherlands, Luxembourg, Switzerland, Hungary and Ukraine. This work is now somewhat dated, and does not include much information other than spatial data and, in most cases, references to sources of evidence. Feugère claims there are 104 sandal *fibulae* in his catalogue (1984: 375). If one counts them carefully, however, the number is actually 124, as some of his find-locations involve more than one example (1985: 377–380). As far as possible, the brooches in Feugère's catalogue were checked carefully against the references to enhance accuracy. This proved necessary, since comparing the figures in Sellye (1939: plate vii.29) and Hampel (1893: 451 fig.16) revealed that Feugère recorded one shoe brooch from Szöny, Pannonia twice (1985: 379 nos.89 and 90.29). Unfortunately, this study has been unable to access some of the literature to which Feugère refers.

Nevertheless, Feugère's work proved very useful. Further sources of information for France include: Dollfus (1975), Lerat (1979), Pietruk (2005), and the *Artefacts* database.

Collecting data for Swiss sandal *fibulae* began with Ettlinger (1973). This study has been superseded by others from the area: for example, Ettlinger catalogues only two shoe brooches from Augst and Kaiseraugst (1973: 126), whereas Riha's later studies (1979 and 1994) record 17 sandal *fibulae* found there; Ettlinger (1973: 126) mentions one from Avenches, while Mazur catalogues two (1998: 61 no. 345; 2010: 70 no. 769), giving find settings, dimensions and pictures.

Prominent German studies of Roman brooches include Böhme (1972), Rieckhoff (1975) and Rieckhoff-Pauli (1977). These reports on brooches from each individual location give details of decoration, condition and size for each shoe brooch. Additionally, Böhme's footnote 279 (1972: 39) contains copious information on further sandal *fibulae*.

Heeren and van der Feijst published a study of Roman (and other) brooches from the Low Countries, particularly around the lower Rhine basin (2017: 2). They claim 16 shoe brooches from the Low Countries (2017: 157) but give details for only four, which include size in the form of scale drawings, but do not mention colour. The authors state explicitly that a complete record is impossible (2017: 3). Nevertheless, they have omitted a type 2 shoe brooch from Vechten which is in the Rijksmuseum van Oudheden, Leiden and, according to the museum website, was discovered in 1941. In addition, the Portable Antiquities Scheme of the Netherlands includes details of two sandal *fibulae* which are not included by Heeren and van der Feijst. A further shoe brooch from Voorburg is also lacking.

Tache's catalogue of Roman era brooches in private collections includes 25 sandal *fibulae* with photographs and dimensions (2015: 46–47 and plates MTF116–117). This work is useful for studying form and colour. However, since Tache gives no find-locations, the shoe brooches can neither be added to a distribution map, nor used in the analysis of find settings. The same is true for a number of sandal *fibulae* found by French metal-detectorists or sold online.

As can be seen from the above, the level of detail recorded for each sandal *fibula* varies widely. Nevertheless, any shoe brooches found by this study were catalogued because they could all contribute something to the analysis of this representation of feet and footwear, if only the type or the find-location.

7.2 Typologies

In order to populate the database, this study needed a system of categorisation for the different shapes and styles of sandal *fibula* to enable comparisons between the different forms and to aid analysis. This was not straightforward, as there is no one, standard typology. Scholars usually base their typologies on construction and describe sandal *fibulae* as one brooch-type that has several variants, but numbers and distinguishing criteria vary from author to author. Heeren and van der Feijst, who base their typology on chronology, then construction (2017: 25), have just one variant, 57j7, probably because their catalogued sandal *fibulae* are all type 1 (2017: 570). Hull's typology (forthcoming) denotes the type as 275, brooches in the form of a sandal, and sub-divides the category into four variants, mostly based on shape: rounded toe (which seems strange, as none has a particularly round toe), pointed toe, triangular, and without hobnails. Feugère also classifies them as one type, 28b, but distinguishes just three variants, largely categorised by whether or not they have a loop at the heel (1985: 373):

- 28b1: surmounted by a loop or a small protuberance (tinned or enamelled)
- 28b2: enamelled and without loops
- 28b3: smooth, unenamelled

Feugère's method of classification does not take account of the different shapes of sandal *fibulae*, all of which have examples with loops, protrusions, or neither.

Riha identifies three variants according to surface decoration within her group seven (1979: 200–201):

- 7.23.2: a brooch where the hobnails are formed by raised metal protuberances, often square or triangular
- 7.24: a flat, copper alloy plate with a pressed, sheet-metal overlay, the 'Pressblech' technique
- 7.25 figurative brooches inlaid with enamel.

Riha's types are not exclusively sandal *fibulae* but comprise all forms of representational plate brooch.

Mackreth (2011: 178–179) establishes five categories within one group, using a mixture of shape and surface decoration as criteria to identify his sub-types:

- 1.1a: unenamelled
- 1.1b: the 'standard' design
- 1.1c: the enamelled field is broken up by lines
- 1.1d: wide metal border
- 1.1e: very pointed toes

Eckardt's study of Roman shoe brooches in Britain identifies four 'sub-types' based on criteria similar to Mackreth's (2013: 218–220):

1. the most common type, with a pointed toe (corresponding to Mackreth's 1.1b)
2. with a wide border and narrow enamel field (Mackreth's 1.1d)
3. markedly angular with a triangular, pointed toe (Mackreth's 1.1e)
4. 'unusual', which includes unenamelled shoe brooches and those with a curvilinear design instead of hobnails (Mackreth's 1.1a and 1.1c).

Croom bases her typology on Eckardt's, but splits Eckardt's type 4 into two variants:

4. with curvilinear designs instead of hobnails
5. unenamelled (2018: 301).

Although the latter three studies focus solely on Roman Britain, shoe brooch typologies based on these criteria are the most useful, as they are widely applicable and enable clearer distinctions between the different forms. The typology used in this study (Figure 7.3) is, therefore, based on Croom's adaptation of Eckardt's typology:

1. pointed toe: these are indeed the most common, with 265 examples
2. wide border: 28 examples
3. angular: 54 examples, 43 of them from Britain
4. curvilinear: very rare, with only 4 examples, all from Britain
5. unenamelled: 35 examples.

It proved necessary, however, to add a sixth category, 'irregular', to take account of 21 shoe brooches that did not fit into Croom's five types due to their unusual shapes. It has been suggested that some of the 'irregulars' may have been misinterpreted as sandal *fibulae*, and possibly represent daggers (Allason-Jones 2021). However, these have been retained due to their categorisation as shoe brooches by a number of sources (Riha 1979: 200; Pietruk 2005: 129; Gaspar 2007: 216–217; Nickel 2011: 115; Mackreth 2011: 178–179; Eckardt 2013: 223 and 227). A further 40 brooches are labelled 'indeterminate', since it is not possible to tell the shape of the toe because they are heel fragments, or because the relevant literature contains no picture or description (Figure 7.4).

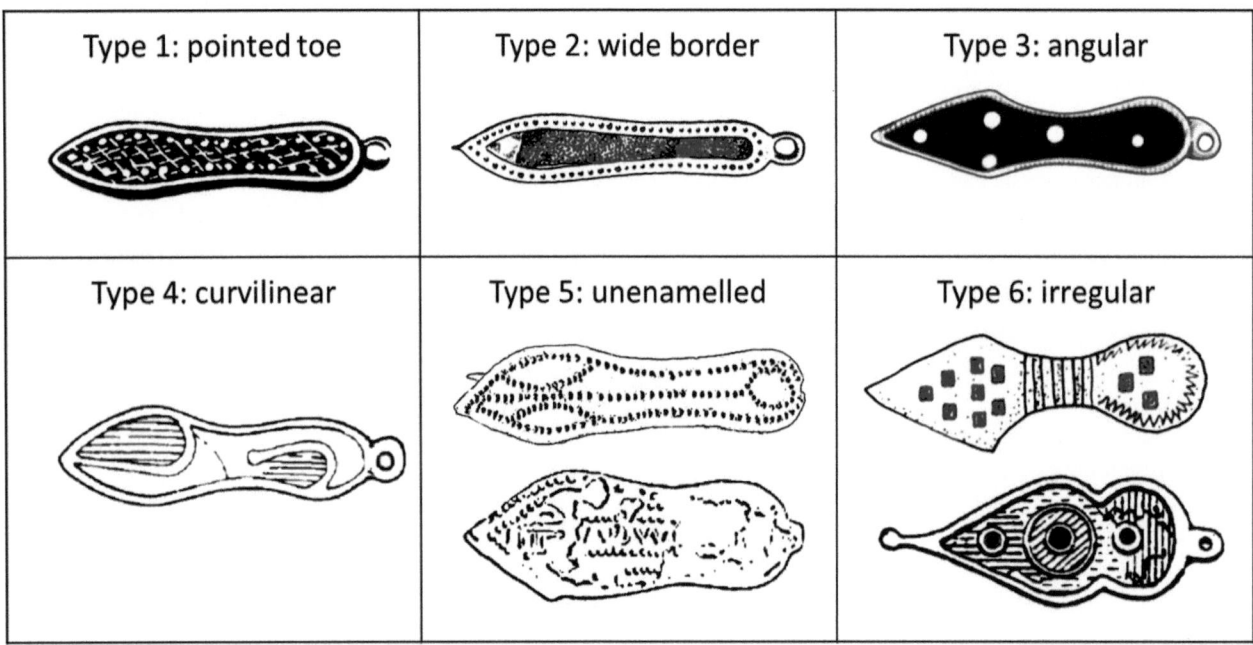

Figure 7.3: Typology of Roman shoe brooches (Author's drawings).

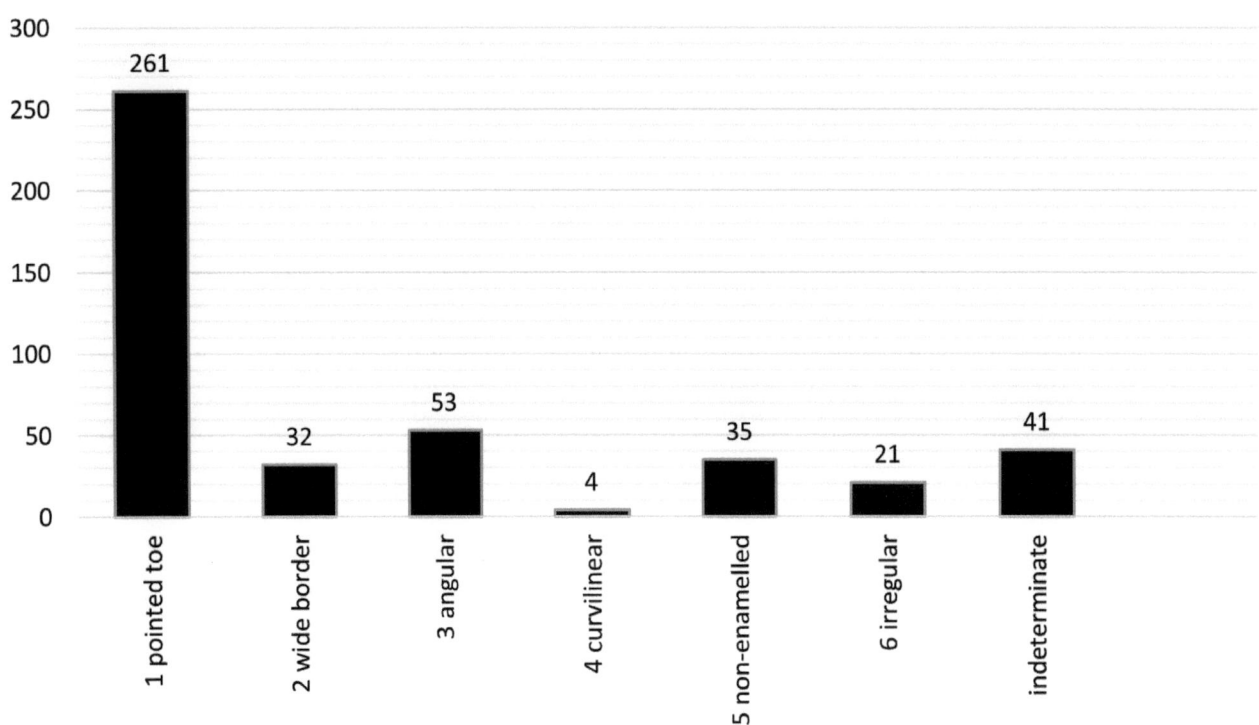

Figure 7.4: Chart to show the proportions of type in 447 Roman sandal fibulae.

There does appear to be some regional variation in types of shoe brooch (Figure 7.5): types 1, 2, and 5 are found across the north-western provinces, while 81% of type 3 brooches are British, which has implications for where these *fibulae* were made. All type 4 brooches are also British, and were probably made in the same workshop, likewise a particular kind of irregular brooch (see Figure 7.3).

7.3 Numbers

The statistics for Roman Britain illustrate that, as stated above, the shoe brooch was not common compared with other types. This section aims to illustrate how common the sandal *fibula* was among Roman brooches. It will also consider the numbers of shoe brooches catalogued by other scholars.

Of the 34,686 Roman brooches on the Portable Antiquities Scheme database at the time of writing (Figure 7.6), just 67 are shoe brooches (0.2%). Only one of about 250 brooches (0.4%) from the Roman site of Arbeia, South Shields, is a sandal *fibula* (Croom 2018: 301). Even in Nornour, where a greater concentration of shoe brooches was found, the statistics are still only nine out of 329,

Roman sandal fibulae: a case study

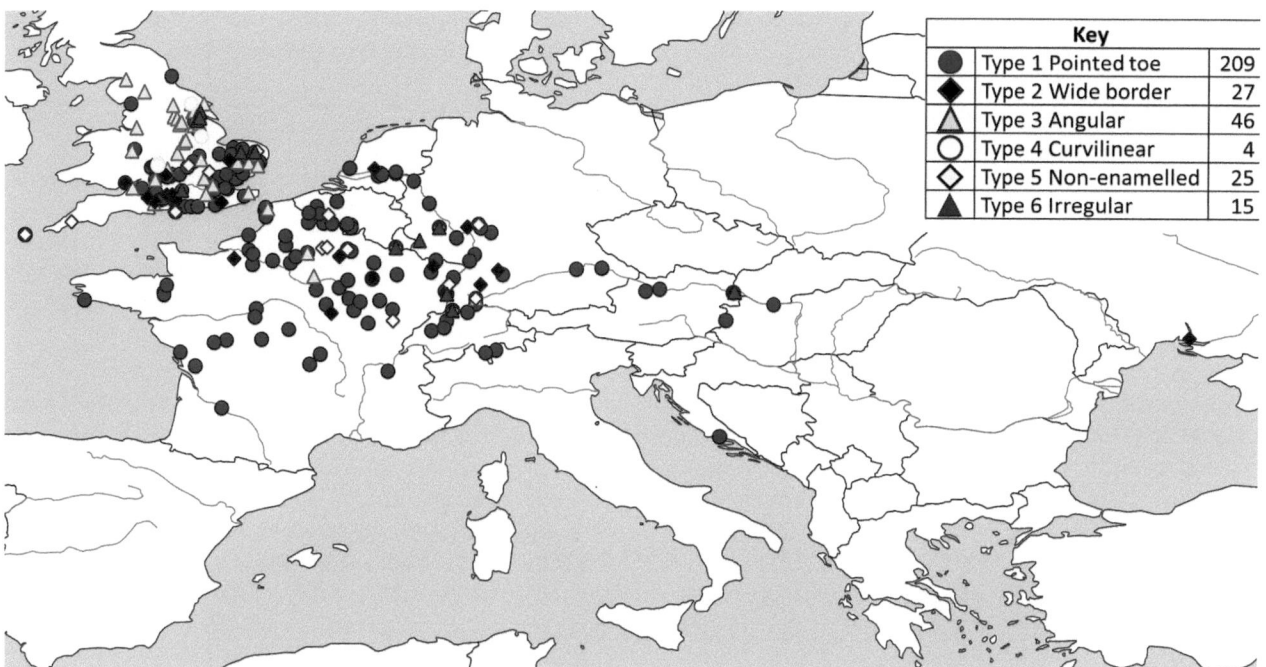

Figure 7.5: Distribution map of 324 Roman shoe brooches of a known type with a known find location.

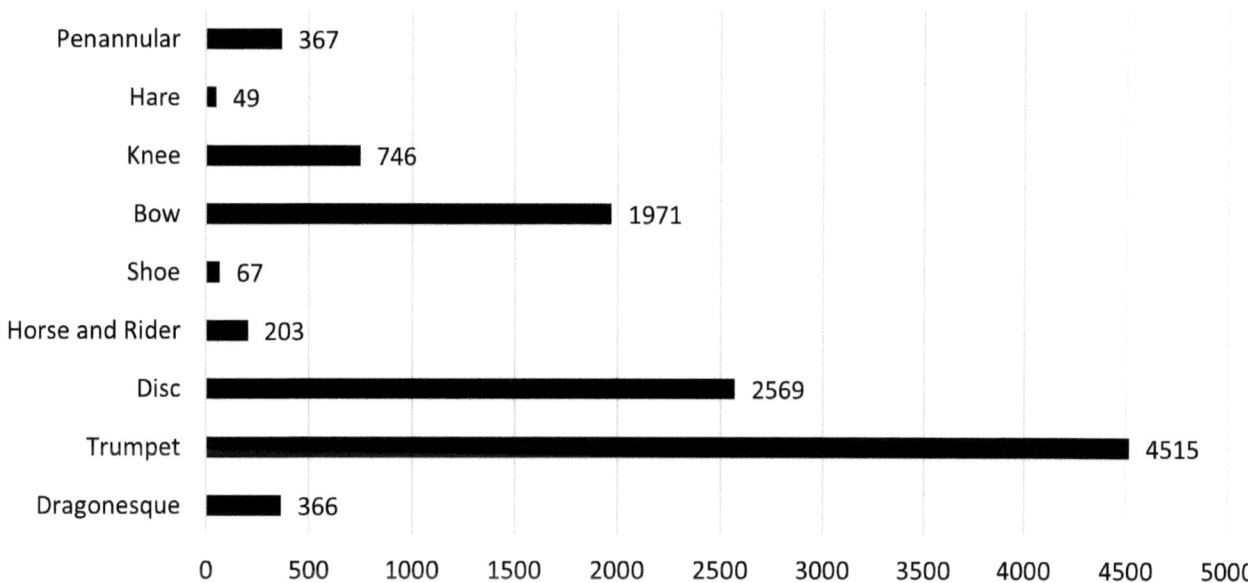

Figure 7.6: Chart to show comparative numbers of different Roman brooches from the PAS database.

or 2.7% (Butcher 2004: 29). The numbers for the north-western provinces are similar. Feugère estimates a total of eight to ten thousand Roman era brooches in his catalogue (1985: 12) but only 124 are sandal *fibulae*, a mere 1.5%. Riha's studies of the Roman brooches from Augst and Kaiseraugst, Switzerland, have produced a catalogue of 3,027 (1994: 202). Among them are just seventeen sandal *fibulae* (0.6%). It is possible that further shoe brooches could have been melted down and recycled. There may also be more sandal *fibulae* in private ownership that we do not know about. Shoe brooches are rare, minority objects but the small number in comparison with other brooch types may indicate that they had a special value.

The shoe brooch is, however, the most common skeuomorphic type of Roman brooch (Johns 2012: 177; Croom 2018: 303). Croom claims that, in Roman Britain, shoe brooches are the second most common representational *fibula* after the horse-and-rider (2018: 303). Her statistics for 243 plate brooch types, taken from Mackreth's catalogue (Croom 2018: 308 note 5), show 49 horse-and-rider brooches and 44 sandal *fibulae* (Croom 2018: 304 fig. 14.20), although Mackreth actually catalogues 47 shoe brooches from Roman Britain (2011: 179–180). The Portable Antiquities Scheme database contains 61 sandal *fibulae* to date, compared with 203 horse-and-rider brooches. However, outside Roman

Britain, the shoe brooch appears to be more popular than the horse-and-rider brooch. Feugère's catalogue contains 124 sandal *fibulae*, 20 of them from Roman Britain (1985: 377–378), but only 21 horse-and-rider brooches, 9 from Roman Britain (1985: 414). Riha's catalogue also contains more sandal *fibulae* (17) than horse-and-rider brooches (three) (Riha 1979: 201; 1994: 171). Heeren and van der Feijst record four sandal *fibulae* from the Netherlands, but no horse-and-rider brooches (2017: 570).

7.4 Chronological Distribution

The exact date range of the sandal *fibula* is unclear. Many scholars date them to the second century based on the assemblages with which they were found, or by comparison with other examples known to be second century (Hull 1968: 29; Feugère 1985: 377; Eckardt 2013: 217; Heeren and van der Feijst 2017: 153; Croom 2018: 301), and 399 (89%) of this study's catalogued shoe brooches are broadly second century. Others extend the range into the third century (Ettlinger 1973: 192; Dollfus 1975: 210). There is also an argument that the unenamelled type of sandal *fibula* is earlier, dating from the late first century (Mackreth 2011: 179; Butcher 2004: 29). One of the earlier shoe brooches from Augst has been dated to the Neronian or early Flavian periods due to its accompanying finds (Riha 1979: 200 no.1727). The difficulties in dating sandal *fibulae* are illustrated by the case of a pair found in a grave in Blicquy, Belgium. The brooches are of type 5, unenamelled, which, judging by excavated finds, seems to date to the late first century. The grave they came from, however, dates to the late second century (de Laet *et al.* 1972: 117). The brooches may have been heirlooms or perhaps this type persisted.

There does, however, appear to be a date range from the late first until the early third centuries. This pattern is visible in the data from the corpus, with 42 (or possibly 44) from the first century, the vast majority from across the second (358), and only four from the third century (Figure 7.7).

7.5 Spatial Distribution

Roman sandal *fibulae* are widespread in Britain and the north-western provinces from Gaul to Pannonia including the Rhineland and Switzerland (Böhme 1972: 30; Hattatt 1985: 172; Feugère 1985: 375; Eckardt 2013: 217). The 151 British sandal *fibulae* catalogued in this study were mostly found south-east of the Severn-Humber line (Figure 7.8), but not necessarily in south-east England (compare Eckardt 2013: 220). This study has revealed a cluster of finds near the Humber in north Lincolnshire and 32 shoe brooches found north of the Wirral, compared with ten or eleven in Eckardt's catalogue (2013: 222–227). None have been found in Scotland to date, and only two in Wales, in Caerleon. Eckardt (2013: 225 no. 39) and Mackreth (2011: 15) record only one shoe brooch from this location, possibly because the second brooch is not mentioned by Brewer (1986: 172). However, the author has observed both brooches on display in the National Roman Legion Museum (Figure 7.9). These data for spatial distribution may be biased because of where detectorists tend to search and where excavations have taken place (Cool and Baxter 2016: 9). The numbers of sandal *fibulae* catalogued for modern European countries are: France 124; Germany 32; Luxembourg 19; Belgium 14; and the Netherlands eight. Outside the north-western provinces, Switzerland 35, Austria seven, and Hungary two. There are two in Split, Croatia, and one from Olbia, Ukraine. Additionally, 52 (12%) shoe brooches in the database have no definite find country.

7.6 Distribution by site type and find setting

An analysis of the types of site where shoe brooches were found should help to assess their symbolism. Of the

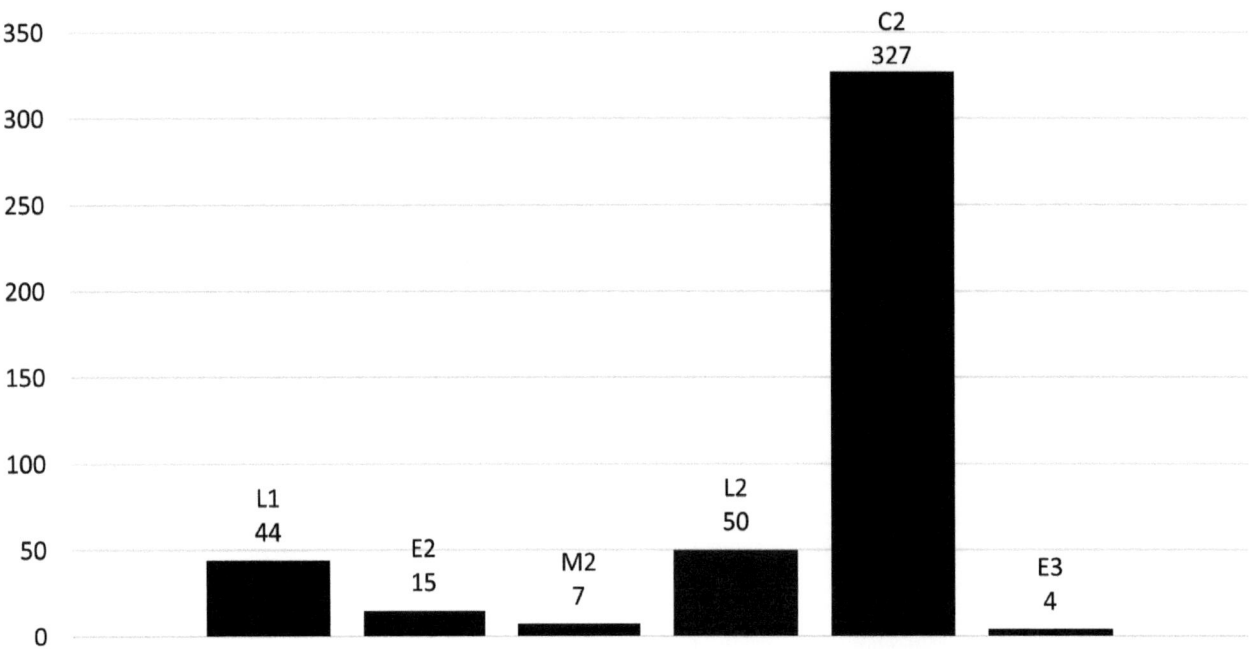

Figure 7.7: Chart to show the date range of 447 Roman sandal fibulae.

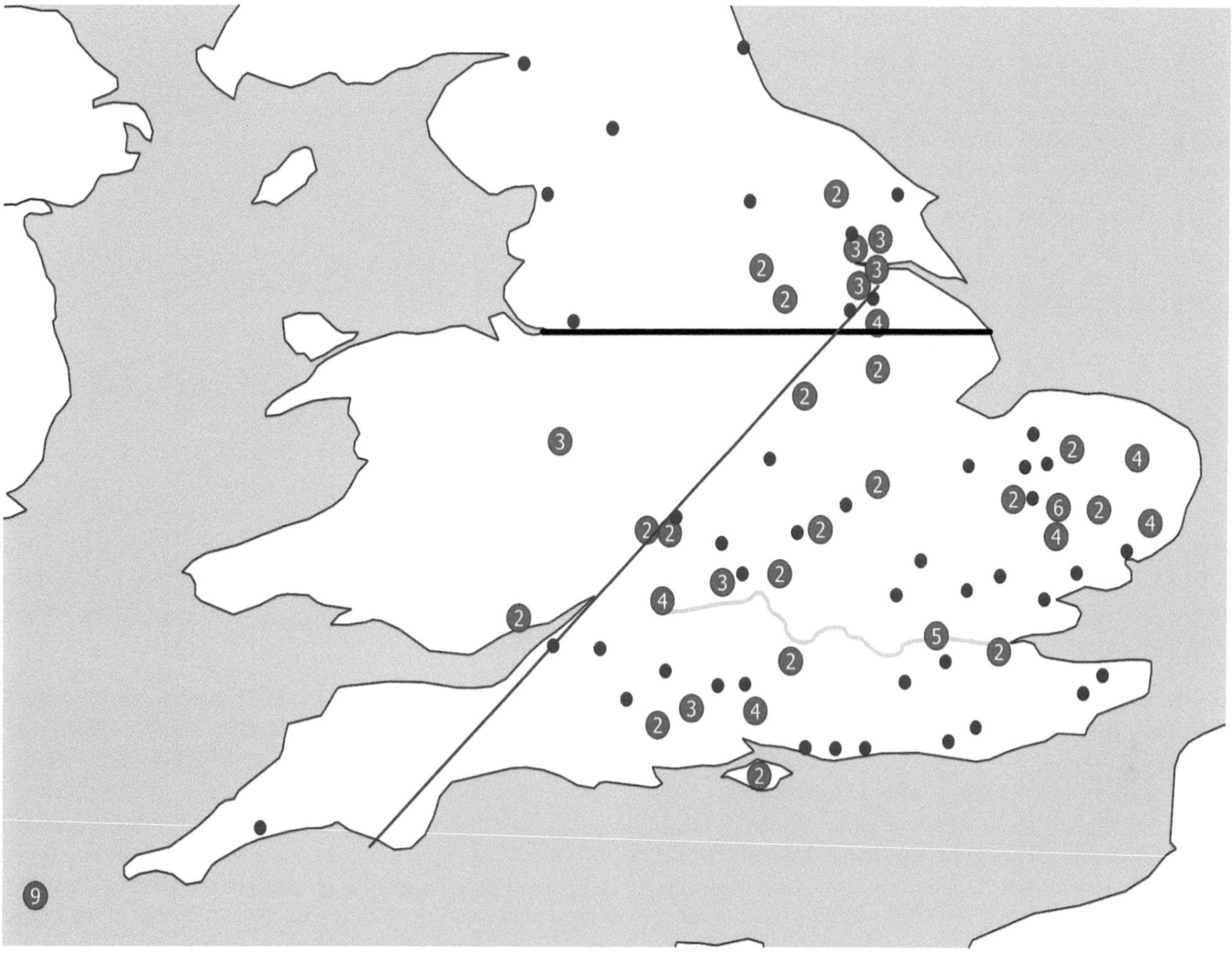

Figure 7.8: Map to show the geographical distribution of Romano-British shoe brooches.

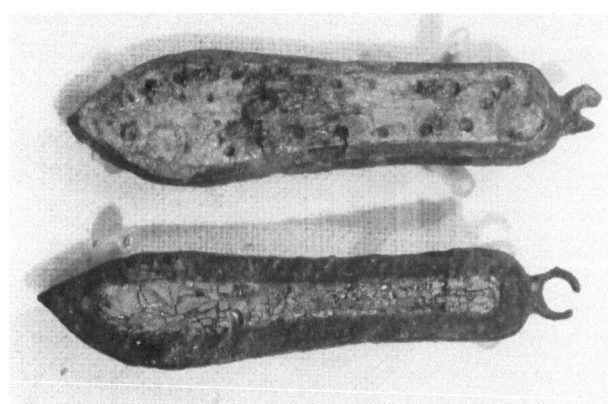

Figure 7.9: Two Roman sandal fibulae in the National Roman Legion Museum, Caerleon (Photo: Author's own).

447 sandal fibulae in the corpus, 188 (or 42%) have no recorded site type (Figure 7.10). Nevertheless, data are available for the site type of 259 shoe brooches. The site types for sandal *fibulae* are categorized as: small town, urban, villa/rural, military (from a fort or its associated buildings), other, and unknown.

The majority of the catalogued shoe brooches with a known find setting are from small-town or urban settings (159, or 65% of those with a known site type). The greatest concentration of sandal *fibulae* from a small-town setting came from the Titelberg, Luxembourg (18), and in a larger urban setting from *Augusta Raurica* (17). Sixteen of these seventeen shoe brooches were found in *insulae* (Riha 1979: 200–203; 1994: 171–174) and one in the theatre (Riha 1979: 203 no. 1754). Five sandal *fibulae* come from London, two from Cologne, and five from Carnuntum, Austria. It is likely that the popularity of sandal fibulae owes a lot to their availability in markets or other places where there was a trade in copper alloy jewellery, and these would have been more accessible in towns.

There are, however, 51 shoe brooches from villa/rural sites (21%) and the 59 PAS finds are likely to have come from such sites too, but we cannot be certain. Even in rural areas some sites account for more than one: three were found at the villa of Biberist-Spitalhof, Switzerland (Deschler-Erb 2006: 438–439) and two from Overbetuwe in the Netherlands (Heeren and van der Feijst 2017: 457, PAN00005552).

Sandal *fibulae* are rare on military sites (Eckardt 2013: 220). This study catalogued 31 and, in some cases, it is unclear exactly where on the military site the brooch was found. The sandal *fibula* from Arbeia Roman fort was sold

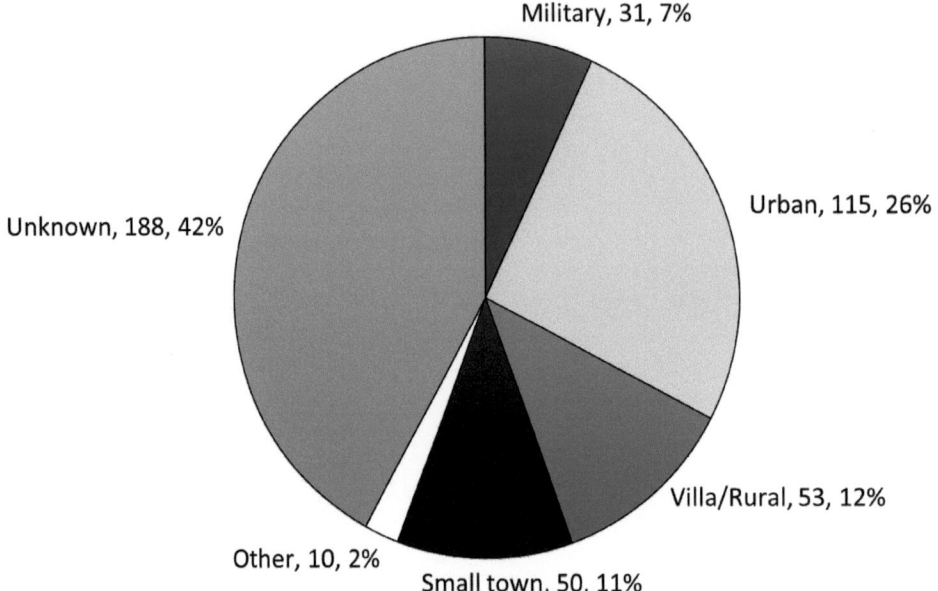

Figure 7.10: Chart to show the site type of 447 Roman sandal fibulae.

to a local antiquary, so its precise provenance is unknown. It could be from the fort, the extra-mural settlement, or the cemetery (Croom 2018: 301). The case is even less clear for the Tullie House sandal *fibula* in Carlisle. Haverfield (1919: 13) says its find-location is unknown while Snape (1993: 118) says it was probably found in Stanwix fort. Malton Museum, Yorkshire, has two brooches connected with the Roman fort, but their website suggests that these may have been votive deposits at a shrine, so they may not be 'military'. There are eight shoe brooches from the German Limes forts of the Saalburg, Hüfingen, Sulz, and Zugmantel. Those from the Saalburg were actually found inside the fort (Böhme 1972: 39). If this type of brooch were worn exclusively by women,[1] this would constitute further evidence of their presence in forts (see van Driel-Murray 1997b). The precise find-location of the Zugmantel brooch is unclear (Böhme 1972: 106). The Hüfingen brooches came from the extra-mural settlement (Rieckhoff 1975), as did those from Sulz (Rieckhoff-Pauli 1977), Taverny, France (Gouyet 1976: 76) and Castleford (Cool and Philo 1998: 55). The other three 'military' brooches are from Eining and Köngen, Germany, and Vechten, Netherlands. This may indicate that, unlike Roman footlamps, the army played little part in the spread of this kind of brooch.

The remaining 10 sandal fibulae are from sites categorised as 'other'. Nine of these were found at Nornour (see section 9.12), while the other came from North Ferriby and is thought to be from a port (Eckardt 2013: 227 no.59).

Data are available for the find setting of 155 shoe brooches, meaning that 292 have an unknown find setting (Figure 7.11). The 50 from religious settings and 24 funerary brooches are discussed below. A sandal fibula from London was found in the Walbrook, a definite 'water' setting, and two found at Mildenhall may be fen-edge votives (Eckardt 2013: 28; 48). Domestic settings account for 39 sandal fibulae, of which 20 are from villa/rural sites, four from small towns, and 12 from urban sites. Two further brooches from the artisanal quarter of Bliesbruck-Spitalhof may also be from domestic find settings, but are included in 'other' because they may be from workshops too (Wilmouth 2014: 17). Seven are from settings designated 'industrial'. In addition to the brooch from North Ferriby, the brooch from Voorburg was found at a port on a Roman canal (Archeologie van Zuid-Holland 2022). Two brooches from Rheinzabern and one from West Stow came from potteries (West 1990: 71). The shoe brooch from Wilderspool was found with an enameller's workshop (May 1904: 73) and one from Biberist-Spitalhof was also found in a metal workshop (Schucany 2006: 457).

Thirty-two shoe brooches were allotted to a category labelled 'other'. Twenty-one of these were found in a setting that related to a military site, and are discussed above. Eight sandal fibulae come from find settings related to public buildings. In addition to the brooch from the theatre in Augusta Raurica, two sandal fibulae are from entertainment venues: one came from the Roman theatre in Vendeuil-Caply, France (Musée archéologique de l'Oise 2016) and another was found in the amphitheatre at Avenches, Switzerland (Mazur 1998: 61 no. 769). One came from the civil basilica at Alesia (Lerat 1979: 72), one from the baths/macellum portico at Wroxeter (Ellis 2000: 155) and one from the bathhouse at Wels, Austria (Greisinger 2014: 8). Ironically, a shoe brooch found in Bath came, not from the Roman baths, but from a site that is a mixture of industrial and funerary (Bush 1907). It is unclear in which part of the site the brooch was found.

The remaining shoe brooches from an 'other' find setting were found in pits or ditches. A brooch from Great Dunmow was found in a pit 594 with some second-century

---

[1] Discussed below.

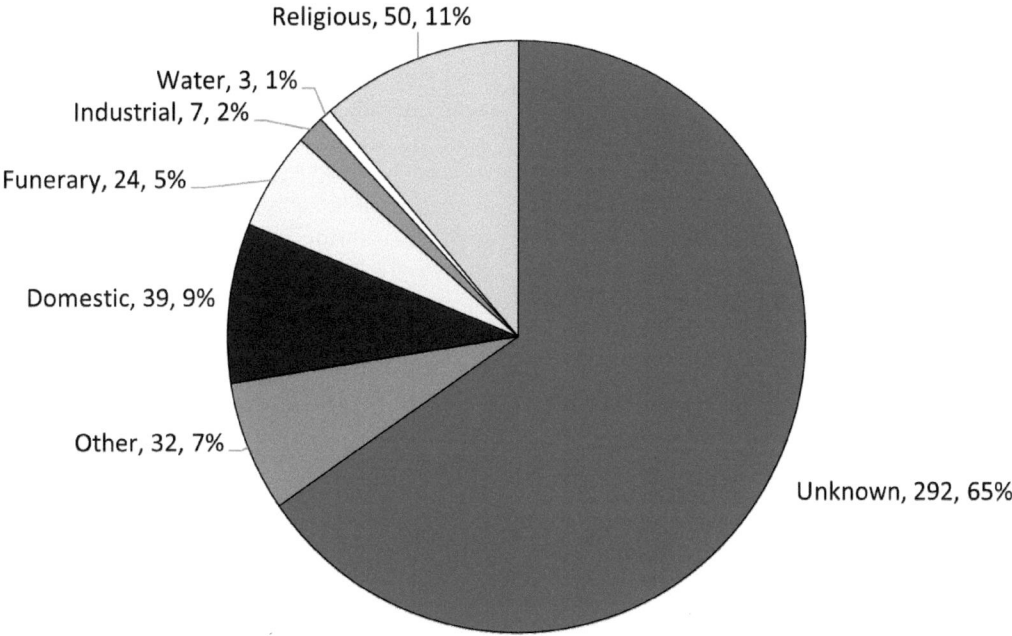

Figure 7.11: Chart to show the find setting of 447 Roman sandal fibulae.

pottery (Wickenden 1988: 11). One from Brebières was found in a ditch (Dananai 2012: 251) but there are no further details. The final example was found in a Roman ditch in Kilhallon, Cornwall (Carlyon 1982: 155). This find is labelled 'other' because little is known about the nature of the site, although the author suggests it may be the defensive ditch around a settlement (Carlyon 1982: 157), or connected to tin mining (Carlyon 1982: 168). The ditch is dated to the mid third century (Carlyon 1982: 155) but may have been in use for longer, since the Kilhallon shoe brooch is of a first-century type (Butcher 1982: 162). No other Roman features were found with the ditch (Carlyon 1982: 155), which was filled with cockle and other shells. Among the shells were pottery, glass, animal bone and copper alloy objects (Carlyon 1982: 157). Carlyon interprets the finds as a rubbish deposit (1982:155). However, there is an argument for this being a special deposit. Layers of deposition were identified and the types of finds that accompanied the shells are thought to indicate ritual deposition. The animal bone groups do not include deer, but there is evidence of ox and horse. Two dog skeletons were also identified (Turk 1982: 165) and these could also indicate a special deposit (Merrifield 1987: 32; Morris 2008: 9). Butcher (1982: 162) seems to be of the opinion that the Kilhallon sandal *fibula* may be of ritual import, as she discusses the magical and religious significance of the shoe brooch. That the pile of shells was sealed with a layer of large, flattish stones (Carlyon 1982: 157) may also be indicative of a ritual for decommissioning the ditch (Thomas 2016: 119). The find setting of this shoe brooch could be interpreted as rural settlement, industrial or religious, hence its inclusion in 'other'.

7.7 How sandal fibulae were worn

Many Roman brooches were worn to fasten clothes together, a sort of antique safety pin (Dollfus 1975: 25; Croom 2018: 302–303). However, it is suggested that the shoe brooch was, like other plate brooch types, too delicate to hold heavy clothing and, therefore, was merely decorative (Riha 1979: 21; Hoss 2016: 36; Eckardt 2013: 217). Nevertheless, the grave-marker of Menimane in Mainz (CIL 13.07067) shows her wearing a pair of brooches pinned to her bodice, which is fastened with three more similar brooches down the front (Allason-Jones 1995: 23; Rothe 2009: 45; Croom 2018: 303). The *stela* of another young woman from Mainz (Harl and Harl 2019a) also shows small plate brooches fastening the neckline of her under tunic (Rothe 2009: 153). Croom suggests that sandal *fibulae* could have been used to fasten linen or light woollen clothing (2018: 303). It seems likely that some people wore shoe brooches as fasteners for light garments and others wore them just as ornaments. We cannot know for certain because of the lack of evidence (Riha 1979: 10).

It is widely thought that women wore multiple Roman brooches (Exner 1941: 46; Riha 1979: 42; Heeren 2014: 453; Croom 2018: 305), possibly due to their dress (Riha 1979: 42; Eckardt 2013: 217; Heeren 2014: 445). There is some evidence from burials of women wearing shoe brooches. The pair of sandal *fibulae* from Cerfontaine is said to come from a woman's tomb. The additional brooches and copper alloy hairpins from Cerfontaine tomb 6 may strengthen this argument (Breuer *et al.* 1952: 104). One might say the same for the assemblage of jewellery from Blicquy tomb 260 (de Laet *et al.* 1972: 117). Nierhaus claims that the brooch from Bad Cannstatt came from a girl's grave (1959: 82), but this is based on one brooch. We should exercise caution when identifying gender on the grounds of grave furniture alone (Philpott 1991: 132).

Many scholars also argue that brooches are not a reliable guide to the gender of the wearer. The sandal *fibula* from

Les Fontaines Salées was originally assumed to have been from the women's baths, as there were two sets of bath buildings and the brooch was part of an assemblage including hairpins, jewellery and toilet instruments (Louis 1943: 38 fig.11). However, the modern interpretation is that these were not separate baths, but that the earlier baths were extended (Rousseau 2004: 7), so the brooch may not have belonged to a woman. Riha says that we are insufficiently informed about which gender wore which types of brooch (1979: 41). Eckardt points out that it is impossible to attribute shoe brooches to either male or female costume (2013: 231). It is difficult to determine whether a particular gender wore a particular type of brooch (Allason-Jones 1995: 24). Of the 23 funerary sandal *fibulae*, only that from Cirencester was definitely found in a woman's tomb (McWhirr *et al.* 1982: Microfiche 1/5 A08 Table 4), so we should not conclude that sandal *fibulae* were worn exclusively by women.

The alignment in which shoe brooches were worn is another question which cannot be answered definitively. Unfortunately, where brooches have been found worn in graves, such as at Great Waldingfield (Ashmolean Museum 1927.350), the precise orientation of the brooches has not been recorded. Croom states that sandal *fibulae* were worn vertically with the toe at the top, and that the loop at the heel confirms this (2018: 303). The brooch engraved with Victory (Tache 2015: 46 no. 1032) seems to support this view, although the wearer may have preferred to look down and see the goddess the right way up for them, so the heel would have been at the top. There are, however, four sandal *fibulae* with inscriptions (three were discussed above; the other below in the apotropaic section). Presumably such brooches would have been worn horizontally so that the inscription could be read easily. A further problem with Croom's conclusion is the use of a heel-loop as confirmation, because not all shoe brooches have a heel-loop. Some duck and chicken brooches, for example one in the British Museum (no. 1866,1203.144), have loops under their tails. If Croom's logic were applied to these brooches, they would be worn with their beaks uppermost, which seems most unlikely. It seems more probable that sandal *fibulae* could be worn in any orientation the wearer preferred. It is worth remembering that foot-shaped artefacts can be used differently or viewed in different ways by different people (McIntosh 2011: 155).

Some Roman plate brooches were worn in pairs, sometimes joined together by a fine chain (Riha 1979: 42; Heeren 2014: 445). It is suggested that sandal *fibulae* could have been worn in pairs (Eckardt 2013: 217; Croom 2018: 303) but this is by no means certain. Very few pairs of sandal *fibulae* have been found, and those that have are mostly from Roman burials in present-day Belgium. One pair joined with a chain was found in grave 260 in Blicquy (de Laet *et al.* 1972: 117) and another pair in tomb 6 in Cerfontaine (Breuer *et al.* 1952: 105), although there is no mention of a chain in this instance. An exceptional brooch in the shape of a pair of soles joined together was auctioned online and may also constitute evidence for wearing pairs of sandal *fibulae*. A single brooch from Vertault, France, was found with a chain attached (Albert and Fauduet 1976: 218; Feugère 1985: 379 no. 56). This is sometimes cited as evidence of a pair of brooches (Albert and Fauduet 1976: 217–218) but we do not know what was on the other end of the chain. It may not have been another shoe brooch, since the attached chain has led to comparisons with amulets that could be suspended from a necklace (Albert and Fauduet 1976: 217).

Not all shoe brooches had loops at the heel, so could not have been fitted with chains. These may still have been worn in pairs, but it has also been suggested that they were worn singly (Coeuret 1981: 11). It may be that some pairs were divided like deposited shoes: the owner kept one as a reminder of a vow and left the other one (van Driel-Murray 1999a: 136). It seems, however, that some shoe brooches were worn in pairs and some were not.

7.8 Left or right

As has already been discussed, chirality is an important quality for Roman culture due to the right side being auspicious. Shoe brooches can represent left or right feet, but assessing which can be problematic. Croom (2018: 301) suggests that sandal *fibulae* might represent footprints, but they are generally thought to show the sole of a shoe (Riha 1979: 203; Feugère 1985: 377; Hattatt 1985: 172; Mackreth 2011: 179; Eckardt 2013: 217). It can therefore be difficult to tell whether a shoe brooch is left or right-footed because they are the wrong way up when viewed.

As an experiment to assess this difficulty, a picture of a sandal *fibula* from the British Museum (no. 1997.0701.1) was tweeted which, if viewed as a sole, is clearly a right foot because of the curve towards where the big toe would be (Figure 7.12). However, of the 51 comments received, 24 said right, 24 left, and three could not tell. Clearly, the process is confusing. There are even some instances where this study disagreed with Eckardt's identification of a brooch's chirality: for example, she interpreted the brooch from Alcester (2013: 222 no. 4) as right and this study as left (Figure 7.13); she identified two brooches

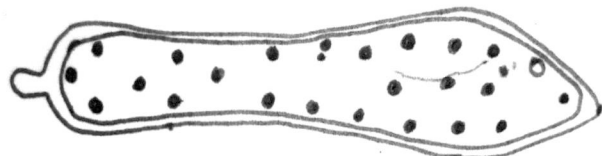

Figure 7.12: The tweeted sandal fibula.

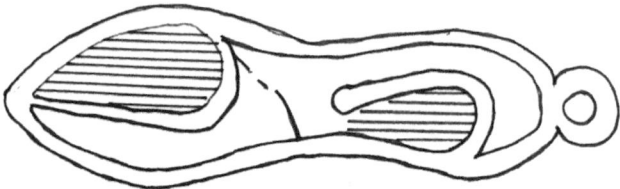

Figure 7.13: Type 4 shoe brooch from Alcester.

from Cirencester (2013: 222 nos.5 and 6) as left, and this study as right (Figure 7.14). In order to assess the less obvious chirality of shoe brooches, this study developed a technique of viewing an original picture next to a flipped image (Figure 7.14). By comparing the two configurations, it became much easier to ascertain which way looked correct. Nevertheless, the chirality of some brooches remains unidentifiable because they are symmetrical or too fragmentary. The difficulty of assigning chirality to shoe brooches may demonstrate that it was not important to the makers or the wearers.

This study's corpus contains 176 right feet, 188 left, while 82 are indeterminate, and one depicts a pair. This shows that, unlike Roman footlamps, there is no marked preference for left or right shoe brooches (Eckardt 2013: 221), which should not be surprising if they were worn in pairs. Even if one considers the chirality statistics for different site types, there is no significant preference (Figure 7.15).

7.9 Ornamentation

Most of the sandal *fibulae* in the corpus are copper alloy decorated with champlevé enamel, where the colour is contained by a raised metal rim. Some of the rims feature a twisted pattern that may represent stitching (Figure 7.16). Unfortunately, enamel sometimes falls out of its copper alloy frame: 89 brooches in the corpus are missing their enamel. Enamel can deteriorate in soil (Hattatt 1985: 29; Bateson 1981: 68; Bayley and Butcher 2004: 48–49) meaning that its original colour cannot be determined accurately (Bayley and Butcher 2004: 48–49). In 56 corpus brooches the original enamel colour is unclear, or not recorded.

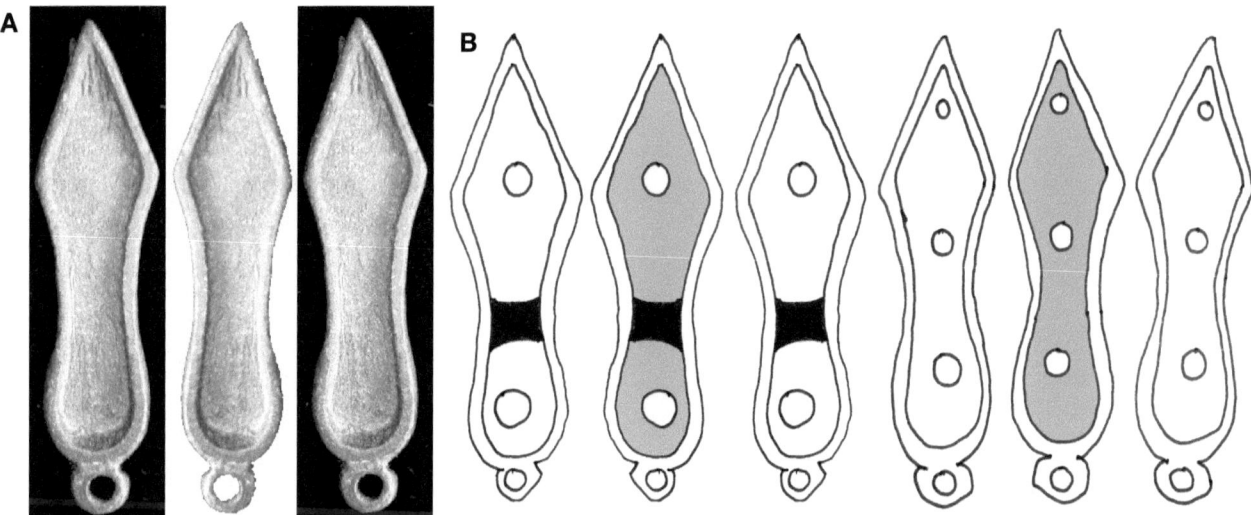

Figure 7.14: PAS LEIC-84F493 original and flipped identifiable as left sole; sketches of Cirencester brooches both identifiable as right soles (the flipped images are darker).

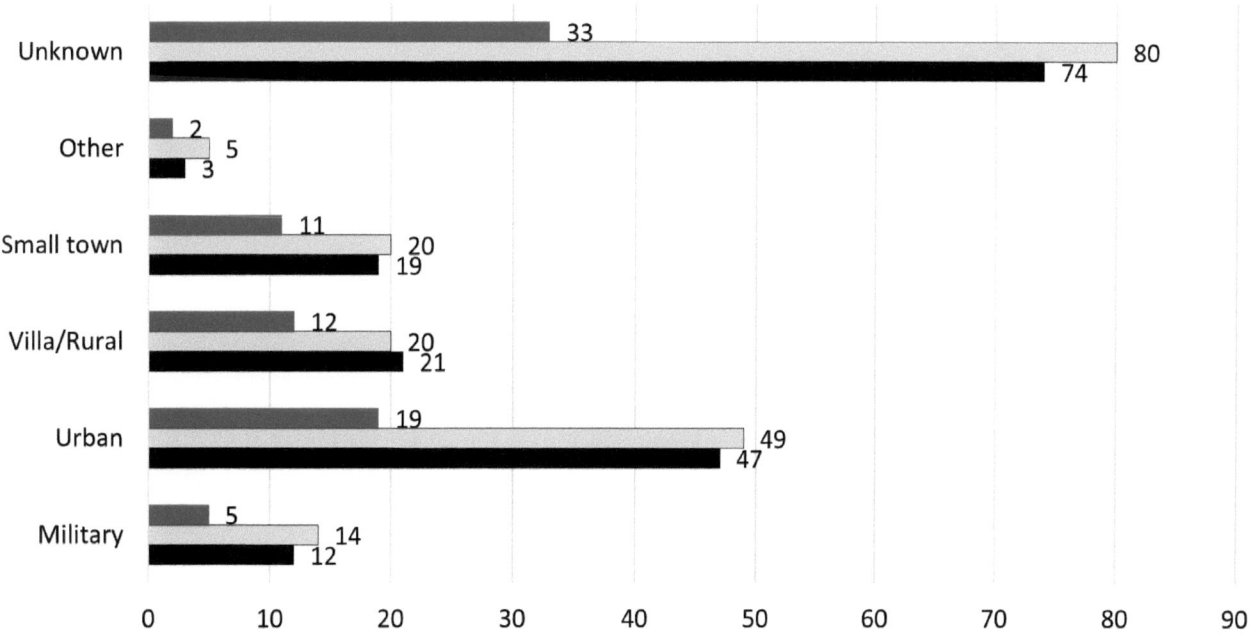

Figure 7.15: Chart to show the proportions of chirality in each site type for 447 Roman sandal fibulae.

The most common Roman-era enamel colour is blue (Bateson 1981: 68; Eckardt 2013: 217). This is true for the corpus overall (73 brooches: see Figure 7.17), but the proportions of enamel colour vary according to brooch type. Of the 261 type 1 brooches, 51 are orange and 34 green, while only 26 are blue, although that rises to 37 if the 11 turquoise brooches are included (Figure 7.18).

Among the 32 Type 2 brooches, the most common colour is red (10 examples) and just three are blue. The majority (36) of the 53 Type 3 brooches are blue, and three of the four Type 4 brooches are blue and red. Because these brooches are so similar, it seems likely that the fourth one was also red and blue, but the two enamel colours are now decayed (Mackreth 1994: 168). Four Type 6 brooches identified by the PAS as representing a type of slipper (FAKL-7D38E8 and NLM-CEF2A4), are also blue and red and, like the Type 4 brooches, were all found in Britain.

Earlier sandal *fibulae* tend not to be enamelled. They are sometimes tinned or silvered to make them look shiny,

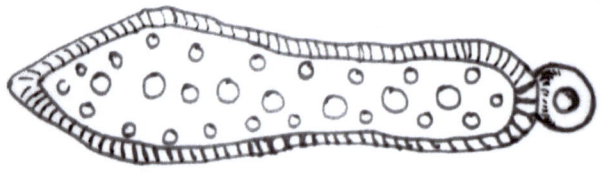

Figure 7.16: Shoe brooch from London showing twisted rim design. (Author's drawing).

and often have hobnailing patterns punched into the plate surface. One unenamelled sandal *fibula* is exceptional in its decoration, in that it is engraved with a figure of Victory. No find setting or location is available for this brooch (Tache 2015: 46; plate 116.1032), so its symbolism is difficult to read. It could be a prize, or perhaps had religious significance.

Some early shoe brooches are decorated using the Pressblech technique, where an embossed metal overlay is brazed to a copper alloy plate which has been deliberately scored to facilitate adhesion (Feugère and Lambert 2010: 163). Four examples are known. One, in the Historisches Museum, Basel, has a very worn, and therefore illegible, inscription (Riha 1979: 201 fig. 32b). It is, however, remarkably similar to an inscribed brooch from Laon, France (see Figure 7.3). Only the copper alloy plate of the third example remains (Tache 2015: 46 no. 1043). The final example is from Kilhallon, Cornwall. This still has a little of the overlay with signs of embossing, but not of an inscription (Butcher 1982: 162 fig.5.1).

Some shoe brooches are decorated with metal inlays and raised copper alloy blocks, which can be triangular or square. Five sandal *fibulae* in the sample illustrate this method, all of which are Type 6, 'irregular', because their soles are an unusual shape. Riha describes them as an oriental sandal type and the example from Augst has square, reddish hobnails (Riha 1979: 200 no. 1726). A brooch from the Martberg, Germany (Nickel 2011: 115

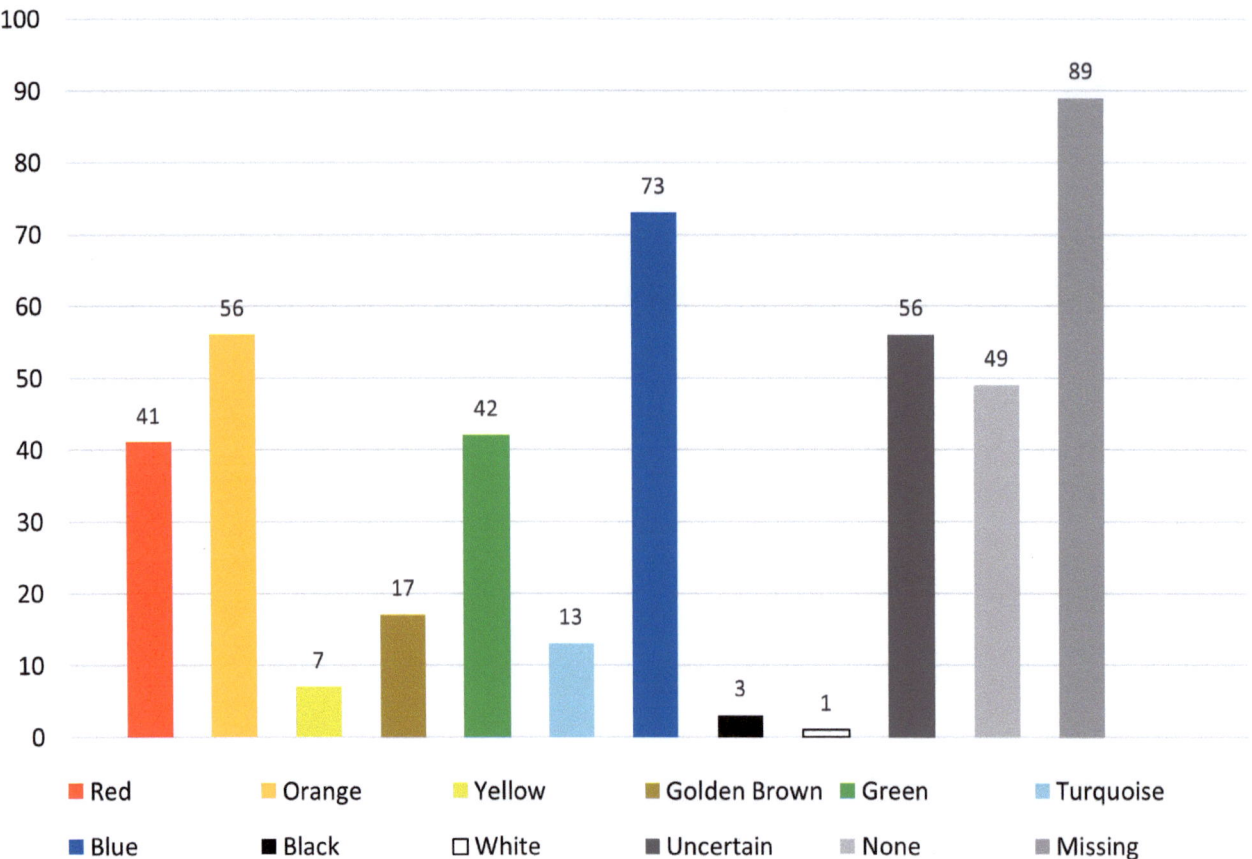

Figure 7.17: Chart to show the enamel colour of 421 Roman sandal fibulae.

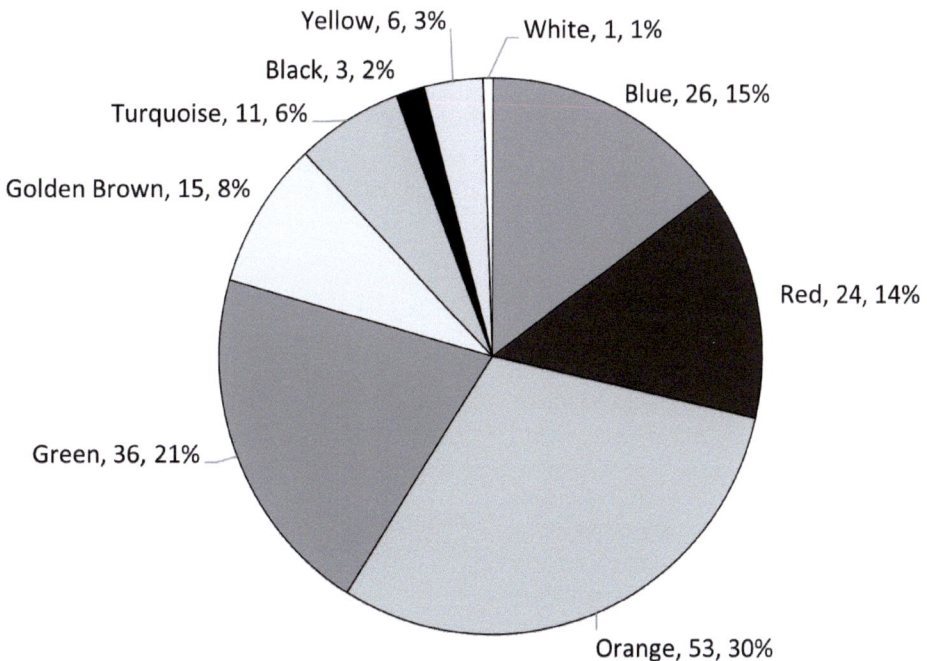

Figure 7.18: Chart to show the colour proportions for 247 Type 1 Roman sandal fibulae.

no. 21), has comparable hobnails, as do a gilt brooch from Carnuntum, Austria (Pollhammer 2019), and one with green nails from the Titelberg, Luxembourg (Gaspar 2007: 217).

A common decorative feature is a heel loop, possibly for attaching a chain, or a protrusion which may be deliberately unpierced, or poor copies of a brooch with a heel-loop, or simply unfinished. Some shoe brooches have neither. This ornamentation formed the basis of Feugère's sub-division of his type 28 (1985: 373). Scholarly opinion is divided on the relative proportions of sandal *fibulae* with heel-loops. Croom claims that 80% of Romano-British shoe brooches in good enough condition to be certain have them (2018: 303). Of Eckardt's 61 catalogued Romano-British sandal *fibulae*, 40 (or 66%) definitely have heel-loops, six (10%) have a protrusion and five (8%) are smooth (2013: 222–227). Of the 151 Romano-British shoe brooches in this study, 95 have loops (63%), compared with 43 that do not: 21 have a protrusion (14%) and 22 have neither (14%). The remaining nine brooches are fragments where the heel is missing. In the database as a whole, 225 (50%) shoe brooches have loops, 67 (15%) have a protrusion and 107 (24%) are smooth. There are 48 (11%) sandal *fibulae* where the information is not recorded or the brooch is too fragmentary to tell. The statistics in this study for heel-loops on Romano-British sandal *fibulae* are more in line with Eckardt's findings than with Croom's.

7.9.1 Hobnailing on sandal fibulae

The symbolic significance of hobnailing was discussed in detail in Chapter 3, where we learned that the designs followed trends and may have carried religious or apotropaic meanings. This section examines whether it is certain that the spotted decoration on sandal *fibulae* does represent hobnailing. It also considers why this Roman shoe-making technology might be depicted in enamel, a surface-decoration technique from the north-western provinces. The religious and amuletic properties of shoe brooches and their imitation of hobnailing are treated later in the chapter.

Many shoe brooches are decorated with spots produced by casting circular copper alloy studs that end level with the enamelled surface (Bayley and Butcher 2004: 213) or by inserting fine glass beads or canes of a contrasting colour into the enamel (Figure 7.19; Böhme 1972: 39; Riha 1979: 38; Hattatt 1985: 172; Bayley and Butcher 2004: 47). This technique can be seen on other types of enamelled Roman brooch (Böhme 1972:39; Croom 2018: 301) and, one might argue, may therefore not depict hobnailing. It is, however, the opinion of many scholars that the dots represent hobnails (Forrer 1942: 84; Böhme 1972:39; Ettlinger 1973: 127; Riha 1978: 203; Hattatt 1985: 172;

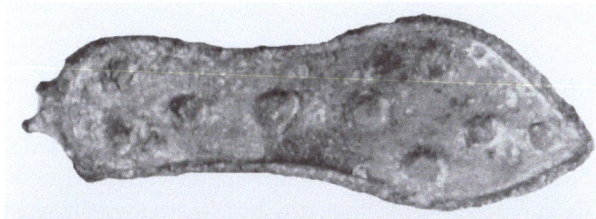

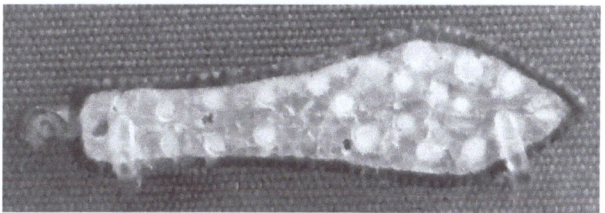

Figure 7.19: Different techniques for depicting hobnails (Photos: Sussex Archaeological Society and Author's own).

Deschler-Erb 2006: 441; Crummy 2007: 226; Mackreth 2011: 179; Eckardt 2013: 217; Hull forthcoming). Confirmatory evidence comes from many of the earlier, unenamelled shoe brooches which feature hobnailing designs (Figure 7.20), so the enamelled version is an adaptation and continuation of this type of decoration. Some of the frames around the enamelling have a punched design depicting hobnails (Figure 7.21). There are also sandal *fibulae* where the pattern of spots resembles actual hobnailing designs, especially circles under the ball of the foot (Figure 7.22). By contrast, Type 3 sandal *fibulae* tend to have a token number of spots, usually three or five (see Figure 7.14). The idea of hobnailing may be more important than the number of dots.

This decorative scheme is striking because, although hobnailing was one of the shoe-making technologies that made Roman footwear radically different from the footwear of Iron Age communities (van Driel-Murray 2016: 141), enamelling developed in the north-western provinces (Bateson 1981: 19; Bayley and Butcher 2004: 213), which is where the majority of sandal *fibulae* were found. Brooches from the Saalburg and Zugmantel were made locally with Roman materials, but according to Germanic traditions (van Driel-Murray 2009c: 817). Romano-British culture, as reflected in its jewellery, combined elements from the traditions of the local population and the Graeco-Roman world (Johns 2012: 23). Shoe brooches with their hobnailing patterns may therefore demonstrate a synthesis of technological ideas, a form created and developed on a Roman base, but in an original format (Feugère 2015: 703; Hoss 2015:144).

It is hard to categorise the fusion of Roman and regional manufacturing and decorative technologies demonstrated by these artefacts. If one factors in their geographical distribution, wearing sandal *fibulae* might show resistance in that they represent a strand of 'native art persisting under Roman rule' (Laing 1999: 90). On the other hand, the combination may express an acceptance of at least some 'Roman values' (Webster 2001: 217). A third possibility is that Roman hobnailing was fashionable (van Driel-Murray 1999a: 132) and shoe brooches provided another way of signalling modishness. One should also consider the apotropaic function of nailed Roman footwear represented by sandal *fibulae* as a reason for the synthesis of ideas.

7.10 The apotropaic qualities of shoe brooches

Amuletic jewellery, intended to offer the wearer some kind of protection, has always been widespread (Johns 2012: 5). This study has already discussed the talismanic qualities of

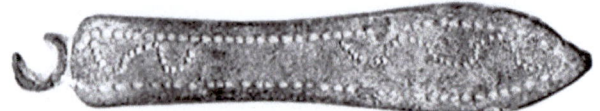

Figure 7.20: Un-enamelled shoe brooch with hobnailing design (Photo: Artefacts FIB-4169).

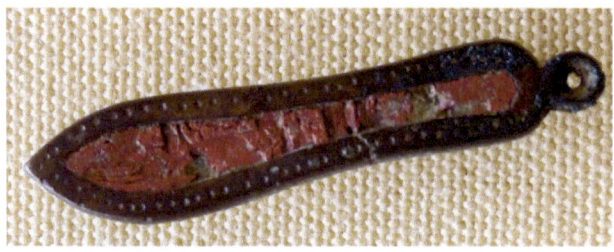

Figure 7.21: Shoe brooch with hobnailing around the rim (Photo: Author's own).

Roman foot- and shoe-shaped artefacts. Possibly because it represents footwear, or because of its hobnailing, or both, the Roman shoe brooch is considered an example of an apotropaic ornament (Nierhaus 1959: 35; Walke 1962: 217; Dollfus 1975: 209; Riha 1979: 42; Butcher 1982: 162; Carlyon 1982: 162; Puttock 2002: 83; Croom 2018: 306). Different scholars suggest various apotropaic functions for sandal *fibulae*. The most common use, as for footlamps and shoes deposited in graves, is as protection on a journey (Puttock 2002: 83; Johns 2012: 178; Eckardt 2013: 217; Croom 2018: 306). A shoe brooch from Saint-Germain, Aube is inscribed '*ave adianto*' (Feugère and Lambert 2010: 164), which could be interpreted as wishing well to a traveller. This may be an actual journey, or to ensure a 'safe and auspicious passage' through life (Eckardt 2013: 231; Croom 2018: 306). It could also be to ease the difficult journey into the Underworld (Walke 1962: 217; Puttock 2002: 83; Eckardt 2013: 231), particularly because the shoe brooch may be associated with Mercury, in his role of *psychopomp* (Crummy 2007: 227).

It has also been suggested that sandal *fibulae* were used in love magic (Nierhaus 1959: 49; Ettlinger 1973: 127) by analogy with the mediaeval and later Germanic custom of giving shoe-shaped drinking vessels as love tokens (Forrer 1942: 213). It is possible that a shoe brooch from Laon supports this argument: it is inscribed with the phrase '*ave vimpi*', being Latin for 'hello' and Gaulish for 'beautiful' (Feugère and Lambert 2010: 163). This wording is known on two further brooches, one from Cirencester and one from Reims (Feugère and Lambert 2010: 163), and other Roman brooches have inscriptions which are messages of

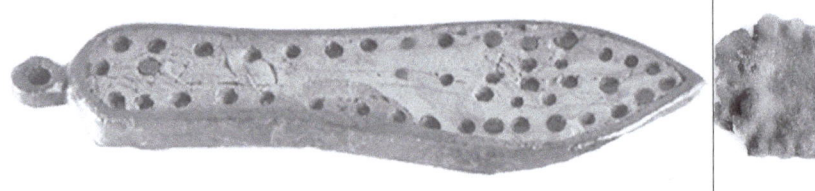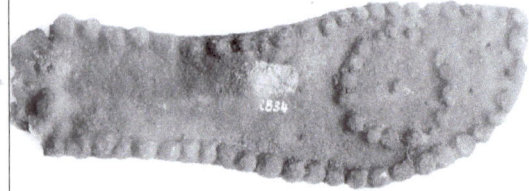

Figure 7.22: Shoe brooch from Sanxay compared with a real hobnailing pattern from Vindonissa (Photos: Author's own).

flirtation or love (Feugère and Lambert 2010: 161–162). The Laon shoe brooch may have been a love-token (Feugère and Lambert 2010: 164), likewise the other *fibulae* of this type. If sandal *fibulae* do represent footprints, and could therefore be seen as a physical reminder of the donor even in their absence (Croom 2018: 306).

Nevertheless, this study is sceptical about the use of sandal *fibulae* in love magic because the arguments appear to be projecting more recent traditions back onto the Roman era. The apotropaic function of shoe brooches to protect the wearer from bad luck, especially on a journey, whether that be actual or metaphorical, seems much more plausible because it echoes the symbolism of Roman footlamps and actual footwear deposited in burials.

7.11 Sandal fibulae in funerary settings

The deposition of Roman footwear in burials has already been discussed, and footlamps have been linked to this custom. Some authors suggest that brooches were common in early Roman imperial graves (Philpott 1991: 129; Jundi and Hill 1998: 129; Dollfus 1975: 19). This does, however, appear to vary according to region (Heeren 2014: 443; Callewaert 2014: 40). The number of brooches in graves declines over time, possibly because of changes in how garments were worn (Philpott 1991: 154; Rothe 2009: 37; Heeren 2014: 443). It is also thought that the inclusion of brooches as grave furniture may be more to do with being worn than with deliberate deposition (Philpott 1991: 141; Heeren 2014: 443).

Only 24 sandal *fibulae* are recorded from funerary settings, about ten percent of known find settings. This does not compare favourably with footlamps, where 42 percent come from funerary settings. However, their scarcity may emphasise the significance of their selection for burial (Crummy 2007: 228). As with footlamps, there are problems with the recording, and availability, of details for funerary shoe brooches. Like the finding of brooches, there are regional variations in the use of sandal *fibulae* in graves.

7.11.1 The data for funerary fibula finds

Very few Romano-British shoe brooches were found in burials. One from Great Waldingfield, Suffolk (Ashmolean Museum AN1927.350) is recorded as having been found on the breast of a skeleton (Eckardt 2013, 225, no. 36). Unfortunately, there are no further details of the exact position the brooch was found in, or the sex of the skeleton (Croom 2018: 305). A brooch from the London Eastern Cemetery was probably from a disturbed burial but redeposited in grave B341 (Barber and Bowsher 2000: 253), and there are no details for either deceased's gender. A third sandal *fibula* came from the Bath Gate Roman cemetery, Cirencester, in 1970. It was found in grave CS70.1 (Mackreth 1982: Microfiche 2/5 B03), which held the body of a woman aged between 35 and 50, who was buried with a coin in her mouth (McWhirr *et al.* 1982: Microfiche 1/5 A08 Table 4). The coin is illegible but is dated third to fourth century (Reece 1982: 129). Again, there are no details of the brooch's precise placement, but it is dated to the second century (Mackreth 1982: Microfiche 2/5 B03), making the burial later than the brooch. This suggests that the brooch could have been curated or that sandal *fibulae* may date to later than usually thought.

There is a distinct lack of recorded detail for most of the nine funerary sandal *fibulae* from France, which makes interpreting their symbolism problematic. Some French finds do have accompanying information, but it is often only partial. A Gallo-Roman cemetery discovered at Kergadec, near Combrit, included a sandal brooch, which was found with fragments of *terra sigillata*, part of a statuette in white clay and a coin of Antoninus Pius (Sanquer 1977: 354). There are, however, no particulars relating to the burial itself. Two different tombs in the Denon sand-quarry, Bavay, produced sandal *fibulae*, but no record survives of which of the five Bavay shoe brooches they were (Rorive 2019). One came from cremation burial 790, and was found with a small copper alloy bracelet, a copper alloy lenticular spatula, two copper alloy rings, some fragments of glass, a fragment of mirror, and a cattle-horn sawn along its length (Rorive 2019). The other was discovered in inhumation burial 815 together with four further *fibulae*: two enamelled disc brooches, a fish-shaped brooch, and an Ettlinger type 35 *fibula*. There were also three copper alloy rings, a ring with a glass intaglio, and a stamped *terra rubra* cup (Rorive 2019). Despite the detailed lists of grave furniture there are, again, no records of the deceased, although the bracelets, mirror and multiple brooches may suggest the latter two burials were female.

The remaining two French shoe brooches were found in much later burials. The Lavoye sandal *fibula* was found in tomb 139 of a Merovingian cemetery dating to the second half of the seventh century (Joffroy 1974: 44; 70; 94). It may have been curated as a valued antique, or dropped by an earlier occupant of the site and redeposited. The shoe brooch from Lusiau près Lizy came from the inhumation grave of a woman (Pilloy 1864: 213). Pilloy himself (1864: 214) identifies it as a possible strap-end, as it was found near another belt-fitting, but Feugère (1985: 379 no. 42) classifies it as a sandal *fibula*. Judging by the drawing (Pilloy 1864: plate A no. 13), the brooch appears to be of an early, unenamelled type, whereas the cemetery is described as Frankish (Pilloy 1864: 208). According to Pilloy (1864: 213), Roman finds are common in Merovingian graves so this brooch may also have been curated, a behaviour noted elsewhere (Thomas 2016: 111).

Seven of the catalogued funerary shoe brooches were found in Belgium, and four of these provide the evidence suggesting some sandal *fibulae* were worn in pairs. The pair from Blicquy was found in cremation tomb 260, which had been disturbed (de Laet *et al.* 1972: 117). Along with the sandal *fibulae* were found a sheep or goat's foot, interpreted as the remains of a funerary meal, the base of a vase, a disc brooch, a copper alloy ring, and a bracelet (de Laet *et al.* 1972: 117). The shoe brooches are of an early, unenamelled type dating to the late first century, but the tomb is dated to the late second century (de Laet *et al.* 1972: 117). This may be another instance of curation. No mention is made of the deceased's gender but the bracelet may hint at a female.

The other matching pair is from cremation grave VI, Cerfontaine. The deceased is identified as female (Breuer *et al.* 1952: 104) based on the grave furniture. The shoe brooches were found in an ovoid urn that also contained cremated bone, two nails, a copper alloy Hod Hill brooch, a pair of enamelled disc brooches, a coin (possibly of Domitian) and two copper alloy hairpins (Breuer *et al.* 1952: 104–105). In the tomb were also a fine ware dish and a vase, or drinking vessel (Breuer *et al.* 1952: 104–105), possibly for a funerary feast.

Other Belgian finds are not so well recorded. The shoe brooch found in Flavion is described as a curiosity (Marmol 1862: 34). The antiquarian report lists what was found in each grave, but only mentions *fibulae* and is not specific as to type, so it is not possible to determine from Marmol's catalogue in which grave the sandal *fibula* was found. Two further shoe brooches, one of them a fragment, were found in two different tombs in Strée. The complete brooch has no grave number, while the fragment is from tomb 69 (Ba*stelae*r 1877: 183). Tomb 69 also contained an urn, a jug, more broken pottery, glass and bronze, another brooch, some nails, and a medallion of Nero (Ba*stelae*r 1877: 67).

Some details of the German funerary shoe brooches are also missing. The brooch from Rottweil is said to have come from a burial, but there are no particulars (Planck 1975: 180). Like the shoe brooches from Lavoye and Lizy, the *fibula* from Zellhausen was found in a much later Merovingian or Carolingian cemetery (Weber 2016: 5), and may have been redeposited or included by accident, as there is evidence of a pre-existing Roman settlement on the site (Weber 2015: 7; 12).

However, the sandal *fibula* from cremation grave 72, Bad Cannstatt is well recorded. It was found with a jug, sherds of two *amphorae*, *terra sigillata*, a folded beaker, and a melted glass vessel. The tomb also contained three metal plates from a small wooden casket, and six iron nails, all of which were burnt, as was the sandal *fibula*, (Nierhaus 1959: 82), and were probably pyre goods. The deceased is assumed to be female due to the brooch and the small casket (Nierhaus 1959: 82).

The last two funerary shoe brooches were found in Switzerland. The Locarno *fibula* comes from cremation grave one, dating to the early second century (Guerra 2009: 170). It was found with three urns, a glass vessel, a beaker, a jug and a small bowl, an iron buckle, and some nails (Simonett 1941: 70). There is no indication of the deceased's gender, nor does Simonett attempt to speculate about it. The shoe brooch from Santa Maria in Calanca was found in grave three with four other brooches, one possible brooch, two finger-rings, and a glass bead (Rageth 1968: 11). There is no evidence of human remains (Rageth 1968: 11). Six brooches and a ring were found in what is interpreted as the area of the deceased's chest (Rageth 1968: 11; 7 fig.8), possibly showing where they were worn.

From the scant data available, it would appear that most of the sandal *fibulae* from funerary settings were either worn by the deceased as part of their clothing, or redeposited. Seven came from five cremation burials, hence it is impossible to tell where they were worn. However, only the brooch from Bad Cannstatt is recorded as being burnt, so the other shoe brooches in cremations were probably deposited separately. Sandal *fibulae* may have been chosen because they were the favourite brooches of the deceased, or were considered the most appropriate by the people arranging the funeral.

The lack of detail for burials becomes an issue when considering whether sandal *fibulae* were worn exclusively by women. Indeed, there is no solid evidence that shoe brooches are found exclusively in women's graves. So, if sandal *fibulae* were mostly worn, not deposited, in graves, and if they are not indicators of gender, what might they signify in funerary settings? Pudney (2011: 127) suggests that brooches may have been deliberately buried with the deceased as a way of officially ending their lives. Thomas also says that brooches in burials may have been points of remembrance or forgetting (2015: 119). This applies to brooches in general, rather than specifically to sandal *fibulae* in particular. The apotropaic qualities of footwear deposited in graves to provide protection on the journey to the Underworld make it likely that the inclusion of shoe brooches in burials lie in their amuletic function (Riha 1979: 42).

7.12 Shoe brooches and religion

Of the 155 Roman sandal *fibulae* from a known find setting, 50 from 25 sites have associations with temples, shrines or other votive deposits. This section discusses the sites where these brooches were found and what we can learn from them. It will consider which deities, if any, the brooches may symbolise and suggest that the apotropaic qualities of shoe brooches may have made them particularly appropriate as religious offerings.

Many of the religious sites from which the sandal *fibulae* come do not have a specific dedication, and may well be where several deities were worshipped. A shoe brooch from the sanctuary at Tremblois, Villiers-le-Duc provides one such example, as several statues were found there (Musée du Pays Châtillonnais 2019). All three sandal *fibulae* from the temple in the Forêt d'Halatte were found within the *cella* (Devillers 2000: 275). The dedication of the temple is unknown (Devillers 2000: 127), although some scholars suggest that one statue of a pregnant woman might be Isis (Devillers 2000: 127; 138), which would accord with the association of Isis and footlamps. Single shoe brooches were found in the eastern sanctuary of the Titelberg (Gaspar 2007: 218), and the Gallo-Roman temples at Viel-Évreux (Dollfus 1975: 209) and Margeride (Feugère 1985:

379). Again, the dedications of these religious sites are unknown. The sanctuary at Sanxay, near which a single sandal *fibula* was found, may have been dedicated to Apollo, although the reconstruction of the inscription is conjectural (Formigé 1948: 73). Five brooches were found in the Gallo-Roman religious site at Népellier, Nanteuil-sur-Aisne (Lambot 1983: 44). No dedication is mentioned for this site. However, many weapons such as swords and spear-heads were found on the sanctuary site (Lambot 1989: 35), so it might have been dedicated to Mars.

Other shoe brooches have links to Mars. Four come from *Fanum Martis*, a Roman settlement near Valenciennes. The town is named for its temple to Mars (Bersu and Unverzagt 1961: 162), whose exact location is unknown, and the brooches may have come from the baths thought to have been attached to the temple (Bersu and Unverzagt 1961: 182). One sandal *fibula* comes from Allonnes, Sarthe, which has a Gallo-Roman temple to Mars Mullo (Aubin 1981: 342). The sandal *fibulae* most definitely associated with Mars are the four found in the temple area of the Martberg (Nickel 2011: 117–118). The Gallo-Roman temple is dedicated to Mars (CIL 13.07661). Hobnailing on shoe brooches is often linked to that on military footwear (Deschler-Erb 2006: 441; Hoss 2015: 144; Heeren and van der Feijst 2017: 411). On the other hand, some scholars argue that, by the second century, when the shoe brooch was at its height, nailed footwear was no longer associated just with the military (Eckardt 2013: 221; Croom 2018: 302). The author's research (2017) has shown, however, that images of *caligae* continued in Roman art until the third century, so this would seem an appropriate offering to Mars.

There is also evidence for the association of shoe brooches with Mercury. Crummy suggests that footwear is a defining characteristic of Mercury (2007: 226) and that sandal *fibulae* are among his symbols (2007: 225). The argument is supported by Eckardt (2013: 221), but queried by Heeren and van der Feijst (2017: 411) and Croom (2018: 306). Sandal *fibulae* have been found near temple 10, Colchester, dedicated to Mercury (Crummy 2007: 227; Eckardt 2013:221) and in the *cella* of a temple to Mercury in Vindonissa (Lawrence and Deschler-Erb 2018: 184). A further shoe brooch was found in Berthouville (Display board, MAN, France) near the Gallo-Roman temple dedicated to Mercury Canetonensis (Babelon 1916: 38). A votive deposit from the Walbrook, London, included a sandal *fibula* and a *caduceus*, Mercury's staff (Crummy 2007: 227; Eckardt 2013: 221). The association with Mercury fits with the idea that shoe brooches afforded protection on a journey, especially to the Underworld, as he was both patron of travellers and psychopomp.

In addition to temple sites, some shoe brooches have been identified as votives, especially those from watery settings, like that from the Walbrook. A pit in property 3, part of the sacral landscape at Springhead, yielded a sandal *fibula* found with, among other items, two votive figurines of Fortuna, and a horse (Schuster 2011: 183). The *thermae* at Les Fontaines Salées formed part of a sanctuary complex dedicated to the deities of the springs (Rousseau 2004: 6). A shoe brooch found in one of the rooms surrounding the apodyterium (Louis 1943: 39) not in the temple, was probably lost rather than deposited.

Eckardt (2013: 28; 48) suggests that two brooches from Mildenhall may be fen-edge votives. The sanctuary of the source at Chamalières produced many *ex voto* objects (Vatin 1969: 104), a shoe brooch among them. A brooch from a ditch at Fontenay has been interpreted as part of a votive deposit, which also included a statuette of Venus, the burial of two young sheep, accompanied by a third burnt with a bowl (Daveau and Yvinec 2002: 132, 146). The authors suggest that the votive character of the ditch is related to its situation at the liminal corner of the enclosure (Daveau and Yvinec 2002: 146), thus requiring apotropaic protection. They also claim that the way the ditch was dug evokes ritual cavities containing offerings intended for the chthonian deities (Daveau and Yvinec 2002: 146), a category which would include Mercury. This ditch may be comparable with that excavated at Kilhallon (discussed above).

A shoe brooch from Wroxeter may also have been deposited ritually. It is known to have come from macellum portico pit F561 (Mackreth 2000: 155). These pits may have been for rubbish disposal or dug for another purpose and only used secondarily for waste (Ellis 2000: 344). Pit F561 also included glass vessels, pottery (Ellis 2000: 61) and a dog skeleton (Meddens 2000: 329), which may signal structured deposition (Merrifield 1987: 32: Morris 2008: 9). Malton Museum (2019) suggests that two shoe brooches might have been deposited as votive offerings at a shrine, although no reasons are given for this conclusion.

Votive deposition is also likely for two bent sandal *fibulae* from Ashwell and Meopham (Eckardt 2013: 221; Crummy 2007: 227). Not all votive shoe brooches are bent, and not all bent shoe brooches are from votive settings. It is recognised, however, that *ex votos* are often deliberately bent or broken in order to put them out of common use (Nickel 2011: 150). Of the brooches catalogued by this study, 25 are bent, of which five are from known religious settings. There are also ten brooches which may have been bent, and are now broken, two of them from the sanctuary at Népellier. It is therefore possible that the other bent or broken shoe brooches were used ritually.

The greatest concentration of sandal *fibulae* on a single Romano-British site is from Nornour, where nine were found (Butcher 2004: 10). There is some disagreement about the interpretation of the more than 300 brooches found there (Butcher 2004: 14). Hull suggests it is easier to believe the deposited brooches show manufacture than a votive deposit connected with a shrine (1968: 28). Subsequent excavations found no evidence of scrap metal, slag, enamel, or the high temperatures needed for making jewellery (Butcher 1977: 43–44). Fulford (1989: 249) argues that the large number of brooches was due to shipwreck based on the homogenous nature of the objects deposited on Nornour (1989: 248).

Reece (2011: 256), however, notes that the Roman coins from Nornour are 'unusual both in number and in unbroken sequence' and suggests frequent visitation over time by people from Roman Britain and Gaul. Mackreth (2011: 180) supports Fulford's interpretation, which was first mentioned, and immediately dismissed, by Butcher, who concludes that the 'strongest alternative possibility is that they were votive offerings at a shrine' (Butcher 1977: 44), particularly as they were accompanied by votive statues (Butcher 2004:17). While there is no structural evidence for a shrine on Nornour (Fulford 1989: 247; Butcher 1977: 44), there is wide acceptance of this interpretation (Crummy 2007: 227; Schuster 2011: 228; Thomas 2016: 121; Croom 2018: 303). Eckardt (2013:227) goes so far as to say that votive deposition at Nornour is certain. The shoe brooches may have been offered on Nornour as tokens for a successful voyage (Butcher 2004, 10; Croom 2018: 304). This is in keeping with the apotropaic qualities of shoe brooches as protection on a journey. However, care is needed with the assumption that representational brooches were chosen for their association, since most showed none, and it is probable that the brooches were simply personal offerings (Butcher 2004:10; Croom 2018: 306). Nevertheless, people had to travel long distances to reach Nornour, suggesting that the deposited shoe brooches were of personal significance, hence their choice as votives (Thomas 2016: 121).

7.12.1 Why were shoe brooches appropriate religious offerings?

Like actual footwear, some sandal *fibulae* appear to have been deposited as votives, particularly in watery places such as rivers or springs. In this context, they may have been chosen merely because they were precious objects, but they could also be substitutes for, or symbols of, footwear.

Shoe brooches may have been made as visible symbols of specific cults or gods, a kind of badge to show the owner's allegiance to a certain deity (Johns 1995: 104; Allason-Jones 2015: 71; Croom 2018: 305). The brooch engraved with the goddess Victory (Tache 2015: 46) may be one such brooch. There is some evidence that sandal *fibulae* may have been symbols of Mercury and Mars.

Some forms of Roman plate brooch, including sandal *fibulae*, may have been sold at religious sites as a sort of pilgrim souvenir (Johns 1995: 104; Allason-Jones 2015: 79; Eckardt 2013: 221). A shoe brooch was found in the accommodation for pilgrims to the sanctuary at Sanxay (Formigé 1948: 48). Such badges may have been taken away and worn, or deposited at the shrine (Johns 1995: 104; Allason-Jones 2015: 79), although this interpretation is influenced heavily by later Christian practice. The apotropaic association of shoe brooches with protection on a journey may have made them particularly appropriate for pilgrims.

7.13 Conclusions

This case study of 447 Roman sandal *fibulae* has shown that they were worn across the north-western provinces, but were rare compared with other kinds of Roman brooch. Jundi and Hill suggest that regional concentrations of particular types of brooch might correspond to political or tribal units (1998:129). However, the relative scarcity of shoe brooches and their widespread geographical distribution would tend to indicate that they were not used as emblems of local, group identities. We cannot regard them as definite indicators that the wearer was female (Eckardt 2013: 231), nor is it possible to say that all shoe brooches were worn in pairs. Their relative rarity may also rule them out as items of fashion.

It is likely that there was no single reason why people bought or wore sandal *fibulae* (Croom 2018: 307). Whether the brooch makers meant them to be purely decorative, or made them with a specific function in mind, it is probable that the wearers imbued them with their own symbolism (Croom 2018: 307). To some they may have just been amusing objects. Shoe brooches may have been used as badges for showing the owner's beliefs and, even if they were not made specifically for this purpose, their owners may have chosen to see them in that light (Croom 2018: 306). There is further evidence that they might, as Crummy (2007: 225) argues, have been connected with Mercury, and some indications of an association with Mars, possibly due to their military-style hobnailing. Sandal *fibulae* were certainly used as votive objects, but not necessarily because they were shoe brooches. The same may be said of sandal *fibulae* in funerary settings. Clearly their significance was different in some respects from that of Roman footlamps.

Nevertheless, like Roman footlamps, Roman shoe brooches seem to be a symbol for protection or warding off evil (Croom 2018: 306). Their apotropaic qualities, due in part to their hobnailing, may have made them amulets to ensure safety on a journey, particularly the journey through life (Eckardt 2013: 231; Croom 2018: 306) and possibly that into the Underworld (Walke 1962: 217; Puttock 2002: 83; Eckardt 2013: 231). Since there is no marked preference for left or right soles, the shoe motif may have been a strong enough talisman (Eckardt 2013: 231).

This case study has shown that the significances noted for other Roman foot-shaped artefacts also apply to sandal *fibulae*. These little brooches were considered appropriate as ritual objects, both for funerary and religious practices. They provide yet another example of Roman use of feet and footwear as apotropaic objects, and may symbolise a whole individual, whether human or divine. They also add to the evidence for the importance of Roman hobnailing.

What is important for this study is that the majority of shoe brooches come from the north-western provinces, while none are known from Italy, and only a handful were found in more southerly regions. Sandal *fibulae*, therefore, provide evidence that the social significance of representations of feet and footwear seen in earlier, more widespread case studies, is also valid for the north-western provinces of the Roman Empire.

8

The social significance of Roman footprints

Actual Roman footprints preserved in ceramic fabric, many of them with hobnails, and representations of footprints, occur across the Roman world. This chapter examines the social significance of these footprints. To help assess the meanings of human footprints on Roman ceramic building materials (CBM), the chapter begins by examining carved stone footprints, which have been found associated on both religious and secular sites. The chapter evaluates how far these *vestigia* can be said to represent the presence of a deity, a worshipper, or a pilgrim. The footprints may also be votive offerings to a deity in thanks for a service, or in fulfilment of a vow. A careful consideration of these *vestigia* and their inscriptions will help to further our understanding of Roman footprints. Roman stamp matrices or seals in *planta pedis* (footprint) form are reasonably common and can be found impressed into all kinds of goods. This section focuses on the use of footprints as signatures, as a kind of *pars pro toto* for the owner or user. It will also consider what religious and apotropaic meanings the footprint frame may have added to the seal or stamp by discussing the inscriptions and other symbols. Next the chapter considers the use of representations of footprints in the form of CBM stamped with *plantae pedis*, especially those of military origin. It considers why this design may have been chosen to sign pieces of CBM, and discusses the possible meanings of such makers' marks, including the footprint as a signature, as a sign of power and, possibly, as an apotropaic symbol, alongside the inclusion of hobnailing. Only then will human footprints in Roman CBM be considered. The chapter assesses whether they may have been made deliberately, to what extent they were part of the manufacturing process, and examines any votive or other significances they may have had for their makers.

8.1 Footprints carved in stone

One Roman representation of footprints that has been widely researched is those carved into stone, usually marble. Examples of these are found across the Roman Empire, especially in North Africa and Spain, but also within the north-western provinces. The footprints, *vestigia* in Latin, are found in temples and shrines, such as those attached to theatres and amphitheatres, and in secular contexts. They can be bare or wearing sandals, which may be a way to tell divine footprints from human (Dunbabin 1990: 91). This study assembled a corpus of 67 sets of carved Roman-era footprints. Some depict one foot, for example three in the Musée des Antiquités in Alexandria, all of which are bare right feet dedicated to Serapis (2020). Others show two feet, sometimes as a pair, like the sandalled feet from Fréjus (Lemoine *et al.* 2013: 44), but also with one footprint larger than the other, or with the feet pointing in opposite directions (Figure 8.1). Pairs can also have one foot further forward than the other, as if walking. Another variant of these plaques depicts two pairs of feet, often facing each other. Sometimes there are more than two pairs. The *vestigia* can point downwards, away from a temple, or upwards, towards a temple. Examples of this can be seen in four of the plaques from the theatre temple in Italica, which were found in situ. The meaning of the different orientations is debated. The plaques are mostly dedicated to Isis and Serapis, but dedications are also known to Caelestis, Nemesis, Bellona, Bona Dea, and Jupiter (Dunbabin 1990: 86).

Footprints as a part of religious iconography are not only known from Roman contexts. Pre-dating this era are

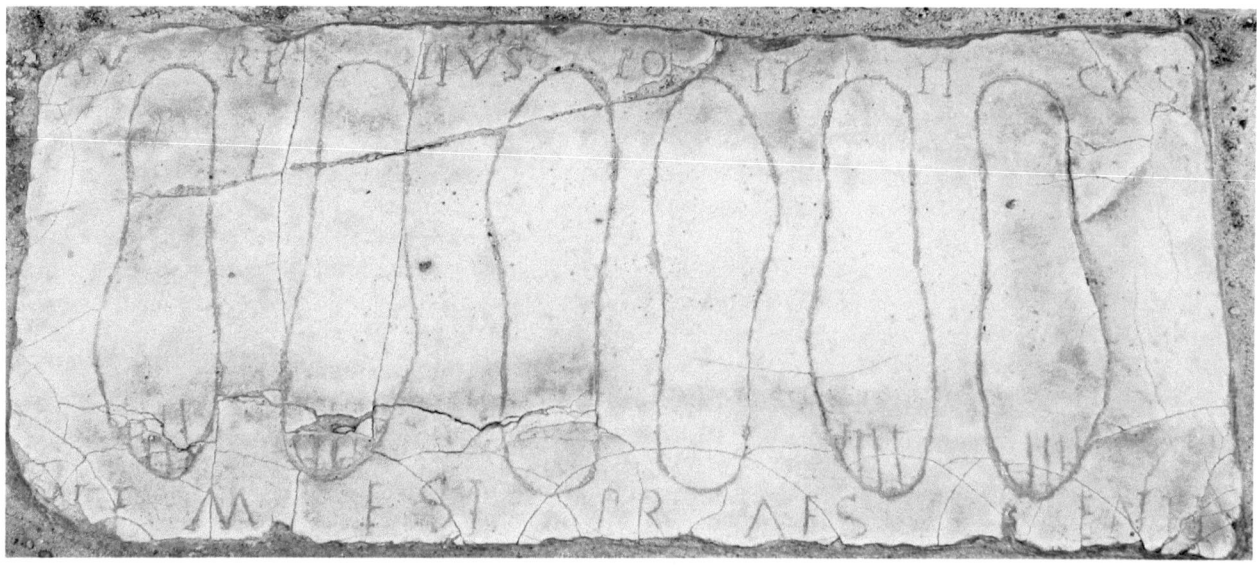

Figure 8.1: Replica plaque with vestigia, Italica, Spain. (Photo: Author's own).

footprints carved into ancient Egyptian temples, such as those at Karnak and Luxor (Castiglione 1970: 105–108). These date to the New Kingdom, 1550–1069 BCE (Revell 2016: 209). Footprints at the Syro-Hittite temple to Ishtar are from the mid-eighth century BCE (Takács 2007: 359). Footprints of the Buddha date from around the first century BCE (Thomas 2008: 310) and are hence roughly contemporary with Roman *vestigia*. The giant footprint on Sri Pada, or Adam's Peak, in Sri Lanka is claimed by several religions. It is said to be the footprint of Shiva by Hindus, of Buddha by Buddhists, of Adam by Moslems, and of Adam or of St. Thomas by Christians (Verhoeven 1956: 132).

The plaques in museums do not necessarily have a recorded provenance, but many, or at least copies, have been left in their original places. There is not enough room here to discuss all of the examples in the corpus. However, this section summarizes academic thinking about carved *vestigia*, examines in detail representations of footprints from present-day France, Germany and Spain, and discusses their significance as markers of presence and as ritual objects.

The variable orientation of the footprints has given rise to a wide discussion of their meaning. On many plaques footprints point in opposing directions, and this has been interpreted as a sign of pilgrimage (Guarducci 1943: 308; Galavaris 2006: 46; Takács 2007: 353; Agusta-Boularot *et al.* 2010: 114; Puccio 2010: 141; Caseau 2012: 121; Lemoine *et al.* 2013: 44). The orientation of the *vestigia* could represent coming or going, and the idea of making offerings for a safe passage, such as the copper alloy plaques from the summit of the St. Bernard pass, which give thanks to Jupiter for going and returning: '*pro itu et reditu*' (CIL 5.6873 and 6875). This votive process for the safe voyages of the emperors Tiberius and Caligula is described by Suetonius (*Tib*.38 and *Calig*.14.2).

Castiglione (1968a: 137; 1968b: 187), however, argues that the footprints do not represent pilgrims. This is because many of the inscriptions show that the plaques were dedicated by inhabitants of the city where the sanctuary stood, or even by priests of that particular temple (Castiglione 1968a: 128). He notes that no *pro itu et reditu* inscription is accompanied by *vestigia* (Castiglione 1968a:128). Instead, Castiglione (1968a: 136) suggests they may have had an apotropaic value, and also that the inverted footprints may depict a movement performed at the end of a ritual (Castiglione 1968b: 189).

Revell (2016: 209) agrees that the *vestigia* do not denote pilgrimage and also that they may relate to ritual practice (Revell 2016: 220). In addition, she suggests that, where one footprint is larger than another, it might symbolise mother and child, possibly Isis and her son, Horus, or Isis and her spiritual children, the worshippers (Revell 2016: 215). However, Revell (2016: 217) does comment that, due to the variability in footprint orientation, it is impossible to give a single interpretation for whom the *vestigia* represent.

Puccio (2010: 16) argues that, if the footprints embody the divinity *pars pro toto*, they also bear witness to the divine epiphany. Nor can it be ruled out that these offerings are *ex votos* in thanks for healing (Puccio 2010: 16). She sums up by describing footprints as either divine or human, with no definite rule to determine the outcome (Puccio 2010: 16).

Dunbabin (1990: 91) discusses a number of interpretations, including *ex votos* for healing, pilgrimage and safe travel, but concludes that the footprints represent the presence of the deity and/or the worshipper in a kind of synecdoche. Footprints that point upwards or towards a temple may commemorate the worshipper's presence in a sanctuary (Dunbabin 1990: 88), while those that point downwards could signify the epiphany, or appearance, of a deity, or their continued presence in the sanctuary (Dunbabin 1990: 96). Takács (2007: 356) also suggests that the footprints could denote the presence of a deity. This seems to be the case for the *vestigia* of Isis described in the second century CE by Apuleius (*Metamorphoses* 11.17; 11.23; 11.24).

Chiarini (2017: 158) interprets carved footprints as an indication of physical presence. She argues that feet were considered the most suitable body part for symbolising the presence of the whole person (Chiarini 2017: 158). Like Dunbabin, Chiarini (2017: 155) suggests that some *vestigia* symbolise the permanent presence of a deity within a sacred space. They also offer a lasting memory of the temporary passage of an individual, often the dedicant, in a given space (Chiarini 2017: 155). She points out that this need not be a sacred space, citing the example of footprints inscribed by *ephebes* (young men), along with their names, on the wall of the gymnasium of Cyzicus to memorialise their attendance there (Chiarini 2017: 158). Similar footprints from the same location were recorded by Worsley and Prowett (1824: 41 fig. 22: CIG 6845). The many footprints, some of which also contain names, inscribed in a later refashioned slab, also from Cyzicus, may be a further example of this (Liddel and Low 2019: 425). In these instances, the *vestigia* function as a kind of signature.

Despite the multiple possible readings of the *planta pedis* plaques, there is clear, scholarly agreement that the footprints represent the presence of a being. A detailed examination of some examples from modern France, Germany and Spain may help us to interpret their significance. A plaque from Les Aiguières, Fréjus, depicts a pair of carved feet wearing luxury sandals. There is no inscription, and the original orientation is unknown. It was found in the rubble of a Roman building whose use has not been identified. The style of sandals is commonly associated with bathing but, since no trace of hypocaust or plumbing has been found, a temple is suggested (Lemoine *et al.* 2013: 44). It is thought that, as the sandals are Egyptian in style, they may be the feet of Isis (Lemoine *et al.* 2013: 44).

Four *stelae* with carved pairs of footprints were found in an oppidum near Cadenet, Vaucluse, which is a sanctuary of indigenous origin transformed in Roman times (Lemoine *et al.* 2013: 44). One bears an inscription in Gallo-Greek, the reading of which is contested (Agusta-Boularot *et al.* 2010: 113). Lejeune suggests an epitaph (1985: 138–140), but it is uncertain whether the carving is of religious or funerary origin (Agusta-Boularot *et al.* 2010: 113). The other three *stelae* bear no inscription and all of the feet point upwards. They are dated to the end of the Iron Age (Agusta-Boularot *et al.* 2010: 113) but could also be early Roman (Guéry and Hallier 1990: 175). In the same area were found four dedications to a local deity called Dexiva (Agusta-Boularot *et al.* 2010: 116), so the *stelae* could also be religious offerings.

A similar *stela* was found immediately adjacent to the north-west corner of the mausoleum of Cucuron (Guéry and Hallier 1990: 173), seven kilometres from Cadenet (Gascou 1990: 199). It bears a pair of feet pointing upwards and is made from the same stone as one from Cadenet (Guéry and Hallier 1990: 173). This may be supporting evidence that the Cadenet stones have a funerary origin (Agusta-Boularot *et al.* 2010: 114). Both the *stela* and the first tomb appear to date to between the late first century BCE and the early first century CE (Guéry and Hallier 1990: 175).

A further funerary monument with *vestigia* that point downwards was found in this region, in Saint-Saturnin-lès-Apt, about 20km from Cadenet (Gascou 1990: 199).

This is pyramidal (Guéry and Hallier 1990: 173) and is inscribed ΟΥΑΛΙΚΙΣ / ΟΝΕΡΕΣΤ / ΑΙΟΥΝΙΑΙ, which Espérandieu (1900: 12) translates as 'Valicius to the daughter of Onerestaius', categorising it as an epitaph. Gascou (1990: 199) also suggests that the inscription could be a dedication to a local goddess. It was found in 1870 and there are no precise details for its find location. However, these three sites with early *planta pedis stelae* show that some representations of feet had a ritual significance in Gaul.

A pair of carved, bare footprints pointing upwards was found in Augsburg near Roman baths (Takács 2007: 367). There is a dedicatory inscription to Isis: *Fl(avius) / Eu/dia/ prac/tus // Isi/di / reg(inae) // ex / vo/to // s(olvit) l(ibens) m(erito)*; 'Flavius Eudiapractus gladly and deservedly fulfilled his vow to Isis the Queen, and put this up' (Takács 2007: 367). The reference to a vow may indicate thanks for healing, or another favour. The carvings have clear toes, indicating bare feet and the right foot includes a snake, possibly an *uraeus*, symbol of Isis (Takács 2007: 367). However, the footprints look different, so one may represent the dedicant and the other the deity. This is clearly a votive offering to Isis and, as the feet point upwards towards the goddess, they may represent the donor's presence in her sanctuary (Dunbabin 1990: 91).

Italica, Spain, has two sites where plaques with footprints have been found (see Figure 8.2). Fourteen are known to

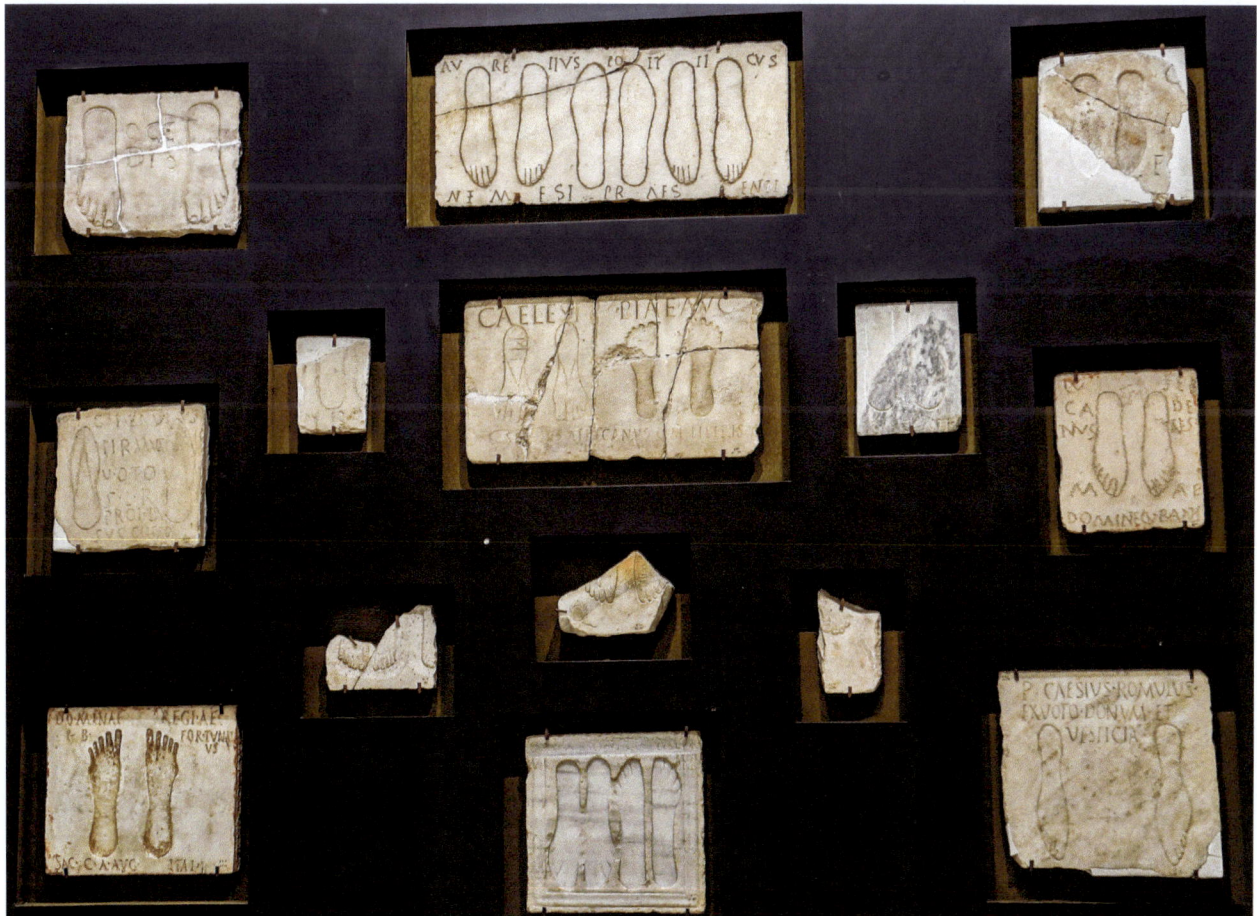

Figure 8.2: Vestigia plaques from Italica (Photo: Author's own).

come from the amphitheatre, from a shrine on the north side of the eastern entrance (Canto 1984: 183; Dunbabin 1990: 91; Revell 2016: 218). There is some debate as to whether the shrine was dedicated to a single, syncretic goddess, Nemesis-Caelestis (Canto 1984: 187), or to two individual deities (Revell 2016: 218) and, possibly, that there were two shrines (Revell 2016: 218). Three of the plaques are dedicated specifically to Nemesis, and one, which just has the word '*praesenti*' may have been to Nemesis, as another plaque dedicated to Nemesis has this form of wording (Canto 1984: 184). However, the epithet is also applied to Caelestis in two inscriptions from Rome (CIL 6.30789; CIL 6.37170) and one from Pozzuoli (Cordischi 1990: 190–191), so it could be dedicated to her. Only one Italica slab mentions Caelestis by name (Canto 1984: 184). It shows a pair of feet in sandals pointing downwards, presumably the goddess, and a bare pair pointing upwards, which may represent the dedicant, Caius Servilius Africanus.

Three fragmentary *stelae* bear no inscription, and three mention the name of the donor, but no deity (Canto 1984: 184–185). Since they were all found in a shrine, these plaques are clearly of religious import, and the inscriptions may help us to interpret the significance of the *vestigia*. One is dedicated *dominae regiae*, which is usually interpreted as 'to the queen of the skies' (Fernandez-Chicarro 1950: 623; Canto 1984: 185). This is usually taken to mean Juno, but could be Isis, or other goddesses (Fernandez-Chicarro 1950: 623). The inscriptions on the other two plaques present some problems in their interpretation.

The dedication on one is:

LV   FE
CA   DE
NVS   LES
M   AE
DOMINE OVRANI
    (Fernandez-Chicarro 1950: 622; Canto 1984: 185).

Between the groups of letters are a pair of bare feet pointing downwards. The problem lies in interpreting the last two lines of the inscription. *Domine* translates as 'lord' or 'master'. However, this has been read as *dominae* (Fernandez-Chicarro 1950: 622; Canto 1984: 185). *Ovrani* has been interpreted as *Ourani(ae)* and *C(aelestis) Urani(ae)* (Fernandez-Chicarro 1950: 622; Canto 1984: 185; Cordischi 1990: 168). *Caelestis* seems reasonable, as the plaque was found in a shrine to this deity. The *M AE* on the penultimate line could be *maestati*, 'majesty' (Fernandez-Chicarro 1950: 622). Canto suggests it should be read as *Domin[a]e Cur[atrici] ani / mae*, 'carer of the soul', based on a parallel inscription from Merida (1985: 146), so this may be a reference to Nemesis (Canto 1985: 146).

The final inscription from the Italica amphitheatre consists of two groups of three letters: QCC DIS. QCC may identify the dedicant as Q[uintus] C[laudius] C[?] (Fernandez-Chicarro 1950: 620; Canto 1984: 185). The DIS can be interpreted as *D[eo] I[nvicto] S[oli]*, a dedication to the sun god (Fernandez-Chicarro 1950: 620), or *D[eo] I[nvicto Mithrae] S[acrum]*, a dedication to Mithras (Fernandez-Chicarro 1950: 620). There is a mosaic footprint at the entrance to the Mithraeum of the *planta pedis* in Ostia (Dunbabin 1990: 93) and two devotees of Mithras in Rome are known to have dedicated a *planta pedis* plaque to Caelestis (CIL 6.80), so an offering to Mithras is possible. Canto suggests that the DIS should be interpreted as *D[eae] I[nvictae] S[acrum]*, arguing that the epithet '*invicta*' is well known for Nemesis, and that there is a painted inscription to *Deae Invictae Caelesti Nemesi* from Merida (1984: 185). The stone was found in a shrine to Caelestis and Nemesis, so this is plausible.

The other site in Italica with *planta pedis* plaques is the theatre, where six come from a shrine to Isis in the *portico* (Revell 2016: 216). Three plaques were found in situ, set into the shrine steps, and all depict single pairs of feet (Revell 2016: 217). They all commemorate the fulfilment of a vow and could, therefore, be healing *ex votos*. The two plaques where the feet point upwards are dedicated to Isis: ISIDE DOMINAE / MARCIA VOLUPTAS EX VOTO / ET IUSSU LIBENS ANIMO SOL[vit], and ISIDE / REGIN. / SOTER / VOTUM / S.L.A. (Corzo-Sánchez 1991: 133). The third, with downward-pointing feet, is dedicated DOMNULAE.BUBASTI / IUNIA CERASA / V.S.L.A. (Corzo-Sánchez 1991: 134). Bubastis is the equivalent of Bastet, daughter of Isis, and the diminutive, '*domnula*', may indicate her subordination to her mother (Revell 2016: 217). Another slab, not found in the steps, but in the general area, shows three feet, two pointing downwards and one upwards (Revell 2016: 217). Since the left-hand edge of this plaque is missing, it is possible that there were originally two pairs of feet (Corzo-Sánchez 1991: 134), although Puccio argues that the three footprints are left feet, and not pairs (2010: 15). Since the toes of one of the feet are broken off, its chirality cannot be verified. The plaque is inscribed DI. VI. PRIVATA. IMPERIO. IUNONIS / D.D. (Corzo-Sánchez 1991: 134). The full inscription would have been a dedication to Isis Victrix, made on the order of Juno (Corzo-Sánchez 1991: 135; Revell 2016: 217). Puccio suggests that the foot pointing upwards represents Privata herself, while the downward-facing feet signify Juno and Isis (2010: 15). The remaining two plaques from this site are small fragments that have no surviving inscription, but both show at least one pair of feet pointing downwards (Corzo-Sánchez 1991: 135–136), possibly representing the feet of the goddess (Dunbabin 1990: 91). These are likely to have been dedicated to Isis.

Two plaques with carved *vestigia* come from the temple to Isis in *Baelo Claudia* (Bolonia, Spain) (Revell 2016: 209). Like those from the theatre in Italica, they were found at the bottom of the temple steps (Revell 2016: 206). They both depict pairs of footprints, one slightly in front of the other implying walking, with the feet pointing away from the temple (Revell 2016: 209). The orientation of the footprints may represent the goddess walking out of the temple to greet worshippers (Puccio 2010: 16; Revell 2016: 209). Both plaques are dedicated to *Isis Domina* in fulfilment of a vow (Revell 2016: 209). The slabs were found covered over with mortar, possibly as part of an inauguration rite (Dunbabin 1990:88; Revell 2016: 210). It has also been suggested that they were taken down and covered when the worship of Isis ceased, or because of earthquake damage (Revell 2016: 210).

It is possible too that, as thresholds were regarded as liminal spaces that needed protection (Dunbabin 1990: 106; van Driel-Murray 1999a: 136), the placement of the footprints may have served an apotropaic purpose. Indeed, it is noticeable that many examples were placed near the entrances to sacred spaces. Additional evidence for a protective function comes from Rome. Two pairs of footprints, dedicated to Cybele and turned in opposite directions, were engraved in the marble threshold of the *Basilica Hilariana* (Castiglione 1968a: 128), immediately beyond a mosaic with apotropaic symbols and a prayer to the gods to favour those who enter (Dunbabin 1990: 101). Good and bad luck is associated with Nemesis (Canto 1984: 188), to whom there are *planta pedis* plaques in Italica. Castiglione suggests that the inversion of footprints may have performed an additional apotropaic role (1968a: 137).

Apotropaic plaques with *vestigia* were not necessarily placed at thresholds. Another carved footprint which may indicate an apotropaic function is in Ephesus, on Marmorstraße. It occurs with an ivy leaf, like those associated with Isis, and a bust of Fortuna (also associated with Isis), which all act as symbols of good luck (Dunbabin 1990: 105). Thus it is possible that the *vestigia* had a protective function in addition to their religious significance.

The interpretations of *vestigia* carved into stone plaques are many and varied (Dunbabin 1990: 85; Agusta-Boularot 2010: 114; Chiarini 2017: 147). They are found in religious, funerary and secular spaces, and it is not possible to assign one single meaning to all plaques. Indeed, one plaque, such as that dedicated to Isis by Marcia Voluptas (Figure 8.3), could be invested with multiple meanings (Chiarini 2017: 164). The donation is in fulfilment of a vow, so it could be a healing votive, or the vow could refer to something else. It is a sign of religious belief. It may show that the dedicant was a pilgrim to the shrine in the Italica theatre, or not. Its placement at the bottom of the steps could be apotropaic, as could the *vestigia* themselves, or represent the approach of the worshipper to the temple. The orientation of the footprints and their footwear, or lack of it, may alter the meaning. One plaque may, therefore, have many layers of meaning. It is, however, widely agreed that the footprints represent the presence of an individual, whether human or divine. The manifold possible significances of footprints carved into stone probably apply to other Roman representations of footprints.

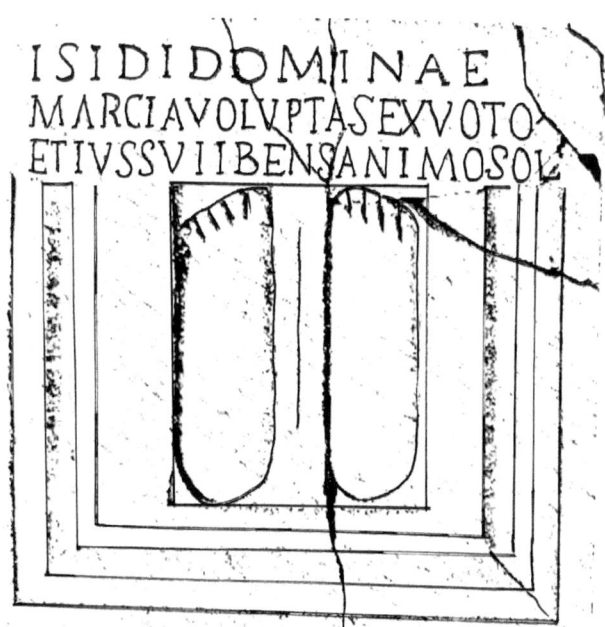

Figure 8.3: Plaque from the Italica theatre threshold dedicated by Marcia Voluptas to Isis.

8.2 Stamp matrices and seals in planta pedis

This section addresses the significances of *planta pedis* stamps. As with other representations of Roman footprints, a corpus was assembled. It catalogues 161 copper alloy stamp matrices, three in terracotta, and one gold, within a foot-shaped frame. One ceramic *planta pedis* stamp matrix, found in the Roman potteries at Holdeurn, near Nijmegen (Figure 8.4), is inscribed for the Tenth *Gemina* (Rijksmuseum van Oudheden Inv. no. e1944/1.76). It was not just CBM that was stamped with foot-shaped seals. Roman stamps and seals were used to mark bread, pottery of all sizes, and other things, linking images of footprints to ideas of ownership, and to signatures.

Stamp matrices vary in length (Rigato 2014: 212 note 44) from two centimetres to over ten, and usually have a handle or ring on the back. The seal end of the stamp can have an inscription, or symbols, or both. Ninety-two of the frames have the outline of a shoe sole, while 35 appear unshod, showing toes. More rarely, four represent whole, shod feet, where the sole of the foot has the inscription or symbols, and the ankle acts as the handle (for example, Figure 8.5). The footwear is uncertain for the remaining 34 stamps, either because it is not recorded or because the image is unclear.

Grünbart (2006: 19–20) divides Roman stamps into three major categories:

1. Those containing single words (the largest group) like αθανασια (immortality), δύναμις (power), ζωή (life), or ὑγια (health).
2. Some with more words, for example εισ θεοσ (one God), Θεού χάρις (God's grace), or καρποί Διός (fruits of Zeus).
3. Monograms or names.

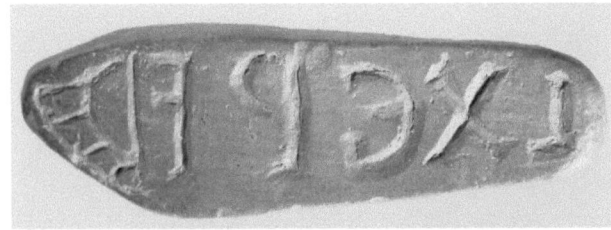

Figure 8.4: Ceramic planta pedis stamp matrix from Holdeurn (Photo: Rijksmuseum van Oudheden).

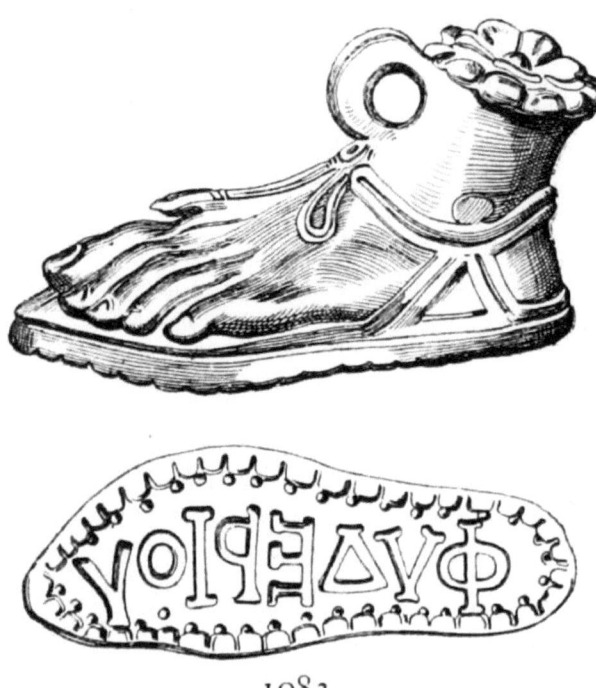

Figure 8.5: Potter's stamp in the shape of a complete foot (Babelon and Blanchet 1895 no. 1083).

To this list could be added a further category: stamps which bear no inscription, only symbols.

Stamp matrices in *planta pedis* form are not rare, but most are unpublished, being antiquarian finds dispersed in museums or private collections (Galavaris 2006: 43). The common use of *planta pedis* stamps is attested by their appearance on Roman pottery. Balestra and Gerri (2011: 120) give some idea of the relative statistics: of the copper alloy stamp matrices from Aquileia, 97 are in a rectangular cartouche and 68 in *planta pedis*. Among the 490 lamps stamped with makers' marks catalogued by Bailey in volumes two and three of his *Catalogue of the lamps in the British Museum*, 198 (40.4%) have *planta pedis* stamps. Such stamps on pottery and lamps may have had the quotidian function of recording which potter had made which pieces, thus providing a means for calculating output and for distinguishing the products of individual workshops in a jointly used kiln (Polak 2000: 42). Being stamped with a certain sign or inscription may have placed everyday objects under the protection of a deity (Caseau 2012: 115) and, as allusions to divine foot-prints (Caseau 2012: 121), foot-shaped frames may add a further level of protection. Alternatively, the additional apotropaic effect may come from the metaphorical protection afforded by the symbol of a shoe (van Driel-Murray 1999a: 131).

Stamp matrices are difficult to date with precision, unless found in a specific archaeological context (Caseau 2012: 117). No definite date is available for 105 stamps (64%) in this study's corpus. Indeed, quite a lot of information is lacking for the majority, which are antiquarian finds, although the inscriptions are documented. Of those with a rough date, one is from the second century BCE, 16 are first century CE, 12 second century, six third, seven fourth, and the remaining 18 from the fifth century.

The statistics for the site types are also affected by the lack of publishing or good recording: 134 out of the 165 (81%) are from an unknown setting. Of the remaining stamps, 29 are from an urban location and two from military sites. This study found no stamps that are known to have come from a rural or villa site, but this does not mean that none did. In addition, one came from a grave, one from a ritual site, and one from the Roman potteries at Holdeurn. The latter is a ceramic stamp and is inscribed, like many of the military foot-stamped CBM, for the Tenth *Gemina*, some of which have also been found at this site.

Inscriptions may bring insight into the significance of the *planta pedis* stamps (Figure 8.6). One is as a signature (Castiglione 1968a: 130–131). This could be a mark of ownership or a maker's mark. The number of names on a stamp might be an indication of status, and therefore ownership or manufacturer. Of the 165 stamps, 27 are inscribed with a *tria nomina*, indicating Roman citizenship (for example, Figure 8.7). These may be the owners of, or merchants in, the items stamped. A further 65 feature names of some description. These may have belonged to, or been used by, slaves (Buonopane 2104: 146) or could have been abbreviations for the sake of convenience (Buonopane 2104: 147).

The other inscriptions on *planta pedis* stamps provide evidence of their further significance. Some of the stamps in the corpus have inscriptions to do with life and health. Seven are inscribed VIVAS (Figure 8.8), two VIVATIS (Figure 8.9) and four with a name followed by VIVAS. Poggi suggests that a stamp from the Roman port at Vada Volaterrana, which is inscribed *PAVLE* should be interpreted as being followed by *VIVAS* because the name is in the vocative case (1876: 60). These stamps wish for life. Three stamps are inscribed ZOH YΓIA and one YΓIA ZOH, wishing life and health (Figure 8.10). Grünbart lists this phrase with quotations from the Bible (2006: 19–20). Elbern (1979: 628) thinks it has more to do with Roman cults other than Christianity. The phrase may have been adopted into Christian culture (Perdrizet 1914: 271; Galavaris 2006: 44; Caseau 2012: 120). There is also a stamp inscribed SALVS. Healing powers can be linked to the feet of Serapis (Dunbabin 1990: 88; Galavaris 2006: 44) and Isis (Caseau 2012: 122). These stamps may therefore have been thought doubly protective of the life

The social significance of Roman footprints

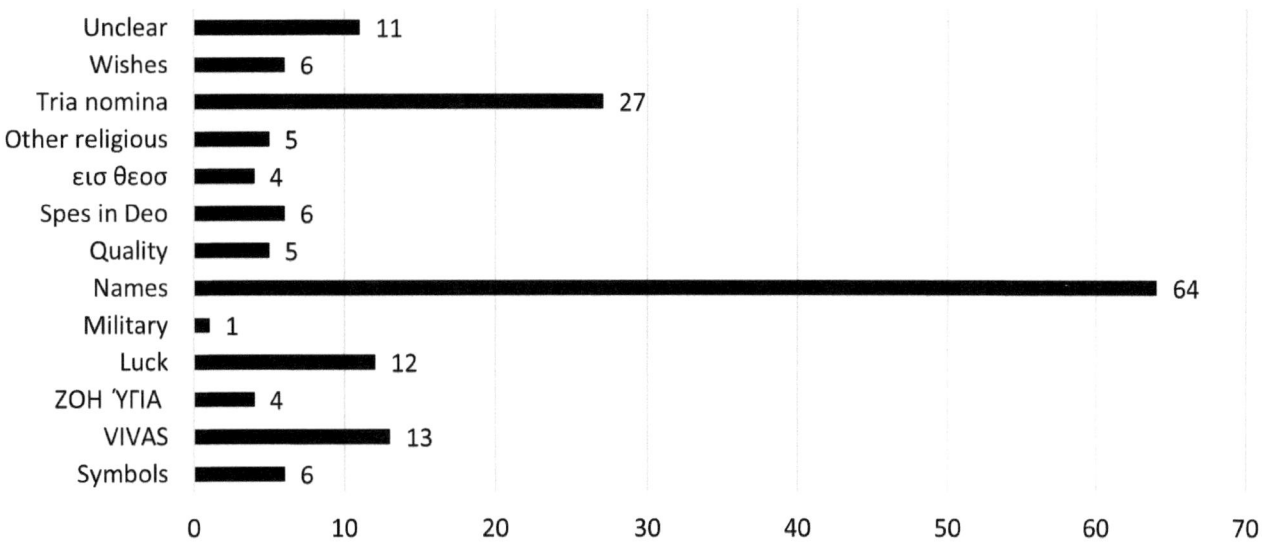

Figure 8.6: Chart to show the types of inscription on 165 Roman planta pedis stamps.

and health of the user and the purchaser of the marked produce.

Further stamps have religious inscriptions. Six read *spes in deo* (Figure 8.11), and one *in deo* (Ashmolean Museum, Inv. No. ANFortnum.FR.322). These are likely to be Christian formulae (Galavaris 2006: 43). However, the five inscribed εισ θεοσ (one god) do not necessarily refer to the Judeo-Christian deity (Figure 8.12), but may also be linked to Serapis (Galavaris 2006: 42; Caseau 2012: 127). A commonly seen extended inscription reads 'εισ θεοσ ὁ νικων κακά' (One god the victor against evil) (Caseau 2012: 127). It has been found on pendants bearing a picture of a rider (Bonner 1950: 46; Caseau 2012: 125). As such, the inscription could be regarded as apotropaic (Caseau 2012: 127), and even more so on a foot-shaped stamp.

Religious symbols feature on some stamps. Three bear a Christogram (Figure 8.13), one of which appears with the word *VIVAS* (see Figure 8.8), and four have crosses (Figure 8.14), which indicate Christianity. These stamps may therefore be of later date. Not all of the religious symbols are Christian. Two of the stamps in the corpus are Jewish, inscribed in Hebrew: both feature the word 'shalom' and one is a full foot with a menorah carved into the ankle (Friedenberg 1994: 18).

One stamp has a *caduceus* and wings, emblems of Mercury associated with other Roman representations of feet from funerary and religious settings.[1] As patron of commerce (Vikan and Nesbitt 1980: 27), Mercury is an appropriate deity to feature on a stamp matrix. Two feature ivy leaves, which are used as punctuation, but are also symbols of Isis. One of these stamps (Figure 8.15) may have belonged to a priest because of the inscribed name (Buora and Lafli 2014: 420).

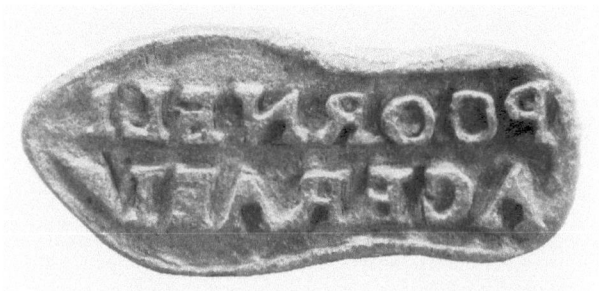

Figure 8.7: Stamp matrix from Venice, Italy, inscribed P CORNELI ACERAEL (Photo: Feugère Artefacts SIG-4018).

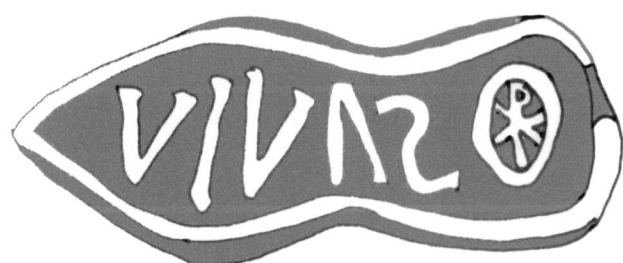

Figure 8.8: Stamp matrix inscribed VIVAS: Staatliche Museen zu Berlin, Inv. No. Misc. 3716.

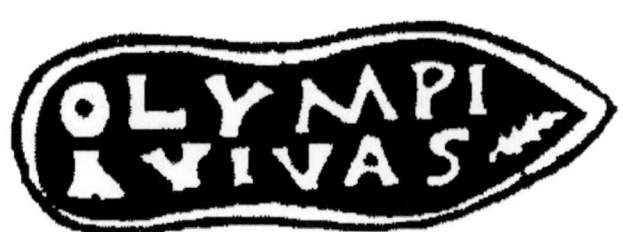

Figure 8.9: Stamp matrix inscribed OLYMPIA VIVAS (Poggi 1876; Pl. 7 no. 106).

---

[1] These are discussed in detail in the chapters on Roman footlamps and Sandal *fibulae*.

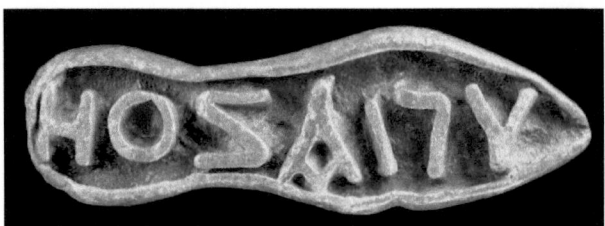

Figure 8.10: Stamp matrix inscribed ΎΓΙΑ ΖΟΗ (Photo: Staatliche Museen zu Berlin).

Figure 8.11: Stamp matrix inscribed SPES IN DEO (Photo: Staatliche Museen zu Berlin, Inv. No. Fr. 1332a).

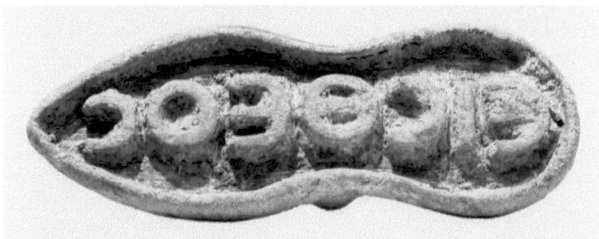

Figure 8.12: Stamp matrix inscribed εισ θεοσ (Photo: Lafli Artefacts SIG-4006).

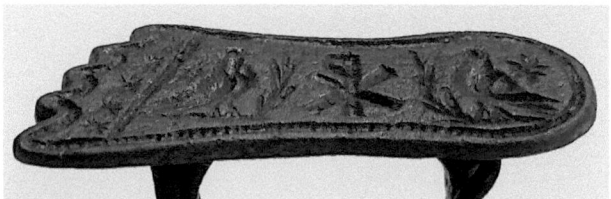

Figure 8.13: Stamp matrix with a Christogram, National Archaeological Museum, Madrid (Photo: Author's own).

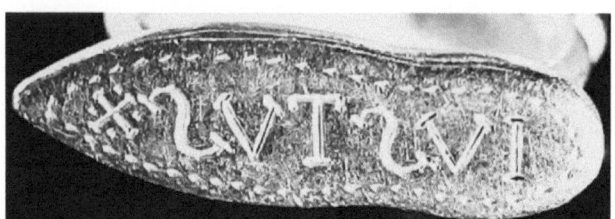

Figure 8.14: Stamp matrix featuring a cross (Photo: Timetravelrome).

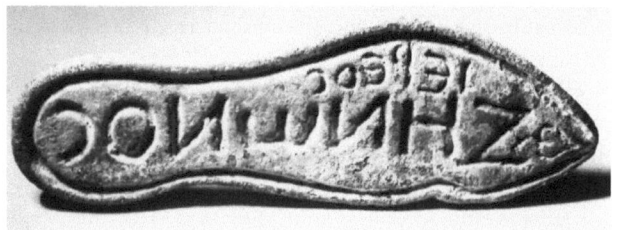

Figure 8.15: Stamp matrix with an ivy leaf at the toe (Photo: Staatliche Museen zu Berlin Inv. No. Misc. 7858).

In addition to the use of stamps as signatures and religious emblems, twelve of the foot-shaped stamps feature an inscription wishing good luck. In this study's catalogue, one is inscribed EYTYXI, ancient Greek for good luck (Grünbart 2006: 22), and two wish for the good luck of Loukis: ευτυχισ λουκισ (CIL 13.10024.305; Ridder 2013: 209). Two stamps in the corpus are inscribed αγάθωνεσ which can be translated as good fortune (van den Hoek et al. 2015: 312). One wishes for the luck of Aurelius: *AVREL / FELICI* (Rigato 2014: 207), and one features the word '*felix*' (CIL 11.6712.182), which may be a name, but is also Latin for auspicious. A whole foot stamp from Pollenzo is inscribed *VTERE FELIX* (Figure 8.16), a common inscription meaning 'use with luck' (Buora and Lafli 2014: 418) and a stamp from Arezzo is inscribed *VT FEL*, an abbreviated form. This formula is also widely used on other small metal objects, such as rings, fibulae, belt mounts, spoons and drinking vessels (Hoss 2015: 143). Three further stamps (CIL 13.1022.295; 15.8575; 11.6712.498) begin *VTER* followed by a letter which may be E or I, or possibly a corrupted F. If the latter is correct, these are also abbreviated *VTERE FELIX* inscriptions. Even if not, it seems likely that the *VTERE* stamps are an abbreviated form of *VTERE FELIX*. *VTERE* stamp matrices are an abbreviated form of *VTERE FELIX*. This group of inscriptions is of apotropaic import, and possibly doubly lucky, because of the amuletic significance of feet to the Romans.

Chirality may also give some indication of the apotropaic significance of Roman *planta pedis* stamps. As already mentioned, the Romans regarded the right foot as particularly auspicious. In the case of the 164 stamps in the corpus, there are four pairs, 38 left feet, 87 right feet, and 35 where it is impossible to tell, usually because there is no image of the stamp and the chirality has not been recorded. The majority (53%) of the stamps do, indeed, depict right feet. Of the twelve foot-shaped stamps which have an apotropaic inscription, the chirality of four is uncertain because no images are available, two represent left feet, and six are right feet.

Roman stamps in the shape of feet and footprints, therefore, have several significances. Firstly, as signatures, where the foot or footprint may stand as *pars pro toto* for the person, impressing their identity. Ideas of ownership and power are associated with feet. Secondly, as religious emblems, either to show a particular religious affiliation, or to invoke a deity's protection, or both. Thirdly, an apotropaic function, protecting property, life and health, or wishing for good luck. These meanings can also be seen in representations of footprints in marble plaques.

8.3 Official *planta pedis* stamps in CBM

Additional evidence for the significance of footprints in CBM might be found in tiles stamped in *planta pedis*.

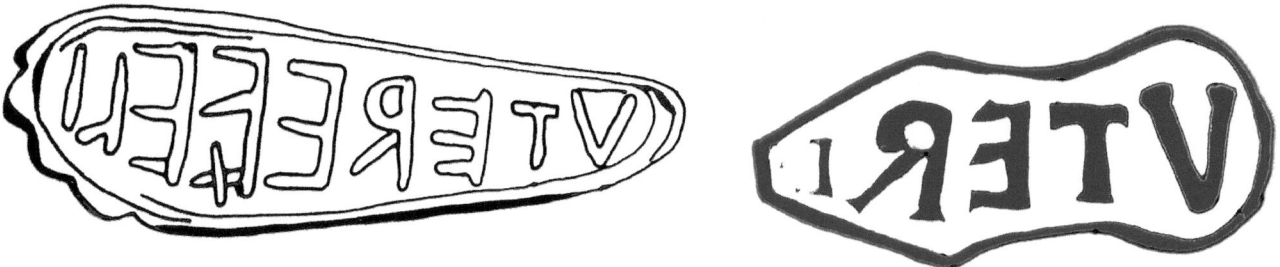

Figure 8.16: VTERE FELIX stamps: Pollenzo (after Ricci 1898); in the Louvre (after Ridder 1913: no. 4052).

These do not appear to be widely recorded, so the data were perhaps not collected systematically and the corpus is not exhaustive. However, details of 153 examples are examples of military Roman CBM with footprint stamps have been catalogued.

The chirality of the *planta pedis* tile stamps is mostly unrecorded, so this has been largely judged from the images. Eleven are indeterminate because the footprint is incomplete, 62 represent left feet, and 80 are right feet. This shows a preference for right feet, which is more in line with Roman superstitions regarding the good luck associated with the right foot than actual footprints in CBM.

Two stamps, which come from the so-called Villa of Titus, are not actually military. They are inscribed CERDO VOLUM L S F for the owner of the property, Lucius Volumnus, and his slave, Cerdo, who was probably the overseer of a tile factory (McCallum et al. 2019: 12). Among the 151 military examples, one has no legible inscription, two are inscribed for the second legion, three for the 14th, three for the eighth and 142 LEGXGPF (LEGIO X GEMINA PIA FIDELIS) or a version thereof for the Tenth *Gemina* (Figure 8.17).

This much larger number shows that planta pedis CBM stamps were important to the Tenth *Gemina* and tiles such stamps have been found where the legion was stationed.

This study has examples from Carnuntum (Petronell), Noviomagus (Nijmegen), Aquincum (Budapest), Vindobona (Vienna), Ala Nova (Schwechat) and Mušov. It is said to be difficult to date the stamps, because the same shapes have often appeared at different times (Janek 2014: 16). Nevertheless, the first appearance in the legion's title of 'Pia Fidelis Domitiana' (Gómez-Pantoja 2000:185), represented by a D, came after Saturninus' revolt against the emperor was quashed in 89 CE. The D disappears from the tile stamps after 96 CE, when Domitian was assassinated and subjected to *damnatio memoriae*. Since none of the stamped CBM in this study features a D, they must be later than that.

The symbol on the shields of the Tenth legion was a bull (Gómez-Pantoja 2000: 172), so the foot stamps may have had a significance other than being a legionary symbol, or were adopted as an 'unofficial' symbol. It might be possible to assess the significance of the military *planta pedis* stamps by considering the ornamentation (Figure 8.18). Of those catalogued by this study, 32 have hobnail representations. The nails may symbolise the army, as soldiers' shoes were heavily nailed (Gansser-Burckhardt 1942: 59; Busch 1965: 172; Rhodes 1980: 107; Keily 2000: 2), and also add to the symbolism of power and authority (Brodribb 1987: 117) as feet and shoes were linked to Roman ideas of domination (Dio Cassius 50.24.3 and 52.34.8; SHA.*Max*.28; SHA.*Prob*.20). This idea is illustrated by Roman statues showing an armed emperor in elaborate boots with his foot on, or

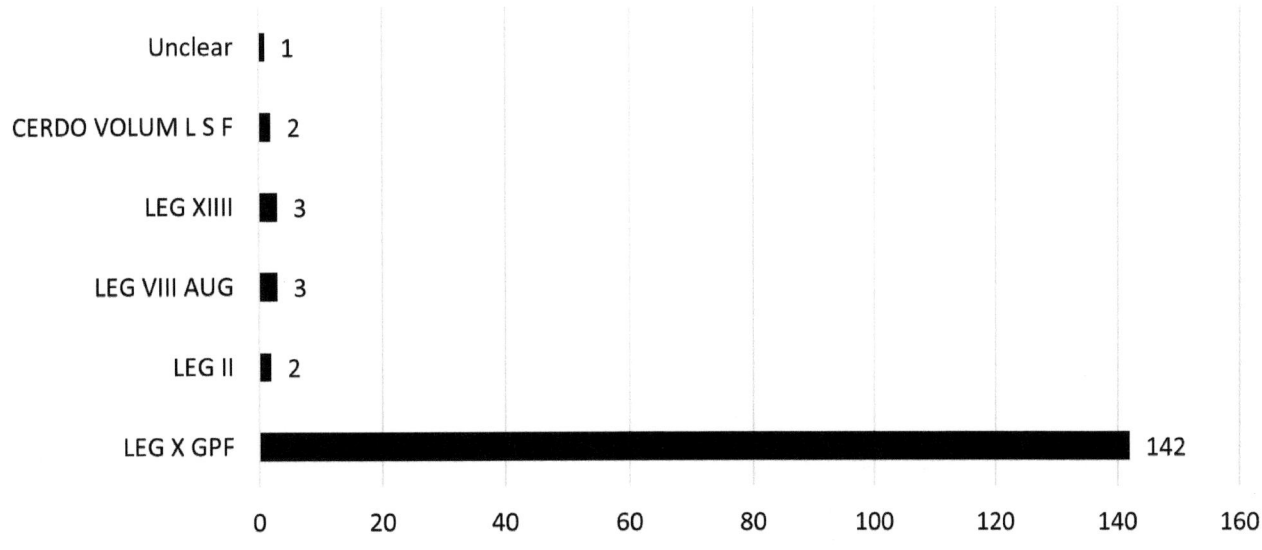

Figure 8.17: Chart to show the frequency of inscriptions on 153 pieces of Roman foot-stamped CBM.

Roman Feet and Shoes

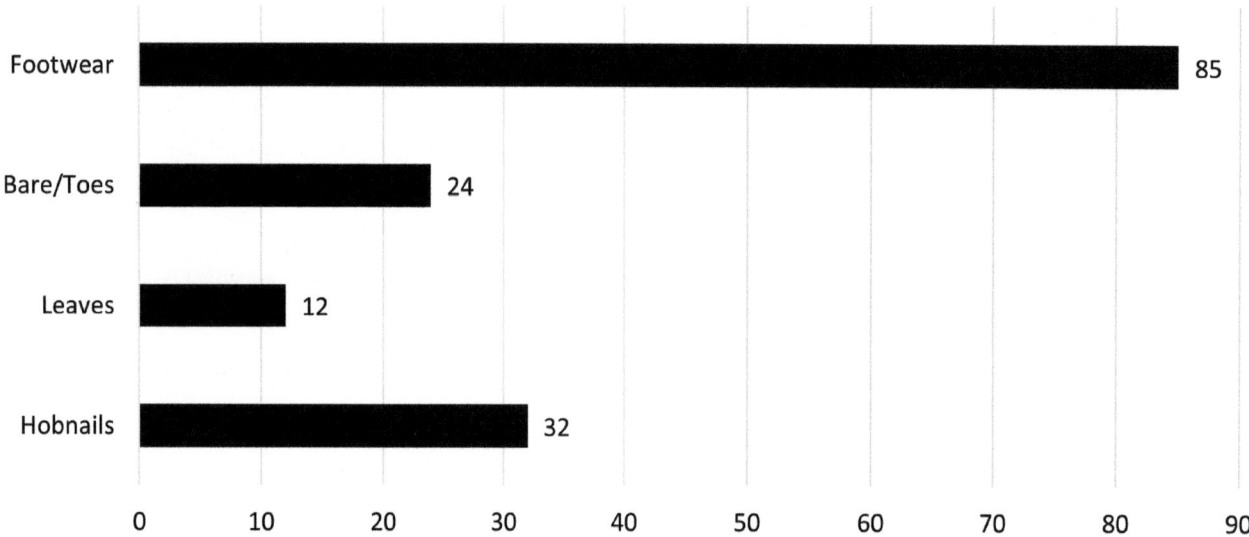

Figure 8.18: Chart to show the ornamentation on 153 pieces of Roman foot-stamped CBM.

next to, a captured non-Roman, for example, a statue found in Crete, but now in Istanbul, from the Hadrianic series from the eastern Mediterranean (Figure 8.19). There is also a possibility that the nailing in conjunction with the *planta pedis* stamps was apotropaic (Forrer 1942: 83), to keep bad luck away from the military buildings, or from the soldiers themselves.

Twelve foot-stamped CBM pieces show a leaf, possibly *hedera*. This plant was used to punctuate inscriptions after 79 CE (Christodoulou 2011: 18), so the leaves may just be there to fill in a space. However, like many Roman carved footprints, ivy leaves are also found associated with the goddess Isis, for example a plaque from Rhodes dedicated to Isis with a crown of ivy leaves (IG XII.1165) and one from Industria, which features a pair of footprints, a sistrum and two *hedera* leaves (CIL V.7488; Takács 2007: 366). There are also 24 military CBM stamps which depict toes and could either be interpreted as being bare feet or wearing sandals. Isis is depicted both in sandals and unshod, so these footprint stamps may be in her honour (Figure 8.20).

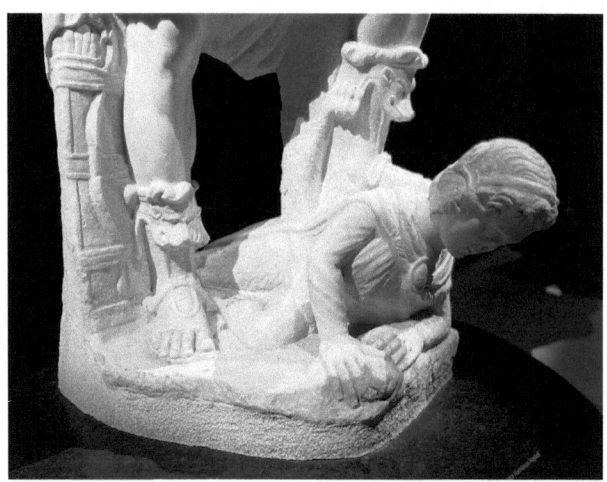

Figure 8.19: Hadrian treading a conquered non-Roman underfoot. (Photo: Raddato.)

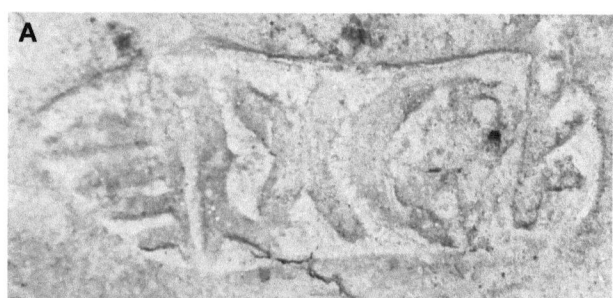
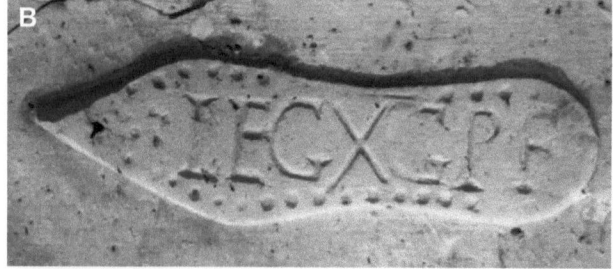
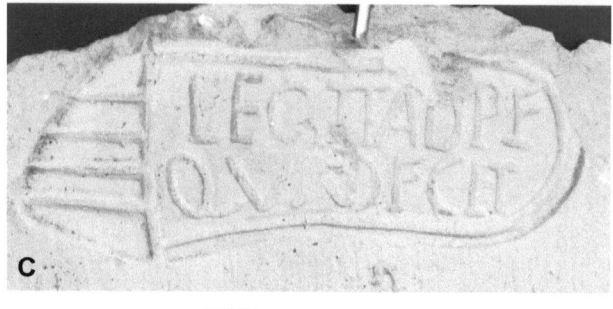
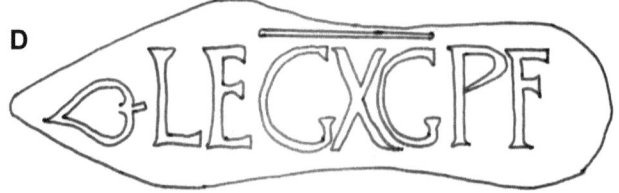

Figure 8.20: Different ornamentation on foot-stamped CBM: Hobnailing, toes and leaves. (Pictures: Erlend Bjørtvedt; Jona Lendering; Carole Raddato).

The foot was also associated with Serapis (Galavaris 2006: 44; Caseau 2012:122). There is some epigraphic evidence of a link between *Legio X Gemina* and Serapis. A military tribune of the Tenth *Gemina*, L. Quirinalis Maximus, dedicated a copper alloy plaque to Jupiter Optimus Maximus Sarapis for the health of Septimius Severus and Caracalla (CIL 3.4560) which was found in Vienna. With it was found another plaque with the dedication *I O M / SARAPIDI / IDEM / MAXIMVS* (CIL 3.4561). Serapis was as important as Jupiter in these inscriptions. Perhaps the *planta pedis* stamped tiles call on the protection of Serapis for the Tenth *Gemina*.

The large *planta pedis* stamps in Roman CBM, therefore, support the arguments for some of the symbolism of actual footprints in Roman CBM. They are a kind of signature, and possibly a sign of power and domination. They may be religious emblems and could have played an apotropaic role.

8.4 Human footprints in Roman CBM

Having examined examples of Roman representations of footprints and discussed their polysemous symbolism, we finally turn our attention to human footprints captured in Roman CBM. As well as accessing some numerical data for CBM from a number of sites (Table 8.1), this study also assembled a corpus of 124 pieces of Roman CBM with human footprints. These comprise examples found in museums, in excavation reports, and on museum websites. While this sample could be regarded as unrepresentative, it does provide examples of a range of footprint types. The database includes such information as site type, chirality, CBM type, placement of the footprints, and footwear type. The data were then analysed to observe any emerging patterns. Most of the footprints are found on *tegulae*, especially those with heavy nailing (Brodribb 1987:125; Jeanne *et al.* 2014:87; Dobosi 2016: 118). Footprints are also found on other flat tiles and bricks (Smith: 8). Because of their tendency to squash if trodden on, it is very rare to find human footprints on flue tiles or *imbrices*, although one was found at 1 Poultry, London (Smith: 8).

One of the first steps in considering the significance of footprints in Roman CBM was to determine how common they are. Roman CBM was manufactured in moulds, then laid out on the ground to dry for about a week, before being stacked and then fired (McWhirr and Viner 1978: 361). Marks such as official stamps, makers' signatures and footprints, whether human or animal, were made while the clay was still wet (Brodribb 1987: 125). The Roman CBM was often produced close to where it was needed in order to reduce transportation costs, but this was not necessarily the case (Darvill and McWhirr 1984: 240; McComish 2012: 57). In fact, recent research by Fulford and Machin shows that early Roman CBM in southern Britain could travel up to 100km (2021: 222). It does, however, tend to be true for CBM used in Roman military buildings (Darvill and McWhirr 1984: 247).

Table 8.1: The proportions of CBM with human footprints on 14 selected sites.

Site	Pieces of CBM	With footprints	%
Alchester	8,097	3	0.04
Boreham	14,101	18	0.13
Brigetio	500	2	0.4
Castleford	1,600	22	1.4
Drapers Gardens	1,943	2	0.1
Elms Farm, Heybridge	87,358	20	0.2
Grange Farm, Gillingham	1,139	4	0.35
Shadwell bath-house, London	2,433	8	0.33
Silchester 1979	314	6	2.0
Silchester 2018	2,000	44	2.2
Tabard Square, Southwark	6,627	4	0.06
Thameslink, Southwark TAA 2 BVK11	1,722	3	0.17
Thameslink, Southwark TAA 6 BVT09	147	1	0.7
Tobacco dock	213	0	0
York	36,000	94	0.26

Working with data from Roman Britain, Warry states that about a tenth of tiles produced by the military have boot marks, but they are rare in civilian production (2006: 16). In order to examine how common the phenomenon is, this study collected data from 14 sites (see Table 8.1).[2] These show that, on most of these sites, the proportion is less than one percent. On the military site at Castleford, the numbers are lower than Warry suggests. Even at Silchester, the site with the most human footprints in CBM, only two percent of the CBM have them. It is worth bearing in mind that most Roman CBM found on the various sites was originally manufactured elsewhere, and some CBM with footprints may have been rejected by the makers as being unusable (Cram and Fulford 1979: 212) so the data may be skewed. It is also very likely that some museums, and excavators, may have kept only the 'interesting' CBM, which would also tend to affect the data (Cram and Fulford 1979: 202; Warry 2006: 16), as would the types of site that are excavated. Tiles with stamps and marks are likely to be recorded on sites as 'small finds' or special finds, while, according to Haynes (2020a), the rest is often discarded as bulk find, with relatively little recording. Nevertheless, human footprints in Roman CBM appear fairly uncommon and might, therefore, be special.

---

[2] Complete data on the examples from these sites were not always available.

One of the aspects considered by this study was the types of site where the CBM was found (Figure 8.21). The majority of examples come from military (44) or urban sites (53), with 22 coming from villa or rural, and five from unknown sites. All footprints on Roman CBM would have been made in a CBM works, and 14 of the CBM pieces in this study were found in such a setting (Figure 8.22). Four are from funerary, and six from religious settings, 20 are domestic in nature, for example from villas, while the provenance of 36 is unknown. There are also 44 from 'other' find settings, 32 from unspecified military buildings and 12 from bath houses.

Those from funerary sites, such as the tile tomb in the Yorkshire Museum, appear to have been reused. This tomb comprises 18 tiles and was found in 1833 near Dringhouses, on the road to Tadcaster. It is formed of *tegulae* and *imbrices*, which are stamped for the Sixth Legion. It is thought that the tiles were erected over the ashes of a soldier from that legion. In the tomb were found the remains of a funeral pile, consisting of charcoal and bones, about six inches in thickness, with several iron nails (York Museums Trust 2020). CBM with footprints may have been chosen deliberately for this grave, considering the apotropaic deposition of shoes in graves and the military associations of footprints.

The length of the footprints can tell us the approximate age and, in adults, the possible gender, of the person who made the impression. Of the 124 pieces in the corpus, 33 are too fragmentary to tell the footprint size, or it is not recorded. Thirty-four contain only children's footprints, four of them toddlers. This may be evidence of child slavery (Christensen 2016; Machin 2018), but it is also

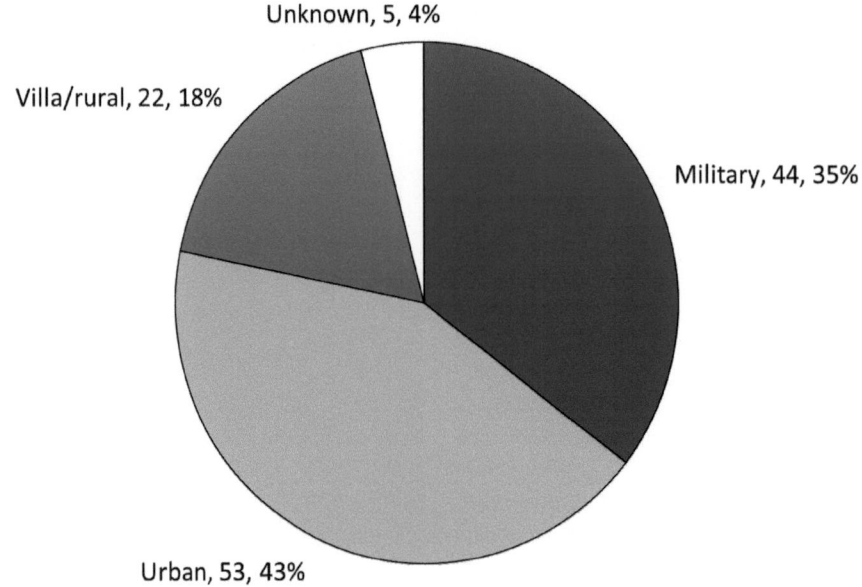

Figure 8.21: Chart to show the site type of 124 pieces of Roman CBM with footprints.

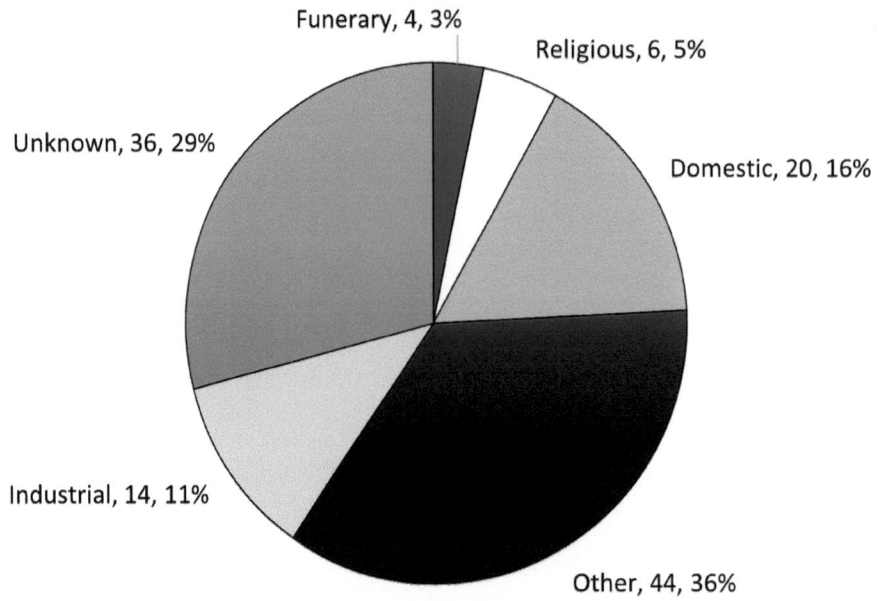

Figure 8.22: Chart to show the find setting of 124 pieces of Roman CBM with human footprints.

possible that the children, especially the younger ones, were playing around the drying CBM. Three pieces, from Vaison-la-Romaine, Alba-la-Romaine, and the Saalburg, have children's walking footprints, and the same child made footprints in two different pieces from Arbeia (Tyne and Wear archives and museums 2020). There are 24 examples where the impressions of the children's footprints are sharp, indicating a lack of movement, and it is possible parents were making a lasting memento of their children. Adult males account for 46 pieces, while seven sport a mixture of adult and child prints. Only four pieces of CBM have footprints of an appropriate size to be women's, although it is possible that some of the impressions deemed to be from teenagers, such as one from Vindolanda, may be women's, since there is some overlap in size between women's and youths' feet (van Driel-Murray 1995: 4). The opposite may also be true, except for the inscribed example from Pietrabbondante. Most of the men's footprints are in heavily nailed footwear, while the women's/youths' footprints are a mixture of barefoot and nailed footwear and the children's footprints are mostly unshod.

Because of changing Roman shoe fashions, the outline shape of the shoe soles can give some dating evidence. Three sets of footprints, a pair in a *tegula* from Corseul (Figure 8.23), one from Luxé, both in France, and a *tegula* from Bedford, show the wide soles popular in the late third and early fourth centuries (van Driel Murray 2001: 194). Many of the heavily nailed footprints have pointed toes (Warry 2006: 16, note 41) which date to the later second century (van Driel Murray 2011a: 345). This contrasts with the rounded end of the traditional legionary *caliga* (Warry 2006: 16, note 41), which disappears from the archaeological record towards the end of the first century (van Driel Murray 2011a: 345). Many of the Romano-British *tegulae* with strong dates are early (Warry 2006: 61), so these later footprints could be evidence for their special nature. Soles with multiple rows of hobnailing are indicative of people doing heavy work (Burandt 2016: 12) and especially of the military (Gansser-Burckhardt 1942: 59; Busch 1965: 172; Rhodes 1980: 107; Keily 2000: 2). Evidence of CBM manufacture in a legionary fort was found in the form of clay adhering to the hobnails on two soles from Vindonissa (Gansser-Burckhardt 1942: 70).

Decorative hobnailing patterns preserved in CBM can also give some indication of date: a CBM fragment found in Austria has an X-shaped pattern on the sole (Figure 8.24) that dates to the late first century (van Driel-Murray 199b: 179). In a *tegula* from Gloucester, there is an S-shaped pattern (Figure 8.25) that was fashionable around 190 CE (van Driel-Murray 2016: 135). A *tegula* from the baths at Heerlen bears a footprint with an asymmetrical S-shape (Figure 8.26) that dates to around 220–230 (van Driel-Murray 2016: 136). Groups of triple nails, such as those in a *tegula* from Aachen (Figure 8.27), are characteristic of the late third and early fourth centuries (van Driel-Murray 2016: 136). It is suggested that this type of hobnailing pattern may have been apotropaic (van Driel-Murray 1999a: 132).

Some of the footprints, therefore, seem to have been made by people wearing their fashionably nailed soles, rather than the heavily nailed working shoes one might expect CBM producers to wear. In the Roman world, the footprint acted as a kind of signature (van Driel-Murray 1999a: 135), so the CBM makers may have been adding their own special and distinctive mark to CBM that was destined for a particular building, such as the footprints destined for the sanctuary in Pietrabbondante (see below).

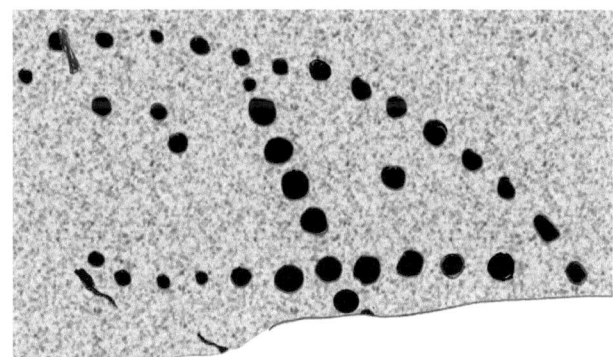

Figure 8.24: X-shaped hobnailing pattern on CBM from Vindobona (Author's drawing).

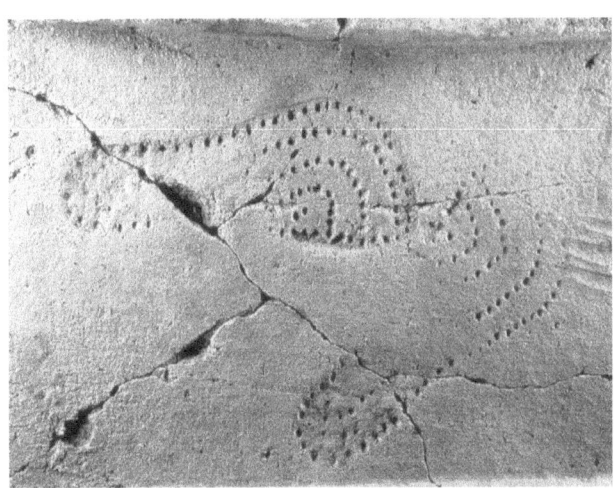

Figure 8.23: Dating evidence: wide soles from Corseul (Photo: Author's own).

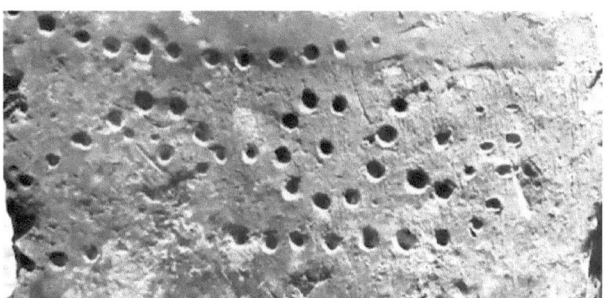

Figure 8.25: S-shaped hobnailing pattern on CBM (Photo: Museum of Gloucester).

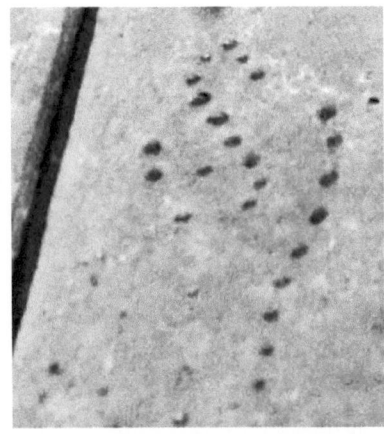

Figure 8.26: Asymmetrical S-shaped hobnailing pattern on CBM from Heerlen (Photo: Author's own).

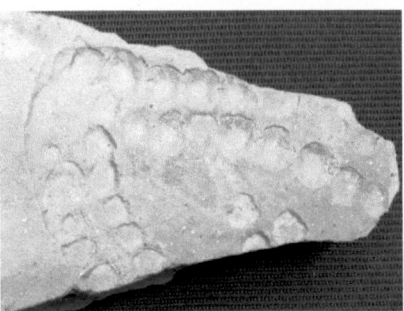

Figure 8.27: Triple nailing pattern from Aachen (Photo: M. Hari).

For this study, one of the most important questions about human footprints in Roman CBM is whether or not they were made deliberately, since this affects their significance. Some scholars regard them as purely accidental, made by people walking or running over the CBM during the manufacturing process (Parker and Rogers 1982: 76; Smith and Betts 1985: 8; Milne and Wardle 1993: 167; Jeanne *et al.* 2014: 88; Dobosi 2016: 117). However, even accidental footprints give a snapshot of lived experience; a transitory moment frozen during manufacture that was then made permanent by firing. Other scholars give the functionalist explanation that the impressions were made deliberately as part of the production process, testing the dryness of the CBM for stacking or firing (Warry 2006: 16; McComish 2014: 273). Brodribb calls the impressions 'quite unofficial' (1987: 155), which is a neutral stance on the question of deliberate marks, since an unofficial mark can still be made on purpose. Perhaps we should note here that the distinction between official and unofficial occurs very often in the Roman world, but it is rarely clear upon what it is based (Haynes 2020a). Christensen (2016) opines that not all human footprints suggest an obvious and accidental reason for their presence.

Looking at the placement of the footprints might help to answer the question. Of the corpus, 42 impressions (34%) are placed centrally on the CBM, the placement of 48 is uncertain because the CBM is too fragmentary, while the remaining 34 footprints are placed around the periphery. The central placement of footprints could be related to testing dryness, as the middle would be the last part of the CBM to dry sufficiently (Warry 2006: 27). Such impressions would be deliberate, but part of the manufacturing process. On the other hand, centrally placed impressions are more prominent and could, therefore, be positioned intentionally and carry more meaning. On 13 pieces of CBM, the footprints (seven adult male, four unclear, one child, and one piece with a mixture of sizes) have been placed adjacent to official stamps or makers' signatures. This would appear to be deliberate placement unrelated to manufacture.

The clarity of the footprints may also provide evidence for whether the impressions occurred accidentally or intentionally (Figure 8.28). Setting aside the five fragments where it is impossible to tell how many prints there are, 30

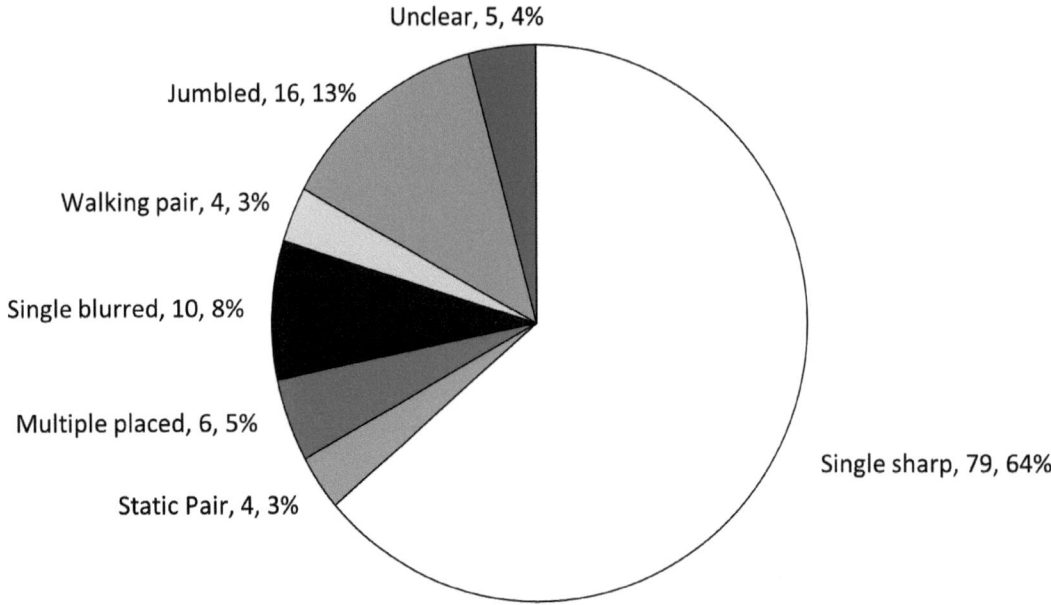

Figure 8.28: Chart to show the clarity of footprints in 124 pieces of Roman CBM.

have footprints that are jumbled, blurred or overlapping. The blurred prints were probably made by moving feet, as walking footprints tend to show 'ghosting' due to foot biomechanics (Vernon *et al.* 2017: 276; Howsam and Brigden 2018: 347). The jumbled prints are probably also a sign of people having to walk across the unfired CBM. Four pieces of CBM have small children's footprints with one in front of the other, possibly indicating walking or running. One piece from Castleford has the imprint of a sock heel (Cram 1998: 236). These are probably all accidental impressions.

However, 79 of the footprints are clear, single feet, and four CBM pieces bear clear, static pairs. These appear to have been carefully placed. Six have multiple footprints, none of which appear to have been blurred by movement, nor is there any other visible indication of motion, such as a noticeably deeper heel impression (Rodgers 1988: 1825). This means that 72% of the human footprints on Roman CBM in this study's corpus could be regarded as deliberately placed. The rest of this chapter will argue that deliberate footprints in Roman CBM were made as more than just a test of dryness, and examine their possible meanings.

Chirality is an important issue when considering the social significance of footprints (Figure 8.29). Roman authors write about lucky right feet and inauspicious left feet, so one might expect most of the footprints in Roman CBM to be from right feet. However, in the corpus, 42 of the 124 pieces (34%) bear single left footprints compared with 30 single right footprints (24%). On the five CBM pieces where the multiple prints are clear enough to tell, there are seven left and only two right footprints. On one piece from Carnuntum (Figure 8.30), all four of the distinguishable footprints are from left feet (Pollhammer 2019: 251). If one leaves aside the 28 pieces (23%) that are too fragmentary, and the 12 (10%) where the multiple prints are too jumbled, to be able to tell the chirality of the footprints, and the eight pairs (6%), we have a ratio of 62% left to 38% right footprints. This is difficult to interpret, since it seems to be at odds with Roman beliefs in good luck associated with the right foot. It could just be a factor of left- or right-footedness. It is possible that the people who made the footprints stood on their right foot for luck. It may also be that, in some provinces, the local population considered the left foot to be lucky. The left foot may have been regarded as part of a contract or vow (van Driel-Murray 1999a: 136), although this is not a watery setting. It is also possible that this could be evidence of resistance, with slaves imprinting unlucky footprints in tiles to 'curse' the roof.

One of the most compelling pieces of evidence for why people left footprints in CBM comes from a roof tile found in Pietrabbondante (Figure 8.31). The *tegula* was found at the large sanctuary site and may have been made for the reroofing of a portico next to temple B (McDonald 2016). The *tegula* bears the hobnailed footprints of two female slaves (or possibly freedwomen), accompanied by inscriptions in two languages, Oscan and Latin. The Oscan inscription reads 'Detfri slave of Herennius Sattius/ signed with a footprint' (Wallace-Hadrill 2008: 90; Richlin 2014: 2; McDonald 2016). The Latin inscription is in a similar vein, 'Amica of Herens signed when we were laying out the tile' (Wallace-Hadrill 2008: 90; Richlin 2014: 2; McDonald 2016). As well as being possible evidence for female (former) slaves' literacy, this *tegula* was deliberately signed by the women and was destined to be placed high up in the roof, where nobody could see it, except perhaps Victoria, to whom the temple was dedicated (Stek 2009: 46). The women may have been adding their voices to prayers for victory over the Romans in the Social War (Stek 2009: 50). They may have been prompting the goddess not to forget the ordinary people, or memorialising their involvement in building the great temple. Certainly, foot impressions on CBM were one way by which ordinary people could stamp their identity on important buildings.

Military CBM producers also seem to have used their footprints as signatures, as shown by a number which overlap, or occur next to, military CBM stamps. In four cases (Figures 5:32, 5:34, 5.39 and 5.44) the footprint

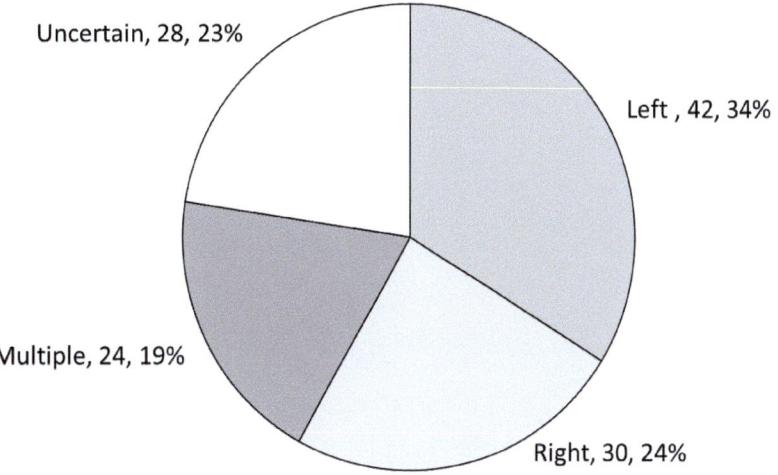

Figure 8.29: Chart to show the chirality of footprints in 124 pieces of Roman CBM.

Roman Feet and Shoes

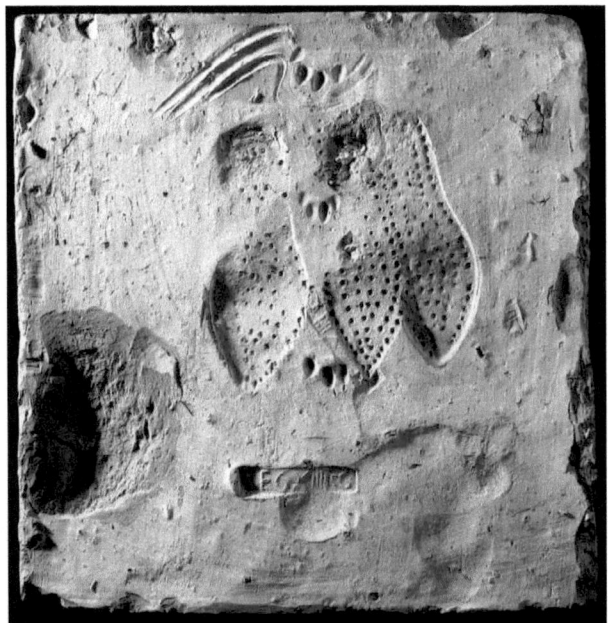

Figure 8.30: Roman tile from Carnuntum with multiple footprints (Photo: Dan's Roman History).

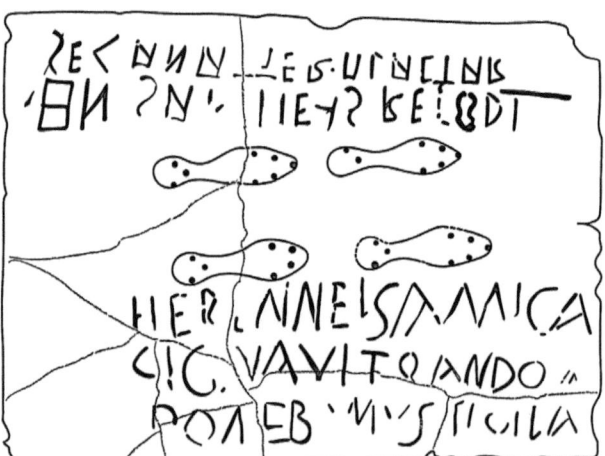

Figure 8.31: Roof tile with footprints from Pietrabbondante. (Author's drawing).

appears to come first, followed by the stamp. This may signify 'official' approval, or perhaps a 'stamp of approval' from the works supervisor and the clerk/*magister*. A brick from Jerusalem is stamped Legio X Fretensis near a left boot-print (Israel Museum inv. no. 1994-2406). A square tile from Svištov, Bulgaria, has the impression of a nailed left shoe that is more central than the Legio I stamp it accompanies (Biernacki 1976: 134). A *tegula* from Caerleon bears two footprints, the left one of which clips the cartouche of the Legio II Augusta (Figure 8.32). Another, from Carnuntum, has a right footprint near a Legio XIIII stamp (Pollhammer 2019: 251). A Legio XIIII stamp with a fragmentary footprint comes from the military tile works at Vindobona (Mosser and Adler-Wölfl 2015: 57). A fragment from Strasbourg (Joconde 2018) is stamped Legio XIII Augusta, with a footprint close to it. A further fragment from Dover has hobnail impressions over a Classis Britannica stamp (Figure 8.33). Two *tegulae* with bare footprints seem unusual because the other examples wear nailed footwear. A *bessalis* from the Roman baths at Heerlen, is stamped for *Legio XXX* (Jeneson and Vos 2020: 153 fig. 8.20). The other, from the CBM works at Holdeurn, is stamped *VEX EX GER* (Figure 8.34), for *Vexillatio Excercitus Germanici*, a group made

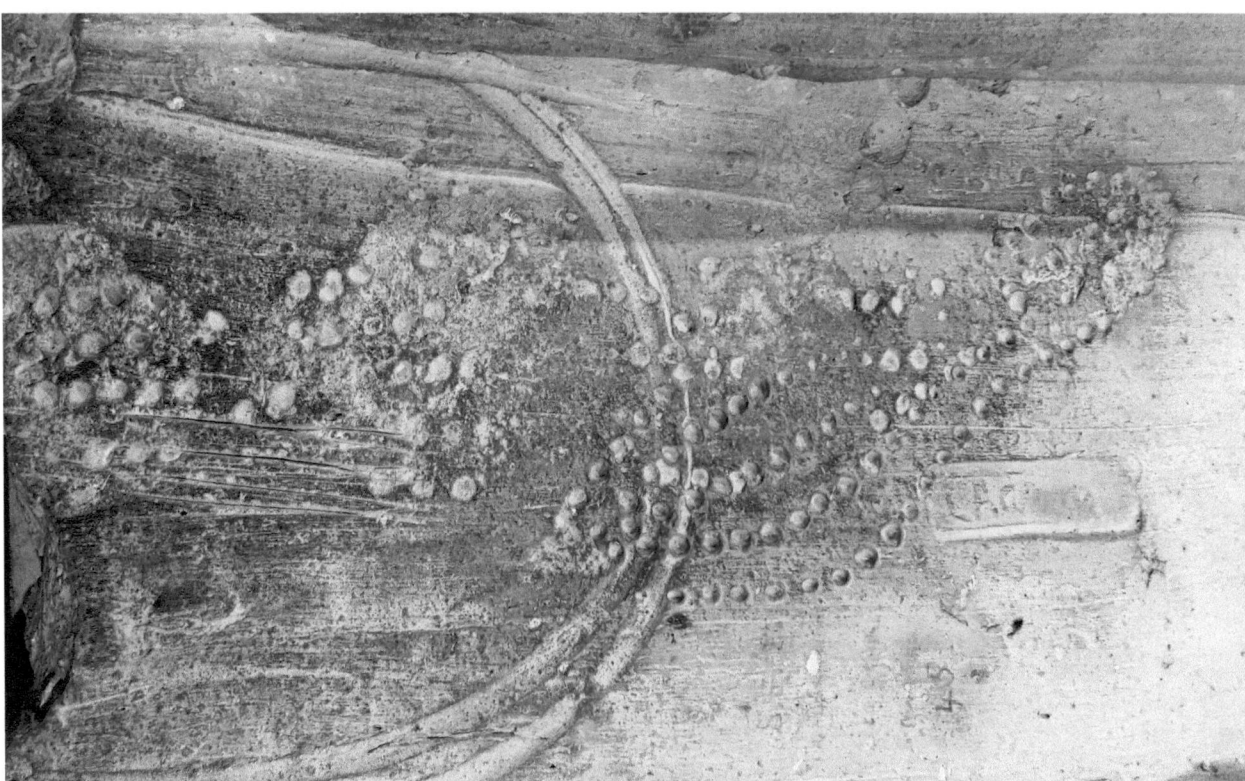

Figure 8.32: A tegula from Caerleon with Legio II Augusta stamp (Photo: Author's own).

The social significance of Roman footprints

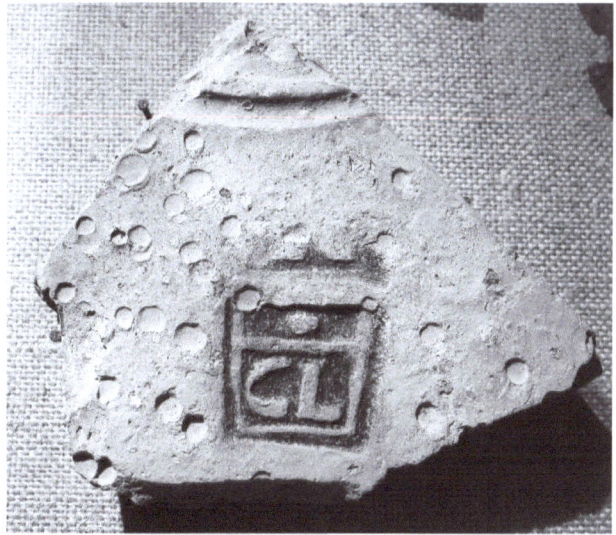

Figure 8.33: CBM from Dover with Classis Britannica stamp (Photo: P. Savin).

up of soldiers from one or more army units to perform a certain task (Collectie Gelderland 2020a). This is quite a small footprint, measuring about 195mm in length. Taking into account shrinkage of about ten percent on firing (Dobosi 2016: 125), we reach an approximate length of 215mm, about the same size as 'Lepidina's sandal' from Vindolanda (van Driel Murray 1997b: 58), so the footprint could belong to a woman or an adolescent. The other prints in this category, however, are from adult males. Because of the proximity of the footprints to the official stamp, it seems likely that the placement of these impressions was deliberate. It is also possible that the owners of the feet were not just testing the readiness of the CBM, but were adding their identity to the important Roman military buildings for which the CBM was being produced.

Human footprints in Roman CBM may, therefore, act as a signature to show the makers' involvement in prestigious buildings. Those included in religious buildings may have brought the tile makers closer to the deity. Those near official military stamps may add to the symbolism of power and authority (Brodribb 1987: 117) since feet and shoes were associated with Roman ideas of domination (see above). Many of the footprints in Roman CBM appear on *tegulae* and the roof was a liminal space in need of protection (van Driel-Murray 1999a: 136; Lawrence 2016). Romans regarded the right foot as particularly lucky (Dunbabin 1990: 105–106) and footwear appears to have provided metaphorical protection (van Driel-Murray 1999a: 131). It is, therefore, possible that the footprints were apotropaic symbols to keep bad luck away from the buildings, or from the makers themselves.

8.5 Conclusions

This chapter has examined the different meanings of Roman footprints, both for archaeologists and for the people who made and used them, using their representations in stone, stamp matrices, and official military marks, as

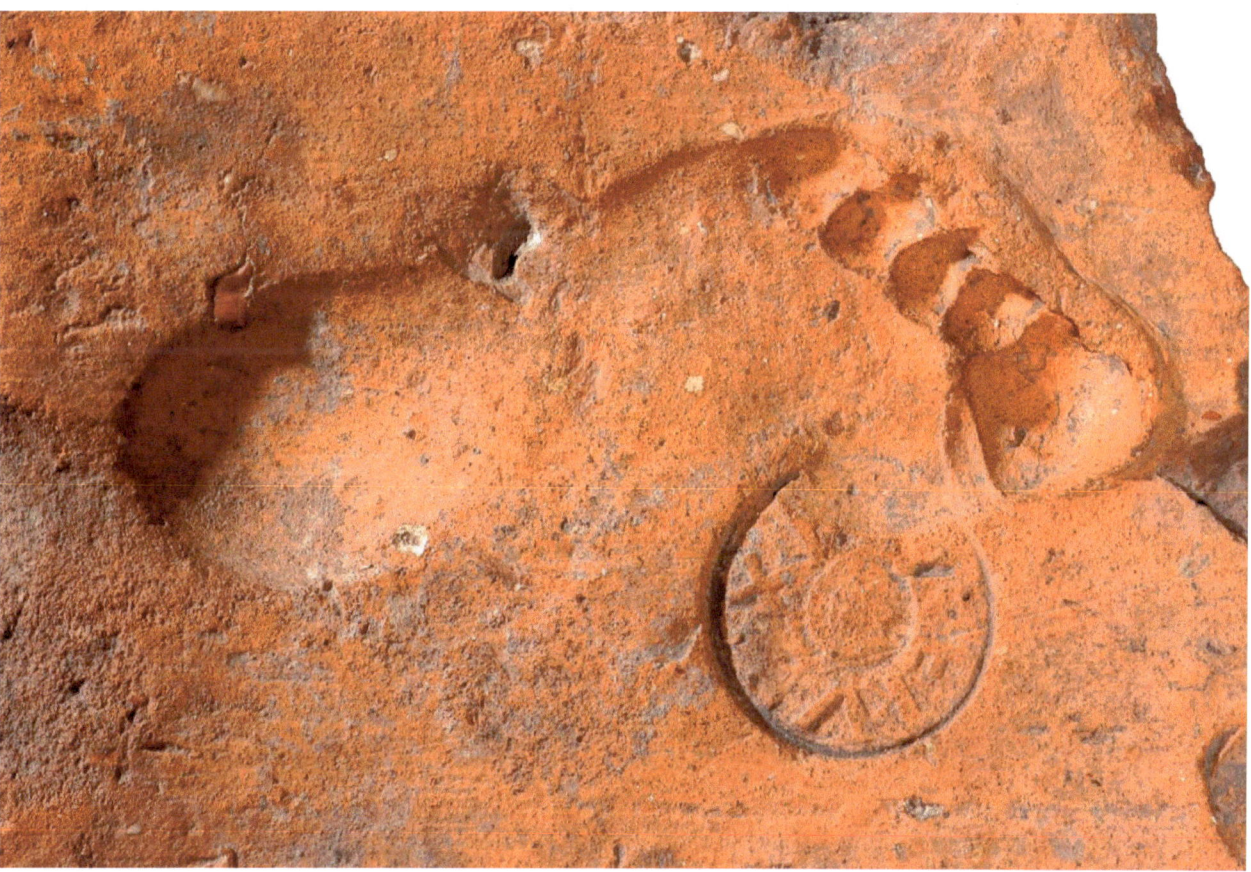

Figure 8.34: Footprint on CBM from Berg en Dal tilery with VEX EX GER stamp (Photo: Het Valkhof).

comparanda in order to discuss the significance of those made in Roman CBM.

Evidence for the idea of the footprint as *pars pro toto* and for memorialisation comes from the *vestigia* carved in stone, such as those from Italica and Dion. In this case, the footprints appear to symbolise the presence of a deity, especially Isis, or of their worshipper, seemingly depending on which direction the footprints point. It is much easier to ascertain the significance of those plaques which include an inscription. These offerings to the deity concerned may just mark the attendance of the donor at the shrine, or they could be an *ex voto* offering, giving thanks for healing or some other favour.

The connection of footprints to healing and divine protection may provide a clue to their apotropaic significance. The inscriptions on *planta pedis* stamps often express a wish for health and life, or good luck, or a deity's protection, and the foot-shaped frame may add to the amuletic effect. The Romans regarded the right foot as particularly lucky, and many stamps are right-footed. Additionally, footwear appears to have provided metaphorical protection. Many of the footprints in Roman CBM appear on *tegulae* and the roof was a liminal space in need of protection, so this may have been one of their functions.

Furthermore, the evidence from Roman representations of footprints appears to indicate a statement of presence along the lines of, 'this is me; I made this' or 'I was here'. Even those impressions that were made by mischievous intent, where the person could not resist stepping on the pristine, damp clay, belong to this category of footprint, as they bear witness to the maker of the footprint having been there. Evidence to support the idea of the Roman footprint as a kind of signature can be seen in the many *planta pedis* stamps or seals, the impressions of which are seen on pottery from across the Roman world. Military tile stamps in *planta pedis* form the signature of the legion or cohort for whom the CBM was manufactured. This is particularly the case for the Tenth Gemina. Footprints may also carry a message of authority and power, or 'treading under foot'.

From an archaeologist's point of view, footprints in Roman CBM tell us something about their makers. The size of the footprints can give an indication of the age and gender of the people who made them. Footprints tend to be adult male size, which is unsurprising, especially for military tiles. There are, however, a number of women's and children's footprints in CBM, which may be evidence of slavery, and certainly of manufacturing practices. In addition, the outline shape of the footwear, and the hobnailing patterns, where these are clear, add to the evidence for dating the tiles, because footwear shapes and nailing designs are known to have changed over time.

The analysis of what footprints in Roman CBM signified to the people who left them is less clear cut. Some of them were most probably accidental, made by people treading on the soft clay while carrying out some tasks or, in the case of small children, playing. As such, what they tell us is that the people were busy. Some deliberate impressions, especially on military CBM, may have been made to test the readiness of the clay for stacking before firing. This is evidence for the manufacturing process, but may carry no further significance.

However, some of the footprints in Roman CBM do appear to have been made deliberately to represent the person who made them in an important building, like the impressions from the sanctuary at Pietrabbondante. In this way, the less important people, who are often invisible, could give themselves a sense of literally being part of a grand building and, in the case of temples, of being closer to the deities concerned. This is a way for ordinary people to memorialise themselves.

By looking at different representations of Roman footprints, we have seen that they carry a variety of meanings. Each footprint may have held a different significance for its maker, owner, or donor. The layers of meaning demonstrated by footprints in stamp or carved form could be applicable to the footprints in Roman CBM, be it religious symbol, signature, sign of authority, memorialisation, amulet, or a combination of all of these. It would appear, therefore, that footprints in Roman CBM should not be dismissed as merely accidents or mischief.

9

Assessing the significance of Roman statue foot-fragments from Britain

This chapter considers why feet that were broken off, or separated from, Roman sculpture, may have been preserved, rather than being melted down and recycled, in the case of copper alloy, or crushed and put in a lime kiln, in the case of stone. It examines whether the foot-fragments fit into patterns of symbolism observed in other Roman foot-shaped artefacts: feet as symbols of a whole individual, whether human or divine; feet and footwear as religious symbols, ritual or apotropaic objects, or symbols of authority and domination. In order to answer the questions, this chapter examines the patterns of spatial, chronological, and find setting distribution, and of factors in the survival of Roman sculpted feet. While considering these questions, it is important to remember that some statues only consisted of carved heads, hands and feet, with the rest of the body modelled on a wooden frame. An example of this is the colossal statue of Constantine the Great in the Capitoline Museums in Rome. One must also note that the ankles are points of vulnerability on a statue, so feet may be broken off more easily.

The data sample for this study was gathered mainly from the *Corpus Signorum Imperii Romani* (CSIR) Great Britain series, looking only at those fascicules which cover Roman sculpture found in Britain (1.1–1.11) because those British fascicules dealing with Roman sculpture from private collections that came mainly from Italy might skew the data, moving the focus away from the north-western provinces. Furthermore, while the sample could have been much larger and from a greater geographical area, relevant data were not readily accessible at the time of the study. Data were also drawn from Aldhouse-Green 1976 and 1978. Admittedly these works are quite old now however more recent data proved difficult to obtain. Bibliographical references were checked carefully and followed up to gain further information.

As well as feet from statues and figurines, this study includes reliefs, altars, and funerary monuments (Figure 9.1). The right foot of pipe-clay figurine of Venus, found in Aldborough in 2019 (Millett and Ferraby 2021), the left foot of a copper alloy figurine from York (York Museums Trust) and a pair of statue feet from Vindolanda (Birley 2007: 138) were also included. All three were found after their relevant CSIR volumes were published.

Relatively few statues have been recorded from Roman Britain (Russell 2019: 129). Nevertheless, CSIR fascicules 1.1 to 1.10 for Britain catalogue 1,061 pieces of sculpture that are humanoid, of which 663 are fragments. As well as cataloguing instances of separated feet, this study considered other sculpted body parts that survived as recorded in the CSIR fascicules (Table 9.1). Feet (72) were the fourth most common type to survive after heads (229), torsos with no heads (81), and upper bodies including heads (78). These data show that there are many more preserved statue heads than feet from Roman Britain. Some of the heads may have been originally carved as busts (Croxford 2003: 88) but that is not to deny the significance of heads in Roman ideology, where they were considered to be the seat of the human spirit (Clarke 1996: 75) and hence were powerful (Croxford 2003: 88–9; Eckardt 2014: 168). On the other hand, it may be that other body parts were more important and were thus not discarded (Fittock 2015: 128). This study ignores the complete sculptures because they cannot inform the preservation of feet. In addition,

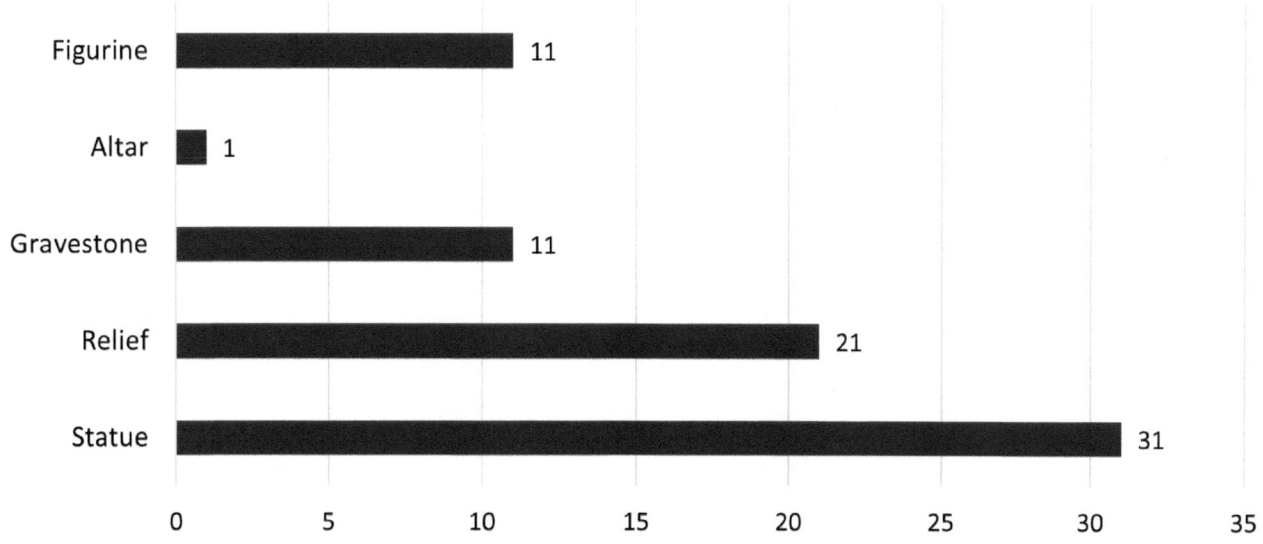

Figure 9.1: Chart to show the proportions of different sculpture types in 75 sets of foot-fragments.

Lindsay Allason-Jones kindly provided the information on three sets of detached feet from the forthcoming CSIR fascicule 1.11. These have not been included in the Table 9.1 statistics, as only details of the foot-fragments were received. There are, therefore, 75 foot-fragments from Roman sculpture in this study's sample.

While this research is akin to Croxford's (2003) and draws from a similar dataset, he focused on heads, arms and hands, not feet. Croxford (2003: 86, footnote 24) collected all published examples of religious images carved or cast in the round from Roman Britain, producing a corpus of 377 which includes 93 feet and 79 bases with feet attached (Croxford 2003: 87). His statistics are somewhat perplexing, as the total number of body parts he records is 1,335. Clearly, he catalogues some of the fragments in more than one category.

Archaeologically, feet are much more easily recognisable than some other body parts, such as kneecaps or elbows, so their preservation may owe something to this. It is, however, likely that there is no single reason why the feet were kept. We should, rather, expect a variety of explanations which range from accidental survival to deliberate, ritual deposition. The major problem in discriminating between these is whether one can tell if the feet were deliberately detached from sculptures during the Roman period. Fragmentation theory recognises five principal ways in which an object may be broken and then enter the archaeological record (Chapman 2000: 23; Croxford 2003: 83):

1. broken accidentally or through use and then thrown away;
2. broken accidentally or through use and then buried;
3. ritually 'killed' by being deliberately broken then buried;
4. broken to disperse some 'power'; the fragments could be distributed to disperse the power further;
5. broken deliberately for use in 'relations of enchainment', for example, instances of iconoclasm.

This study will probably find examples which fit all these categories. Careful consideration of patterning in breakage and deposition is necessary to be able to distinguish archaeologically between these categories. Following a chi square test, which measures the difference between the observed and expected frequencies of the outcomes of a set of variables, Croxford argues that there is a one-in-a-thousand probability of chance being responsible for heads being over-represented in his sample (2003: 88), that is, the heads were deliberately preserved. A similar test on this study's data shows the numbers for feet are too large to have arisen by chance.

9.1 Chronological and spatial distribution

The dating of fragments of Roman sculpture is not always recorded. Of the 75 sets of feet in this corpus, 26 are of uncertain date, 13 of which are antiquarian finds (Figure 9.2). One of these, from York (Rinaldi Tufi 1983: 67 no.113), might be datable to the fourth century by its footwear (Figure 9.3), which resembles the 'Ouse' style (Volken 2014: 263). The actual, leather, 'Ouse style' shoe was found in a well in Skeldergate, York, that was back-filled in the fourth century (MacGregor 1978: 31; 53 no.363). The majority of the sculpted foot-fragments date to the second and third centuries.

The recording of where the sculptures were found is much more thorough: all 75 in the sample have a known find-location. What is striking about the spatial distribution of the foot-fragments is the places where more than one set was found (Figure 9.4). One might expect the most examples to have come from the provincial capital, *Londinium*, and six did. However, eight came from Corbridge and nine from Carlisle, possibly because of their military connections. There are also five from Chester and five from York, important Roman towns. There is a cluster from the more rural area around Gloucestershire, which reflects the possession of statuary by villa owners.

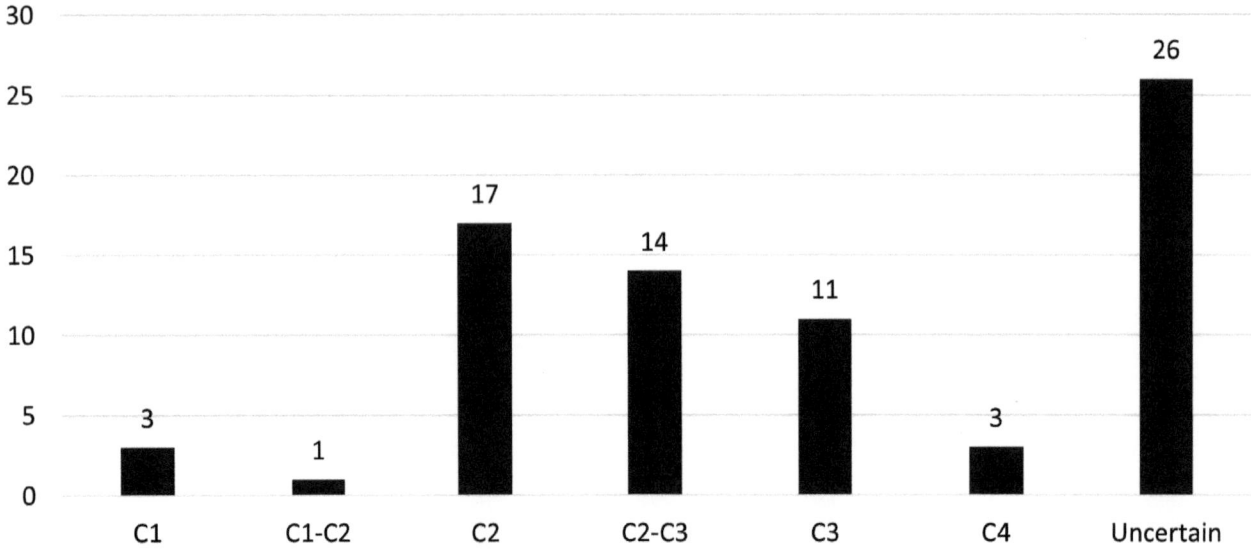

Figure 9.2: Chart to show the dating of 75 sets of feet separated from Roman sculpture.

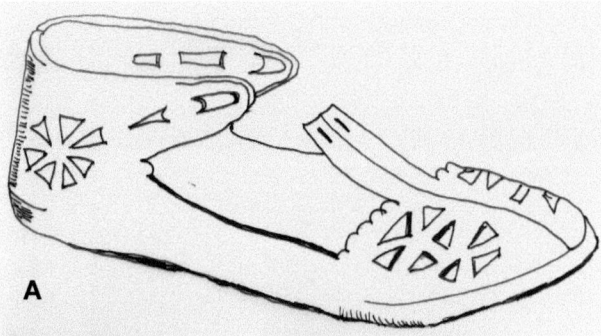

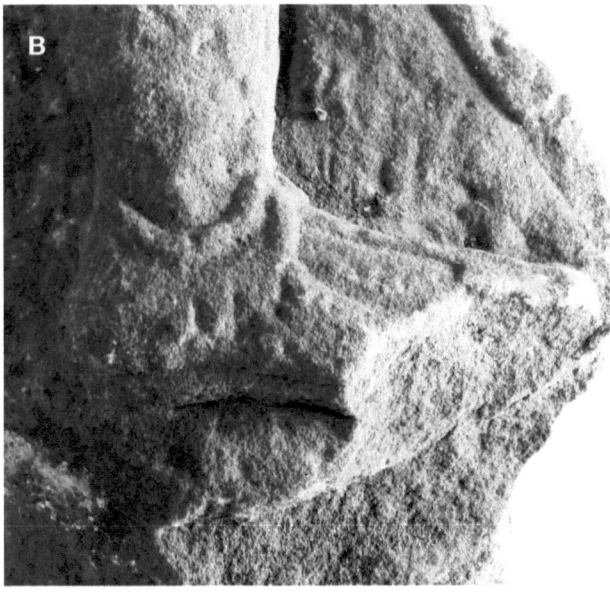

Figure 9.3: The 'Ouse' style (Author's drawing) and detail of York funerary monument (YORYM 2007.6145).

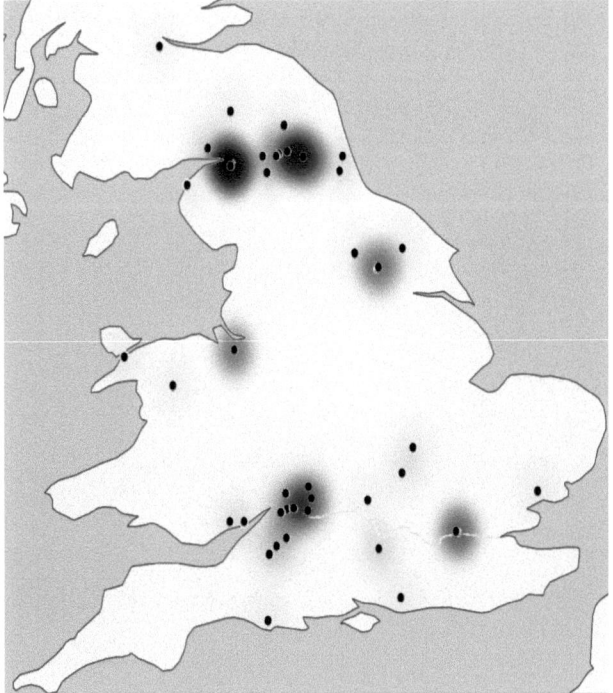

Figure 9.4: Heat map to show the spread of foot-fragments from Roman sculpture.

9.2 Material considerations

The materials from which the sculpture were made may have a bearing on the symbolism of the foot-fragments. Of the 75, four were cast from copper alloy. Two of these were quite large feet found in London, one in Tabard Square (Coombe et al. 2015: 120) and one in Kingsway (Coombe et al. 2015: 121). A third came from a York figurine (Yorkshire Museum Inv. no. YORYM: 2012.377), and the fourth was discovered at Milsington, Scotland (Keppie and Arnold 1984: 17). Five of the examples are carved from marble, of which two came from villas at Woodchester and Bancroft (Henig et al. 1993: 4-5). A further two were found in London (Coombe et al. 2015: 4 and 30), and the last at Maiden Castle (Cunliffe and Fulford 1982: 26). These high-status materials tend to show wealth and power of the people who commissioned and owned the sculptures. However, apart from one of pipe-clay, the remaining foot-fragments were all carved from stone local to the areas in which they were found. This would seem to indicate that the sculptural medium does not necessarily help with the interpretation of the foot-fragments.

9.3 For whom the foot fragments stand

It has been suggested that Roman sculpted feet were preserved because they represented a whole being (Croxford 2003: 92). Chapter 8 of this study discusses carved footprints as a sign of the presence of a deity, or a worshipper, or both (Dunbabin 1990: 95; Chiarini 2017: 155). Chapter 4, on the deposition of Roman footwear in burials and wells, argues that, because actual footwear carries the imprint of the wearer's foot, it functions as a substitute for that individual (van Driel-Murray 1999a: 136). The idea of feet and footwear as synecdoche is, indeed, a recurring theme in this study. With this in mind, it could be informative to examine which deities, and other beings, are represented by the foot-fragments (Figure 9.5).

Nineteen sets in the sample (26%) cannot be attributed to a specific being because there is no evidence for their exact identities apart from the feet. Fragments belonging to statues of gods or personifications can only be identified if they have some distinctive attribute, or are characteristic of the iconography of a deity in terms of appearance, clothing, or movement (Mráv 2016: 180). However, 18 probably represent deities because they have bare feet (Croom 2010: 74). Eleven portray human feet, all of which come from funerary reliefs, and are probably depictions of the deceased. Judging by their footwear, five appear to represent emperors (see Chapter 2.3), who were also considered divine. The two most common deities in this sample, with five sets each, are Victory, all of them from military sites, and Mercury, from a mixture of find settings. There are three each of Diana, often identified by her footwear and accompanying hound, Minerva, Hercules and, more unusually, Vulcan. There are also two of Mars, and one of Mars-Lenus. One might have expected to see feet belonging to Jupiter and Juno, but seemingly none do, unless they have not been identified as such. What

Roman Feet and Shoes

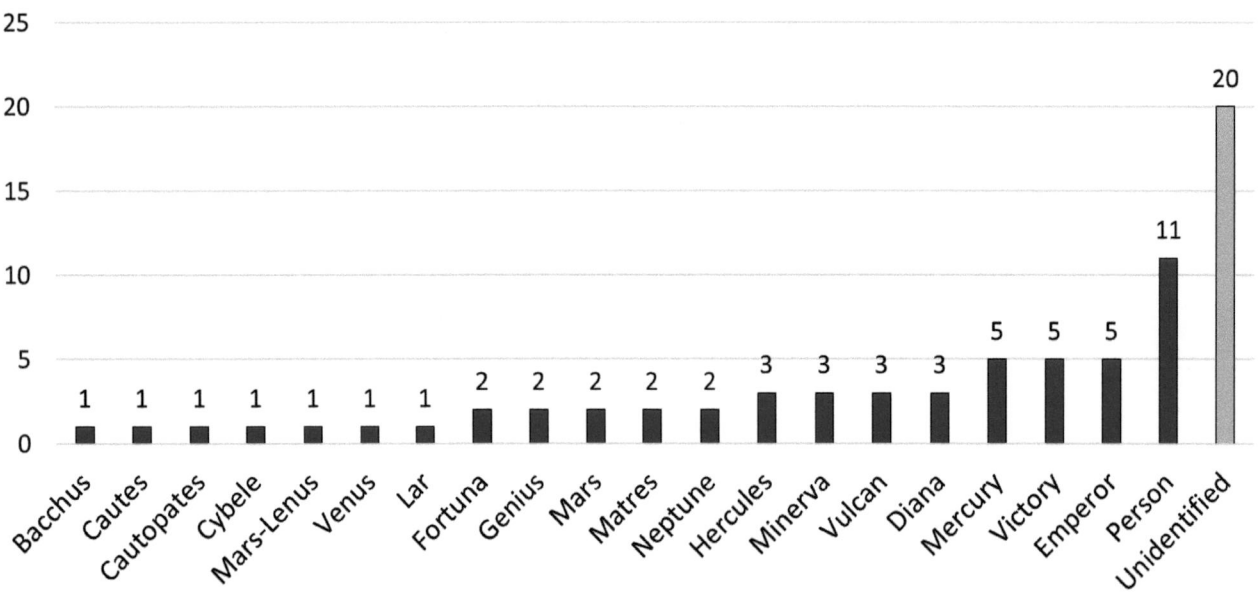

Figure 9.5: Chart to show whose feet are represented on 75 sets of Roman sculpture fragments.

the identification of these subjects of Roman portraiture shows is that the foot-fragments were all either divinities or from a ritual setting.

It may be that the breakage of the sculpture served a function other than mere destruction (Croxford 2003: 93). Not every image may have been broken deliberately to serve a new ritual or social purpose (Croxford 2003: 93), and this will be examined in the next section. However, it may have been thought that the fragments were imbued with the same powers as the whole image, and they could have functioned as apotropaic amulets or personal objects of veneration (Croxford 2003: 93). The proportion of deities in the sample is 62 out of 71, or 86%, if the emperors are included, which might suggest that the feet were preserved because they are divine.

9.4 Distribution by site type and find setting

In addition to analysing spatial and chronological data, and who is represented, this study considered the type of site and setting where the feet were found. Unsurprisingly, the site types with the greatest number of foot-fragments are 'urban', with 34, and 'military', with 26. Only 14 come from a rural or villa site, and one find site is unknown (Figure 9.6). These categories are admittedly vague, but more precision will be provided in the discussion of individual examples below.

The categories used for find settings are: funerary, religious, water, domestic, industrial, road building, unknown, and other. The last one contains seven foot-fragments from an unspecified find setting within a

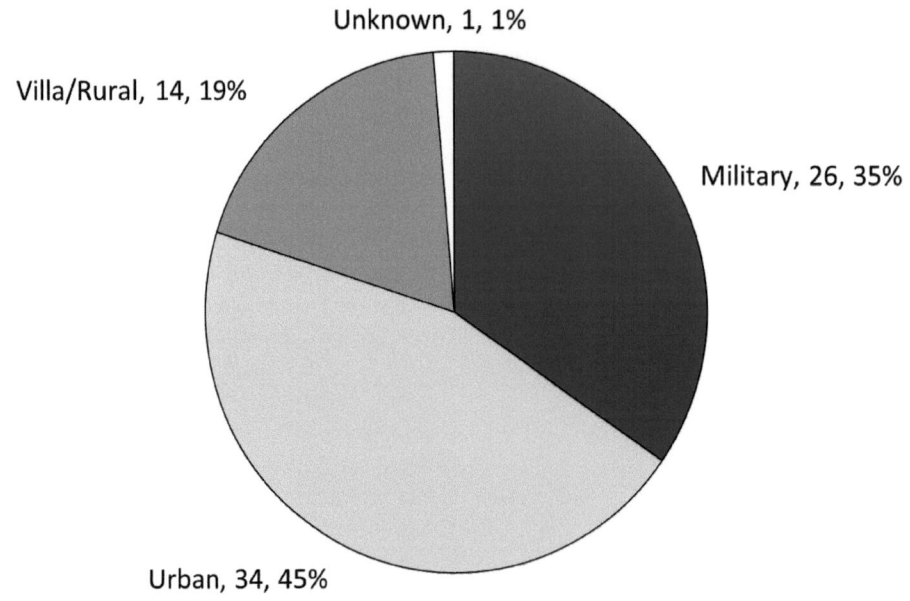

Figure 9.6: Chart to show the site type of 75 sets of feet separated from Roman sculpture.

military site, and the figure of a genius, found in the garden of St. John's House, Chester (Henig et al. 2004: 2). This building stood over the north-west quadrant of the amphitheatre (Wilmott 2007: 37), so this example has been categorised separately as 'amphitheatre' (Figure 9.7). This sculpture might be connected to the Nemeseum, which is to the west of the north entrance (Wilmott 2007: 178), so could be categorised as 'religious'. Ritual sites, such as temples, shrines, burials, and watery places, account for 32 sets of foot-fragments, almost 43% of the sample. For the purposes of this chapter, however, it might be more instructive to discuss the Roman sculpture foot-fragments according to how they were deposited.

9.5 Patterns of deposition

The data analysis of this study's sample showed six broad patterns of deposition (Figure 9.8). In 23 cases (31%) there was not enough information available about where or how the feet were found to be able to interpret why they were preserved (Table 9.2). These are mostly antiquarian finds where the information has not been recorded. We can only speculate as to why these sculptured feet survived.

An example is the deposition of the feet of a relief of Neptune, found in 1911, in the latrine pit in the south-east corner of Housesteads fort (Coulston and Phillips 1988: 32). The relief may have decorated the inside of the buildings, or a water-tank outside (Simpson and Simpson 1976: 136). The rest of the relief was not found with the feet, so this could be deliberate deposition in a watery setting. It may also have fallen into the latrine and not been retrieved, while the rest may have been reused for lime or other building material.

Sometimes the foot-fragments were found repurposed, 11 of them (14%) in the Roman era, often as building stone (Table 9.3). Examples were found used as hard-

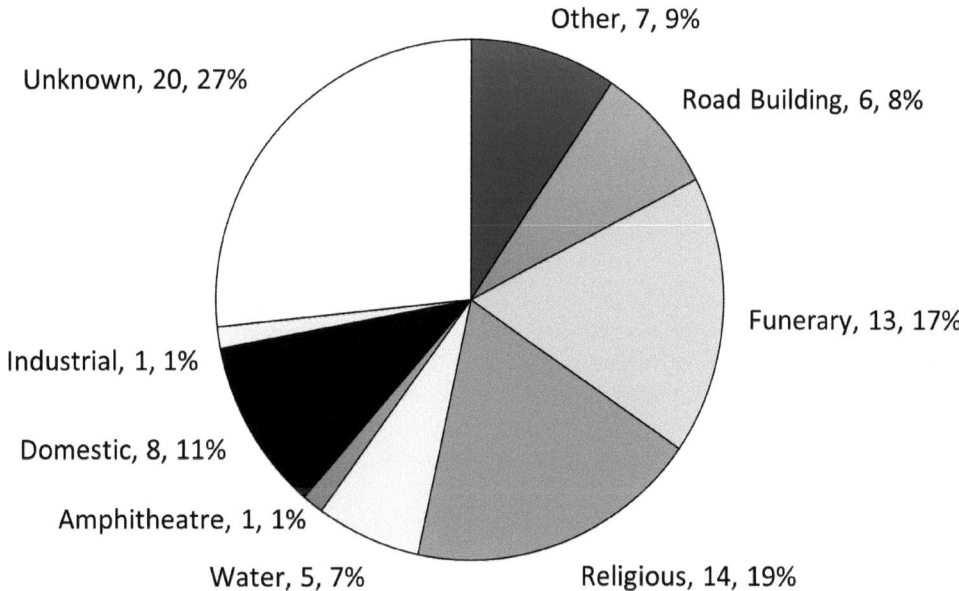

Figure 9.7: Chart to show the find setting of 75 sets of Roman sculpture foot-fragments.

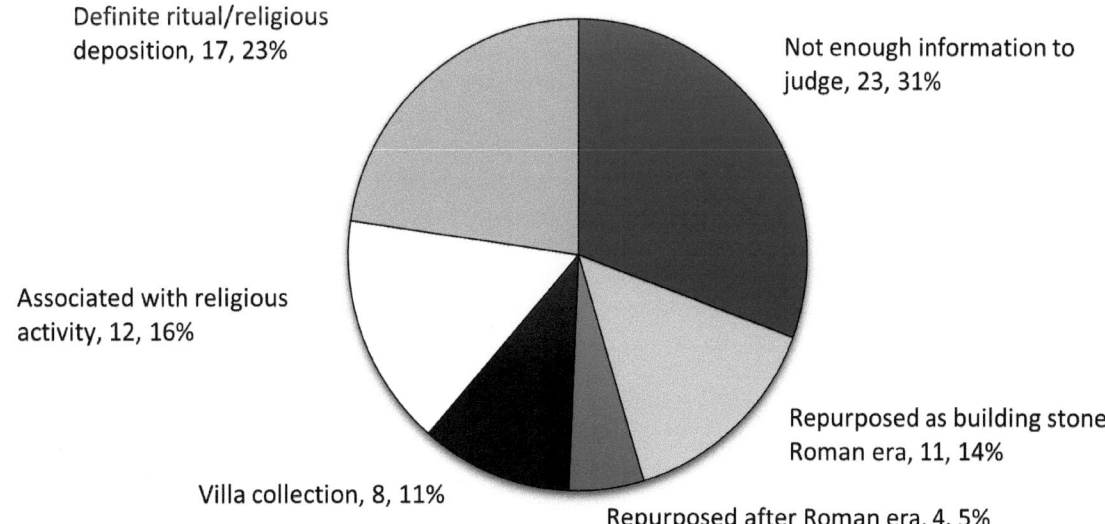

Figure 9.8: Chart to show the patterns of deposition for 75 sets of Roman sculpture foot-fragments.

core, especially six sets from Corbridge which Haverfield describes as 'road ballast' (Haverfield 1914: 514). A fragmentary relief from Carlisle's civilian settlement was reused as post-packing in a late Roman level (Coulston and Phillips 1988: 156 no.471).

In 1870 the lower part of a relief of Vulcan was found at Maryport in post pit [2475] (Allason-Jones forthcoming). The relief is unfinished as well as broken (Coulston 1997: 116; Breeze 2018: 66). Many complete altars, mostly to Jupiter Optimus Maximus, but one dedicated to Vulcan (RIB 846), and other pieces of sculpture, were re-purposed as post-packing in a late fourth-century building with a western apsidal structure, which has been interpreted as a Christian construction (Symonds *et al.* 2014: 21). More recent research, however, suggests that the 'balance of probabilities points to a hall-type building and subsidiary structures', that was adapted 'for an extended period into the 5th century', comparable with the sequence of late halls at Birdoswald (Haynes 2020b: 220).

These feet preserved from Roman statuary show that some examples survived because they were broken and repurposed, and may only have escaped from being classed as rubble because they are recognisable as feet. All the instances in this selection are the feet of deities, however, which may have contributed to their preservation, as may their apotropaic qualities.

Four sets (5%) were repurposed in post-Roman contexts (Table 9.4), possibly due to their value as curiosities or souvenirs, or as useful building stone. A striking example is part of an altar with the feet of a relief of Mercury with his ram and cockerel found in his sanctuary at Uley (Henig *et al.* 1993: 25). The stone was reused in the threshold of a timber building of the fifth or sixth century (Woodward and Leach 1993: 82). There may be an argument that, since feet are in touch with the ground, the foundation of the person, repurposed foot-fragments make an appropriate addition to the foundations of a building. Structure VII, where this foot-fragment was reused, has been interpreted as the baptistery of an early church (Woodward and Leach 1993: 82; Sauer 2003: 61). Since only one known find from the site, a copper alloy plaque, bears Christian iconography (Woodward and Leach 1993: 108–110), much of this argument is based on the apsidal shape of structure VII and a comparison of the Uley building with other Roman basilican churches from southern Britain (Woodward and Leach 1993: 319–321). A similarity to post-Roman timber halls is also noted (Woodward and Leach 1993: 319), and the plan of the structure certainly resembles the hall-type building and subsidiary structures at Maryport (Haynes 2020b: 220 discussed above). This foot-fragment may be an example of early Christian iconoclasm, or just the reuse of perfectly good building stone. If this structure were a church, one might speculate that, since Mercury, as Psychopomp, was associated with death and the afterlife, he may have been considered an appropriate surrogate for Christ (see Woodward and Leach 1993: 325).

Eight sets (11%) were found in Roman villas (Table 9.5) as part of collections of sculpture that demonstrated their owners' status (Caseau 2011: 490) in a domestic setting. Some statuary in this group may also be associated with a shrine, temple or mausoleum on the site, for example, a right foot from Bancroft Roman villa near Milton Keynes may have come from the nearby Blue Bridge Roman temple-mausoleum (Milton Keynes Heritage Association).

Twelve sets (16%), some of which came from military sites, were found associated with religious activity (Table 9.6). For instance, the front part of a larger-than-life copper alloy foot in a sandal came from Tabard Square, London (Coombe *et al.* 2015: 120). This left foot was found in association with Romano-British temples, where it may have stood on a plinth, in a layer that included fourth-century pottery (Killock 2009: 74). The statue may have been an imperial or religious figure (Gerrard and Major 2009: 248). The style of sandal is one usually worn by women and the short length of the foot probably protruded from under a long skirt (Coombe 2015: 196), so this would indicate possibly an emperor's consort or a goddess. Coombe suggests that it could be the foot of Isis (2015: 196). However, the feet of Isis are usually portrayed bare, or in a form of *solea* that resembles modern flip-flops. This foot could have been recycled for its valuable metal content, but was preserved, possibly because of its religious significance.

The last category comprises 17 (23%) sets of statue feet that were deposited in settings that were demonstrably ritual or concerned with religious observance (Table 9.7). Foot-fragments that survive on gravestones may well have done so because they still represent the deceased. This is an instance where the feet definitely belong to a human being rather than a deity. Examples come from Colchester western Roman cemetery (Huskinson 1994: 29), Botchergate, Carlisle (Coulston and Phillips 1988: 165), Chester (Henig *et al.* 2004: 17–26), and the Driffield Estate, York (Rinaldi Tufi 1983: 67).

The feet of a relief of a standing figure were found in an area of known cemetery about 150 metres north-east of Caer Gai Roman fort (Brewer 1986: 7–8). The base is inscribed *Iulius Gaveronis f(ilius) | fe(cit) mil(es) c(o) ho(rtis) I Ner(viorum)* (RIB 418), and an urn with burnt bones was found beneath it. These feet may belong to Hercules and the Nemean lion, or to Bacchus and a panther, indeed, Brewer (1986: 8) argues strongly for the latter. Either might be appropriate for a grave covering. Mercury as Psychopomp also seems particularly appropriate for a Roman grave-marker. He is depicted on a funerary relief from Whiteclosegate, Carlisle, near Stanwix fort (Coulston and Phillips 1988: 159).

Some examples of preserved feet have been found in temples. A statue plinth with a pair of bare feet was found at Vindolanda during the 2005–2006 excavations in Area B within the temenos of a temple (Birley and Blake 2007: 81). The feet of a statue of Cautopates were found at the southern end of the west bench in the nave of the Mithraeum at Carrawburgh (Coulston and Phillips 1988: 42). Unlike the Carlisle feet of Cautes, this statue definitely came from a known Mithraic temple. Richmond *et al.* suggest Cautopates's feet were saved by the stone falling into local peat bog (1951: 41), although the fragment could have been deliberately placed there (Sauer 2011: 509).

A fragmentary relief from the Romano-British temple site at Woodeaton, Oxfordshire, shows the feet of a soldier, probably Mars (Aldhouse-Green 1976: 177; Henig *et al.* 1993: 22). This interpretation is supported by the copper alloy letters M.A.T.I., the copper alloy portrait of Mars, and many votive weapons, especially spears, found at the site (Smith 1995: 189.) The carving of Mars is very small and probably served as an *ex voto*, as did the copper alloy plaque depicting Mars (Henig *et al.* 1993: 22). The exact location of the find is unrecorded but it is known that most votive objects were found around the gateway to the *temenos* (Goodchild and Kirk 1954: 37). The votive Mars relief may have been deliberately broken to put it out of common use (Nickel 2011: 150).

Instances have been found in other demonstrably ritual settings. A pair of separated feet were found in the strongroom under the *aedes* of Segontium Roman fort (Figure 9.9). This piece of Roman sculpture is a relief, possibly of Mars, since the feet are bare and the figure has a cloak, or shield, and a spear (Brewer 1986: 8). The fragment was found in 1922 in a sealed fourth-century deposit under floor III, with an altar to Minerva (RIB 429), a stone inscribed with a V, and part of a human skull (Wheeler 1923: 80). It is possible that the material was simply discarded, and these notable elements within it attracted disproportionate attention. However, the presence of a human skull does point to a special deposit (see Chapter 4.2.1), and the fact that the strong room under the *sacellum* is often associated with cult material finds (Haynes 2021) implies that this could be the careful, ritual preservation of a pair of feet belonging to a deity.

Deposits in watery places, whether natural rivers and bogs, or human-made wells, are increasingly recognised as being ritual (Fulford 2001: 199) and the corpus contains specimens of these. A bog at Milsington, near Hawick, Scotland concealed the gilded copper alloy lower right leg and foot of an equestrian statue (Keppie and Arnold 1984: 17; Figure 9.10). It was discovered in 1880 with another copper alloy object, thought to be a plinth for a smaller statue, or a casing for a large weight (Keppie and Arnold 1984: 17; Hunter 2017). Curle (1932: 324) suggests this was a pedestal for a statue of Victory. It has been assumed that the leg is evidence of looting (Curle 1932: 324; Croxford 2016: 43), although recent research from Germany shows that frontier forts also housed impressive imperial statues (Hunter 2017). Hunter argues that the leg was not hacked off, but carefully dismantled (2017). The leg may have been deliberately deposited in this wet site as a votive offering (Hunter 2017). Indeed, it is not the only known example of this type of sculpture being deposited in a watery place. A similar, left leg was found in Wels, Austria, on the bed of the river Traun, along with part of a copper alloy horse's leg (Harl and Harl 2020). The bed of the river Kulpa in Croatia, near Karlova, also yielded two fragments of large copper alloy sculpture: the head and left foot of Apollo (Mráv 2016: 182). The Milsington leg, then, appears to be a ritual deposit.

Another watery setting, a Roman well beneath Southwark Cathedral, contained the lower leg and foot of a statue of Neptune or Oceanus with a dolphin (Coombe *et al.* 2015: 4). This set of feet was part of a layer of sculpture that sat astride the water table (Hammerson 1978: 210). Hammerson assumes that no ritual significance can be

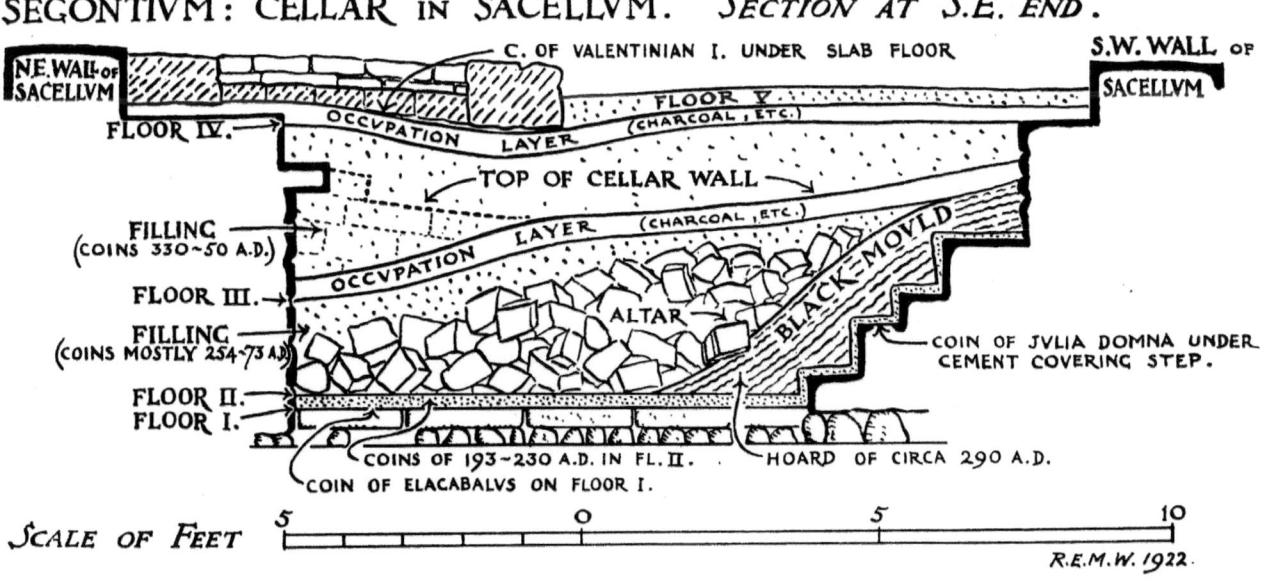

Figure 9.9: Segontium: Cellar in the sacellum: section at south-east end (Wheeler 1923: fig.17).

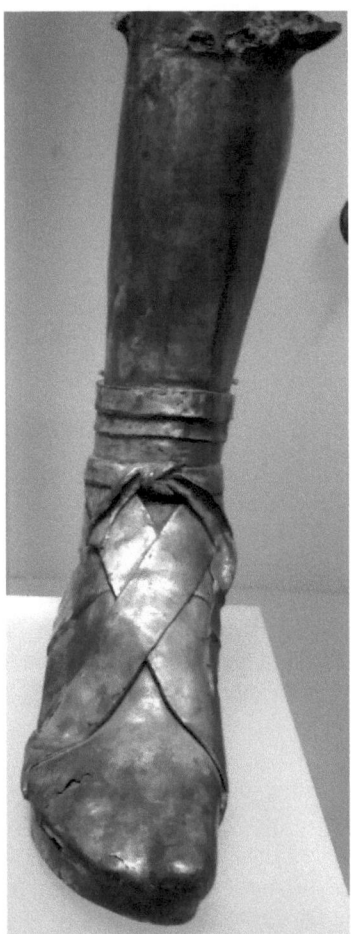

Figure 9.10: The Milsington leg, National Museum of Scotland (Photo: Author's own).

attached to the presence of the skeletons of an old dog and a young cat in the lowest layer of the well (1978: 209) and that the sculptures were just dumped (1978: 210). However, animal bone groups indicate structured deposition, possibly to mark a change in use of the well (Merrifield 1987: 32) and dogs are of particular significance (Morris 2008: 9). Since the deposited sculpture forms a distinct layer (Hammerson 1978: 208 fig.3), this sea-god's foot was probably preserved as a result of ritual deposition, forming the marker for part of the biography of this well.

9.6 Conclusions

This chapter has assessed the evidence for the significance of foot-fragments separated from the rest of the Roman sculpture of which they were a part, looking for patterns of selection, curation and symbolism. It has considered two issues: why the statuary was broken up and why the foot-fragments were retained, when the rest of the image has not been found.

Due to a lack of recording, or of access, or both, it has not been possible to ascertain how or why many of the statues were broken. It does appear, however, that the five principal ways in which an object may be broken recognised by fragmentation theory are represented here.

Doubtless some statues were damaged in the course of their use, or in uncertain times, as those from Corbridge appear to have been, and were disposed of or buried. It would also appear that some feet were taken as part of the 'ritual killing' of statues and carefully deposited, such as the Milsington leg.

Christian iconoclasm has been suggested as a reason for the destruction of carved images. Croxford argues that the many sculptures that have been deliberately fragmented make this interpretation unsound (2003: 93). Caseau says that it is easy to conclude that zealous Christians had a hand in the destruction of statues, but questions whether this was the main motivation (2011: 497). There is little evidence for Christian iconoclasm in this study's sample, which accords with Sauer's findings that, 'Apart from Mithraic art, there is astonishingly little evidence for iconoclasm in Britain' (2003: 60).

Caseau also suggests that some sculpture was broken up to be used as emergency building stone, a practical application which resembles iconoclasm but is not (2011: 498). There is some support for this in our sample, but it does not explain why the repurposed feet were still recognisable. The foot-fragments from Corbridge, for example, could have been crushed up a lot smaller for inclusion in the road. If the statues had been fragmented for purely economic reasons, surely the material would have been recycled in its entirety, with nothing being retained. Whatever the reason for the breakage of the sculptures, it appears that many fragments were not just discarded casually (Croxford 2003: 93).

Perhaps, then, as Croxford suggests, this is deliberate fragmentation to serve a new ritual or social purpose (2003: 93). Fulford acknowledges that such ideas permeate even the record of fairly prosaic acts (2001: 216). Each destructive episode was performed by people who made personal choices informed by notions of the image (Croxford 2016: 45). Russell agrees that there was a process of selection at work (2019: 130). Roman sculpture was polysemous and did not just portray individuals and deities (Gerrard 2015b: 198). It could demonstrate the status (Caseau 2011: 479) and patronage of powerful individuals (Gerrard 2015b: 198). We should, therefore, consider the synecdochical properties of the foot-fragments. When we look at the sample, we see that, with the exception of the grave *stelae*, all the foot-fragments come from sculpture depicting beings regarded by the Romans as divine, whether gods or emperors. The fragments may have been seen as possessing the same powers as the whole image (Croxford 2003: 93). Statuary could be seen as having apotropaic properties (Lavan 2011: 448; Gerrard 2015b: 198; Russell 2019: 131). There are many instances of feet being used as apotropaic symbols throughout this study. The talismanic qualities of statue fragments may point to why feet survived when the rest of the sculpture had disappeared. It seems likely that some foot-fragments were kept as representative of the whole statue, its qualities and powers.

It has to be admitted that no strong pattern emerges as to the significance surrounding the selection, curation or symbolism Roman of statue foot-fragments. As has been argued, some of the foot-fragments do indeed have some kind of demonstrable belief-based significance. Others may just have survived accidentally. The reason for this lack of a strong pattern may be due to the fact that the foot-fragments were made as part of a sculpture and repurposed, rather than deliberately manufactured as representations of feet and footwear. The previous and following chapters demonstrate much clearer patterns of the social significance of Roman representations of feet and footwear.

Table 9.1: The body fragment statistics from CSIR GB series 1.

CSIR GB	Area covered	Head	Eye	Headless	Upper Body	Lower body	Torso	Hand	Finger	Arm	Leg	Feet	Humanoid	Total Sculptures
1.1	Hadrian's Wall E. of North Tyne	40	0	5	22	10	17	4	0	8	10	10	170	355
1.2	Bath and Wessex	32	1	8	2	2	6	1	0	3	0	7	90	135
1.3	Yorkshire	10	0	5	5	1	3	1	0	0	1	7	67	114
1.4	Scotland	14	0	1	3	1	5	1	0	1	0	4	51	124
1.5	Wales	9	0	0	1	1	2	0	2	0	0	4	40	68
1.6	Hadrian's Wall W. of North Tyne	36	0	19	11	19	13	6	1	1	4	14	215	474
1.7	Cotswold Region, Devon & Cornwall	22	1	5	8	8	6	3	1	1	5	11	157	180
1.8	Eastern England	14	0	4	8	2	10	0	2	0	1	3	58	74
1.9	North West Midlands	13	1	8	6	2	5	4	2	2	2	6	85	154
1.10	London and the South-East	39	0	6	12	5	14	7	4	5	3	6	128	174
	Total numbers	229	3	61	78	51	81	27	12	21	26	72	1061	1852

Assessing the significance of Roman statue foot-fragments from Britain

Table 9.2: Cases where there is not enough information to interpret why the feet were preserved

Find Location	Represents	Chirality	Sculpture type	Footwear	Material	Date Made	Site Type	Find Setting	Current Location	Current Institution	Reference number	Literature	Notes
Aldborough	Venus	Right	Figurine	Bare	Other	Uncertain	Urban	Unknown				Millet, M. and Ferraby, R. (2021)	Pipe-clay figurine from Gaul.
Caerleon	Mercury	Pair	Relief	Bare	Stone	Uncertain	Military	Other	Caerleon	National Roman Legion Museum	31.78.	CSIR GB 1.5 no. 5	Found 1908 SW corner of E wing of building on sinistral side of principia. Oolitic limestone
Camelon	Uncertain	Left	Statue	Caliga	Stone	C1 CE	Military	Other	Edinburgh	NM Scotland	FX 312	CSIR GB 1.4 no. 162.	Found 1900 inside fort. Figure half life-size. Local sandstone. Cf sandalled foot from Corbridge (68)
Carlisle	Hercules	Left	Relief	Bare	Stone	C2 CE	Urban	Unknown	Carlisle	Tullie House		CSIR GB 1.6 no. 480	Found c.1970. Local sandstone. C2-C3. No details of exact provenance
Carlisle	Cautes	Right	Statue	Calceus	Stone	C3 CE	Urban	Religious	Carlisle	Tullie House	CALMG: 1894.154	CSIR GB 1.6 no. 483	Antiquarian find, English St. (2m down). Red sandstone. Deo Cauti Iu[lius] / Archietus [d(ono) d(edit)] Only British dedication to Cautes
Carlisle	Deity	Pair	Relief	Uncertain	Stone	C3 CE	Military	Unknown	Carlisle	Tullie House		CSIR GB 1.6 no. 518	Found 1981 on Annetwell St. site. Probably deity due to scale. Local sandstone.
Carlisle	Deity	Right	Statue	Calceus	Stone	C3 CE	Urban	Unknown	Carlisle	Tullie House		CSIR GB 1.6 no. 515	Found Carlisle 1980 on Keays Lane site in late Roman level.
Carvoran Magna	Cybele	Pair	Statue	Bare	Stone	C2 CE	Military	Other	Chollerford	Chesters Museum		CSIR GB 1.6 no. 116	Found 1902 inside fort. C2-C3
Chester-le-Street	Vulcan	Pair	Relief	Bare	Stone	Uncertain	Military	Unknown	Chester-le-Street	Ankers House		CSIR GB 1.11 (forthcoming)	Lower part of a cloaked but otherwise naked figure standing on an anvil. Sandstone.

Roman Feet and Shoes

Find Location	Represents	Chirality	Sculpture type	Footwear	Material	Date Made	Site Type	Find Setting	Current Location	Current Institution	Reference number	Literature	Notes
Cirencester	Diana	Pair	Statue	Calceus	Stone	Uncertain	Urban	Industrial	Cirencester	Corinium Museum	C2751	CSIR GB 1.7 no.23b.	Found Ashcroft 1899 with other statues and an inscription. Oolitic limestone
Corbridge	Victory	Pair	Relief	Bare	Stone	Uncertain	Military	Unknown	Corbridge	Corbridge Museum		CSIR GB 1.1 no.45	Buff sandstone. C2-C3
High Rochester	Uncertain	Left	Statue	Bare	Stone	Uncertain	Military	Other	Newcastle	GNM: Hancock	NEWMA: 1958.50.	CSIR GB 1.1 no. 323	Buff sandstone. C2-C3
Housesteads	Neptune	Pair	Relief	Bare	Stone	C2 CE	Military	Water	Chollerford	Chesters Museum		CSIR GB 1.6 no. 87	Found 1911 in latrine pit in SE corner of fort. Local sandstone. C2-C2.
London	Serapis?	Right	Statue	Sandal	Marble	Uncertain	Urban	Unknown	London	Unknown		CSIR GB 1.10 no.49.	Excavated on the site of Arundel House in the Strand 1972 (ARH72). Last recorded at the Howard Hotel, the Strand. Possibly votive.
London	Deity	Right	Statue	Bare	Copper Alloy	Uncertain	Unknown	Unknown	London	British Museum	1924, 1213.41.	CSIR GB 1.10 no.224.	Over life-sized statue. C1-C3. Kingsway area more than 1km beyond W boundary of Roman city – more likely product of recent collecting than genuine antiquity from Londinium.
Malton	Uncertain	Pair	Figurine	Bare	Stone	Uncertain	Urban	Unknown	Malton	Malton Museum		CSIR GB 1.3 no.115.	No reliable date. Found in the civilian settlement. Limestone.
Silchester	God/Emperor	Right	Statue	Panzer boot	Stone	Uncertain	Urban	Religious?	Reading	Reading Museum	3702	CSIR GB 1.2 no.147.	Found 1882 in or near forum. 1.5 x life-size. Limestone.
Silchester	Uncertain	Left	Figurine	Calceus	Stone	Uncertain	Urban	Unknown	Reading	Reading Museum	3711	CSIR GB 1.2 no.151.	Exact provenance uncertain. Chalk (?)
Stanwix	Victory	Left	Statue	Sandal	Stone	C2 CE	Military	Other	Newcastle	GNM: Hancock	NEWMA: 1856.17	CSIR GB 1.6 no. 104	Found before 1856. Local sandstone.

Find Location	Represents	Chirality	Sculpture type	Footwear	Material	Date Made	Site Type	Find Setting	Current Location	Current Institution	Reference number	Literature	Notes
York	Uncertain	Left	Figurine	Bare	Copper Alloy	Uncertain	Urban	Unknown	York	Yorkshire Museum	YORYM: 2012.377		
York	Fortuna	Pair	Figurine	Solea	Stone	Uncertain	Urban	Unknown	York	Yorkshire Museum	YORYM: 2007.6161	CSIR GB 1.3 no.1.	Found 1831 York nr. Legionary fortress wall NE of multangular tower in St. Leonard's Place.
York	Deity?	Pair	Figurine	Bare	Stone	Uncertain	Urban	Unknown	York	Yorkshire Museum	YORYM: 2007.6152	CSIR GB 1.3 no.111	Found 1954 York, 9 Blossom St. during road works. Limestone.
York	Uncertain	Right	Statue	Uncertain	Stone	Uncertain	Urban	Unknown	York	Yorkshire Museum		CSIR GB 1.3 no.112.	Found Trinity Yard, Micklegate, 1736. Pedestal with illegible inscription and right foot only.

Table 9.3: Foot-fragments repurposed as building stone in the Roman era

Find Location	Represents	Chirality	Sculpture type	Footwear	Material	Date Made	Site Type	Find Setting	Current Location	Current Institution	Reference no.	Literature	Notes
Birrens	Victory	Pair	Relief	Solea	Stone	C2 CE	Military	Other	Edinburgh	NM Scotland	FP 16	CSIR GB 1.4 no. 27b.	Fragment of commemorative slab.
Caerwent	Mars Lenus	Pair	Statue	Bare	Stone	C2 CE	Urban	Domestic	Newport	Museum and Art Gallery		CSIR GB 1.5 no. 13 RIB 309	Found 1904 House XVIII.iiS re-used in dividing wall. Oolitic limestone.
Carlisle	Genius	Left	Relief	Bare	Stone	C3 CE	Urban	Unknown	Carlisle	Tullie House	LAL D 480, ST 17	CSIR GB 1.6 no. 471 RIB 3463	Found 1980, Laws Lane Carlisle in a late Roman level used as post packing. Local sandstone. Possibly base of altar
Carlisle	Deity?	Pair	Relief	Uncertain	Stone	C3 CE	Military	Unknown	Carlisle	Tullie House		CSIR Gb 1.6, no. 518	Relief of human (?) figure - probably deity due to scale. Found 1981 on Annetwell St. site in C3 context. Local sandstone.
Corbridge	Mercury	Right	Relief	Uncertain	Stone	Uncertain	Urban	Other	Corbridge	Corbridge Museum		CSIR GB 1.1 no. 18. RIB 1133	Theodosian level of main E-W street south of east granary Buff sandstone

Find Location	Represents	Chirality	Sculpture type	Footwear	Material	Date Made	Site Type	Find Setting	Current Location	Current Institution	Reference no.	Literature	Notes
Corbridge	Victory	Pair	Statue	Bare	Stone	Uncertain	Military	Other	Corbridge	Corbridge Museum		CSIR GB 1.1 no.41 Haverfield, F.J. (1914): 514 no.58.	Buff sandstone. Road ballast. C2-C3.
Corbridge	God/Emperor	Right	Statue	Caliga	Stone	Uncertain	Military	Other	Corbridge	Corbridge Museum		CSIR GB 1.1 no.152 Haverfield, F.J. (1914): 514 nos.55-57.	Buff sandstone. Road ballast. C2-C3.
Corbridge	Uncertain	Pair	Figurine	Uncertain	Stone	Uncertain	Military	Other	Unknown	Unknown		CSIR GB 1.1 no.151 Haverfield, F.J. (1914): 514 no.59.	Carving now lost. Road ballast. C2-C3.
Corbridge	Uncertain	Right	Statue	Uncertain	Stone	Uncertain	Military	Other	Unknown	Unknown		CSIR GB 1.1 no.153 Haverfield, F.J. (1914): 514 nos.55-57.	Carving now lost. Road ballast. C2-C3
Corbridge	Uncertain	Uncertain	Statue	Uncertain	Stone	Uncertain	Military	Other	Unknown	Unknown		CSIR GB 1.1 no.154 Haverfield, F.J. (1914)	Carving now lost. Road ballast. C2-C3
Maryport	Vulcan	Pair	Relief	Calceus	Stone	C2 CE	Military	Religious?	Maryport	Senhouse Roman Museum	1993.4.	CSIR GB 1.11 (forthcoming)	Found 1870 in Post Pit [2475]. Lower part of a male figure with naked legs wearing open-toed boots. Re-used as packing

Assessing the significance of Roman statue foot-fragments from Britain

Table 9.4: Roman sculpted feet repurposed after the Roman era

Find Location	Represents	Chirality	Sculpture type	Footwear	Material	Date Made	Site Type	Find Setting	Current Location	Current Institution	Reference No.	Literature	Notes
Birrens	Victory	Pair	Relief	Solea	Stone	C2 CE	Military	Other	Edinburgh	NM Scotland	FV21	CSIR GB 1.4 no. 26a.	Fragment of commemorative slab. First reported 1760 built into wall at Hoddom Castle. Other fragments recovered from courtyard of HQ Birrens fort 1895.
Carlisle	Goddess	Left	Relief	Solea	Stone	C3 CE	Military	Unknown	Carlisle	Tullie House		CSIR GB 1.6 no. 516	Found 1981 Annetwell St. in post-Roman context. Probably deity due to scale. Style of sandal indicates female. Local sandstone.
Irchester	Deities	Pair	Relief	Calceus	Stone	Uncertain	Urban	Unknown	Irchester	Chester House Farm		CSIR GB 1.9, no.6c. Woodfield, P. (1978)	Fragments of an octagonal stone with reliefs of the gods of the week. Found 1879 Burrow Fields excavations.
Gloucester	Deity	Pair	Relief	Calceus	Stone	Uncertain	Urban	Unknown	Gloucester	City Museum		CSIR Great Britain 1.7, no.135.	Altar or relief with figure of deity. Unstratified. Built into wall at St. Oswald's priory.
Uley	Mercury	Pair	Altar	Uncertain	Stone	Uncertain	Villa/rural	Religious	London	British Museum	1978, 0102.11.	CSIR GB 1.7 no. 73. RIB 3056.	Found 1978 temple of Mercury. Re-used as post-Roman building stone in C5 building

129

Table 9.5: Preserved statue feet from Roman villas

Find Location	Represents	Chirality	Sculpture type	Footwear	Material	Date Made	Site Type	Find Setting	Current Location	Current Institution	Reference	Literature	Notes
Bancroft Villa	Uncertain	Right	Statue	Bare	Marble	Uncertain	Villa/rural	Funerary?	Milton Keynes	Archaeological Unit		CSIR GB 1.7 no.7.	Possibly from the temple-mausoleum
Chedworth	Diana	Pair	Statue	Sandal	Stone	Uncertain	Villa/rural	Domestic	Chedworth	Site museum	NT 73979	CSIR GB 1.7 no.22.	Found room 5 (probably triclinium). Oolitic limestone.
Chedworth	Lar	Pair	Statue	Calceus	Stone	Uncertain	Villa/rural	Domestic	Chedworth	Site Museum	NT 73980	CSIR GB 1.7 no.43.	Found room 5 (probably triclinium). Oolitic limestone.
Chedworth	Deity?	Pair	Statue	Calceus	Stone	Uncertain	Villa/rural	Domestic	Chedworth	Site Museum	NT 74005	CSIR GB 1.7 no.149.	Only feet remain on a pedestal. Oolitic limestone.
Chilgrove	Fortuna?	Pair	Figurine	Calceus	Stone	Uncertain	Villa/rural	Domestic	Chichester	Novium Museum		CSIR GB 1.2 no.101.	Found 1964 during excavations at Brickkiln Farm, Chilgrove nr. Chichester. Limestone.
Colerne Park	Mater	Pair	Relief	Calceus	Stone	C4 CE	Villa/rural	Domestic	Bath	Roman Baths		CSIR GB 1.2 no.121. RIB 3052	Found 1954. Oolitic limestone. Inscription: Ing(enuus) Fabillí [...]
Wadfield	Uncertain	Right	Figurine	Bare	Stone	Uncertain	Villa/rural	Domestic	Unknown	Unknown		CSIR GB 1.7 no.152.	Found 1863
Woodchester	Youth	Pair	Statue	Bare	Marble	C4 CE	Villa/rural	Domestic	Unknown	Unknown		CSIR GB 1.7 no. 6	Found by Lysons, 1793, room 25. Grey marble. Possibly Meleager or Bacchus.

Assessing the significance of Roman statue foot-fragments from Britain

Table 9.6: Foot-fragments associated with Roman religious activity

Find Location	Represents	Chirality	Sculpture type	Footwear	Material	Date Made	Site Type	Find Setting	Current Location	Current Institution	Reference no.	Literature	Notes
Bath	Female	Left	Relief	Bare	Stone	Uncertain	Urban	Religious	Bath	Roman Baths		CSIR GB 1.2 no.7. RIB 141	Block from architectural façade of four seasons, precinct of Minerva. Found 1790 during building of Pump Rooms. Oolitic limestone. Later Roman period.
Caernarfon	Mars?	Pair	Relief	Bare	Stone	Uncertain	Military	Religious	Caernarfon	Segontium Fort		CSIR GB 1.5, no. 8. Wheeler, R.E.M. (1923)	Found 1922 in strong-room under *aedes* in HQ building with altar to Minerva. Grey sandstone.
Camerton	Female	Pair	Figurine	Calceus	Stone	Uncertain	Villa/ rural	Religious?	Unknown	Unknown		CSIR GB 1.2 no.156. Haverfield, F.J. (1906)	Found 1814-1815 in excavation of large building (temple?). Now lost.
Carrawburgh	Cautopates	Pair	Statue	Calceus	Stone	C3 CE	Military	Religious	Newcastle	GNM: Hancock	NEWMA: 1956.10.48	CSIR GB 1.6, no. 112	Found 1950 southern end of west bench in nave of Mithraeum. Local sandstone.
Cirencester	Mater	Pair	Statue	Calceus	Stone	C3 CE	Urban	Religious	Cirencester	Corinium Museum	1980/109/ 2180	CSIR GB 1.7 no.121. McWhirr, A., Viner, L. and Wells, C. (1982)	Found 1973 roadside building on Fosse Way, SE of Bath Gate (CT107). Seated figure. Nothing remains above knees. Appears single, not in a three. Oolitic limestone.
Corbridge	Minerva	Uncertain	Statue	Uncertain	Stone	Uncertain	Urban	Unknown	Unknown	Unknown		CSIR GB 1.1 no.29 RIB 1134	Buff sandstone. Now lost.

Roman Feet and Shoes

Find Location	Represents	Chirality	Sculpture type	Footwear	Material	Date Made	Site Type	Find Setting	Current Location	Current Institution	Reference no.	Literature	Notes
London	Goddess	Left	Statue	Sandal	Copper Alloy	C2 CE	Urban	Religious	London	Museum of London	LLS02[13563] <3147>	CSIR GB 1.10 no. 223.	From Tabard Square. Associated with Romano-British temples.
Maiden Castle	Diana	Pair	Figurine	Bare	Marble	Uncertain	Villa/rural	Religious	Dorchester	Dorset County Museum		CSIR GB 1.2 no.98.	Found 1936 SW of temple in centre of Maiden Castle among C4 debris.
Vindolanda	Deity	Pair	Statue	Bare	Stone	Uncertain	Military	Religious	Vindolanda	Vindolanda museum	SF10231	Birley, A. and Blake, J. (2007)	Unidentified deity found 2005-6 in pit inside tenemos.
Wallsend	Mercury	Pair	Relief	Bare	Stone	C2 CE	Military	Religious	Newcastle	GNM: Hancock	1894.02.	CSIR GB 1.1 no.202 RIB 1303	Found in allotments about 300m west of fort. Buff sandstone.
Whitley Castle	Hercules	Pair	Statue	Uncertain	Stone	Uncertain	Military	Religious?	Unknown	Unknown		CSIR GB 1.11 (forthcoming) Sopwith, T. (1833)	Found 1803 near NE corner of fort with altar RIB 1199. Sandstone.
Woodeaton	Mars	Pair	Relief	Calceus	Stone	C2 CE	Villa/rural	Religious	Oxford	Ashmolean Museum	1896-1908. R.337	Aldhouse-Green, M.J (1976) CSIR 1.7 no 61 pl.19	Fragmentary stone with relief of Mars. Temple and fairground site. Green Schist

132

Assessing the significance of Roman statue foot-fragments from Britain

Table 9.7: Roman sculpted feet preserved by ritual/religious deposition

Find Location	Represents	Chirality	Sculpture type	Footwear	Material	Date Made	Site Type	Find Setting	Current Location	Current Institution	Reference	Literature	Notes
Caer Gai	Deity	Pair	Relief	Bare	Stone	C2 CE	Military	Funerary	Cardiff	National Museum of Wales	55.411/2-4	CSIR GB 1.5 no. 7 RIB 418	Found 1885 NE of auxiliary fort in area of known cemetery. Thought to depict Hercules and Nemean lion or Bacchic procession with panther. Red sandstone
Carlisle	Woman	Pair	Gravestone	Calceus	Stone	C3 CE	Urban	Funerary	Carlisle	Tullie House	CALMG: 1999.38	CSIR GB 1.6 no. 492 RIB 958	Gravestone of Anicia Lucilla. Found 1852 Botchergate
Chalford	Uncertain	Pair	Statue	Uncertain	Stone	Uncertain	Villa/rural	Religious?	Stroud	Museum in the Park		CSIR GB 1.7 no.136.	
Chester	Man	Pair	Gravestone	Caliga?	Stone	C1 CE	Urban	Funerary	Chester	Grosvenor Museum	CHEGM: 999 6 67	CSIR GB1.9, no.45. RIB 524	Grave-stele of L. Camulius Albanus. Found 1891 North Wall. Mason's tools roughly outlined at feet. Sandstone
Chester	Man	Pair	Gravestone	Calceus	Stone	Uncertain	Urban	Funerary	Chester	Grosvenor Museum		CSIR GB 1.9 no.50. Thompson, F.H. (1969)	Found 1961-2 Linenhall St. Trench 1, layer 2 in a medieval context to do with C3 rebuilding of fortress wall. Sandstone.
Chester	Man	Right	Gravestone	Calceus	Stone	C2 CE	Urban	Funerary	Chester	Grosvenor Museum	CHEGM: 1999 6 136	CSIR GB 1.9 no.58. Haverfield, F.J. (1900): 69 no.136.	Grave stele of a horseman. Antiquarian find from North Wall. Sandstone.
Chester	Woman	Pair	Gravestone	Calceus	Stone	C3 CE	Urban	Funerary	Chester	Grosvenor Museum	CHEGM: 1999 6 123	CSIR GB 1.9 no.77.	Grave-relief of a woman. Antiquarian find from North Wall. Sandstone.
Colchester	Togatus	Pair	Gravestone	Calceus	Stone	Uncertain	Urban	Funerary	Colchester	Colchester and Essex Museums		CSIR GB 1.8 no.61. Hull, M.R. (1958): 253 no.36.	Fragment of a tombstone. Found Western Cemetery, Manor. Rd.

133

Roman Feet and Shoes

Find Location	Represents	Chirality	Sculpture type	Footwear	Material	Date Made	Site Type	Find Setting	Current Location	Current Institution	Reference	Literature	Notes
London	Neptune/ Oceanus	Left	Statue	Bare	Marble	C2 CE	Urban	Water	London	Cuming Museum		CSIR GB 1.10 no.8.	Found 1977 Southwark Cathedral Roman well in crypt (site code SCC77).
London	Ganymede?	Right	Relief	Bare	Stone	Uncertain	Urban	Water	London	Museum of London	80.325/31a	CSIR GB 1.10, no.163.	Carved block from the Screen of gods. Found 1975 Baynard's Castle, Upper Thames St. Roman riverside wall. Barnack Stone
London	Vulcn and Minerva	Pairs	Relief	Calceus	Stone	Uncertain	Urban	Water	London	Museum of London	80.325/32	CSIR GB 1.10, no.164.	Carved block from the Screen of gods. Found 1975 Baynard's Castle, Upper Thames St. Roman riverside wall. Barnack Stone
Milsington	Emperor	Right	Statue	Calceus	Copper Alloy	C2 CE	Villa/ rural	Water	Edinburgh	National Museum of Scotland	X.1920.1	CSIR GB 1.4 no.45. Hunter, F. (2017)	Equestrian statue - probably imperial. Gilded. About 50cm tall. Statue carefully dismantled. Found in a bog with another copper alloy fragment.
Stanwix	Mercury	Pair	Relief	Sandal	Stone	C2 CE	Military	Funerary	Carlisle	Tullie House	CALMG: 1936.30.1.	CSIR GB 1.6 no. 481 RIB 952	Found 1936 90 m. west of the Near Boot Inn, Whiteclosegate, Carlisle, with a jar and the base of a cinerary urn. Inscribed DM / CIS.
Wroxeter	Man	Pair	Gravestone	Caliga	Stone	C1 CE	Urban	Funerary	Shrewsbury	Shrewsbury Museum	SHYMS: A/ 1994/ 001/005	CSIR GB 1.9: 47. RIB 292. Wright, T. (1872)	Found Roman cemetery 1861. Memorial to Titus Flaminius of 14th Gemina
York	Man	Right	Gravestone	Caliga	Stone	Uncertain	Urban	Funerary	York	Yorkshire Museum	YORYM: 2007.6145	CSIR GB 1.3 no.113. RCHM (1962) Eburacum: 128	Found 1860 or before Driffield Estate, Mount School, York at intersection of 2 Roman roads. Gritstone. Footwear dates it to before AD 200.

10

Discussion and Conclusions

This work has examined why the Romans chose foot iconography for decorative objects, considering *en route* the ideological significance of feet and footwear in the Roman world and what we might learn from shoe-shaped Roman artefacts about the identity and beliefs of the people who owned them. The evidence came from a corpus of 1,492 Roman representations of feet and footwear across 12 categories (Figure 10.1). The study examined the deposition of actual footwear in 18,465 Roman graves and 1,311 Roman wells to explore its ritual significance. It considered the significance of Roman hobnailing patterns and how this was extended to depictions of hobnailing. While there are many studies of Roman lamps and brooches, for example, specific studies of small groups of foot- or shoe-shaped artefacts are very rare, and nobody has studied them in such great detail as this before. The study built on previous research by synthesising, and adding to, earlier findings, and has, therefore, filled a substantial gap in our knowledge.

This chapter presents an overview of the study's findings in terms of the chronological, geographical, and find-setting distribution of Roman foot- and shoe-shaped artefacts. It discusses the major strands of significance: the ritual use of foot-shaped objects, including funerary, religious, and other votive use, feet as *pars pro toto*, and their apotropaic role. It will be seen that there is a considerable amount of overlap between these three strands. The chapter also summarizes the significance of chirality and hobnailing, and considers how far the evidence from Roman authors for the significance of footwear applies to the north-western provinces.

10.1 Chronological distribution

The corpus of foot-shaped artefacts contains 1,492 items dating from as early as the second century BCE and as late as the fifth century CE. It should be noted that, of these, 243 (16%) have an uncertain date, either due to lack of recording, or lack of dating evidence with the find. On average, the majority of the corpus artefacts date to the second century CE, with most of the rest from either the first or third centuries CE (Figure 10.2). This is, however, an over simplification, since the date range tends to vary for different objects (Figure 10.3). Lamps in the shape of feet peak in the first century, and again in the fourth. Sandal *fibulae* are predominantly second century, while jugs where the handle terminates in feet are principally from the third century, and most knife or razor handles ending in a foot are late third and early fourth century. It is also worth remembering, as we have already seen, that foot-shaped artefacts featured in Ancient Egyptian, Ancient Greek, and Iron Age European iconography. Such items also continue after the Roman era, for example, a double-sole-shaped stamp in the Ashmolean Museum that dates to the fifth or sixth century (AN1873.131).

We have also seen evidence for the curation of sandal *fibulae* into the seventh century. Roman foot-shaped

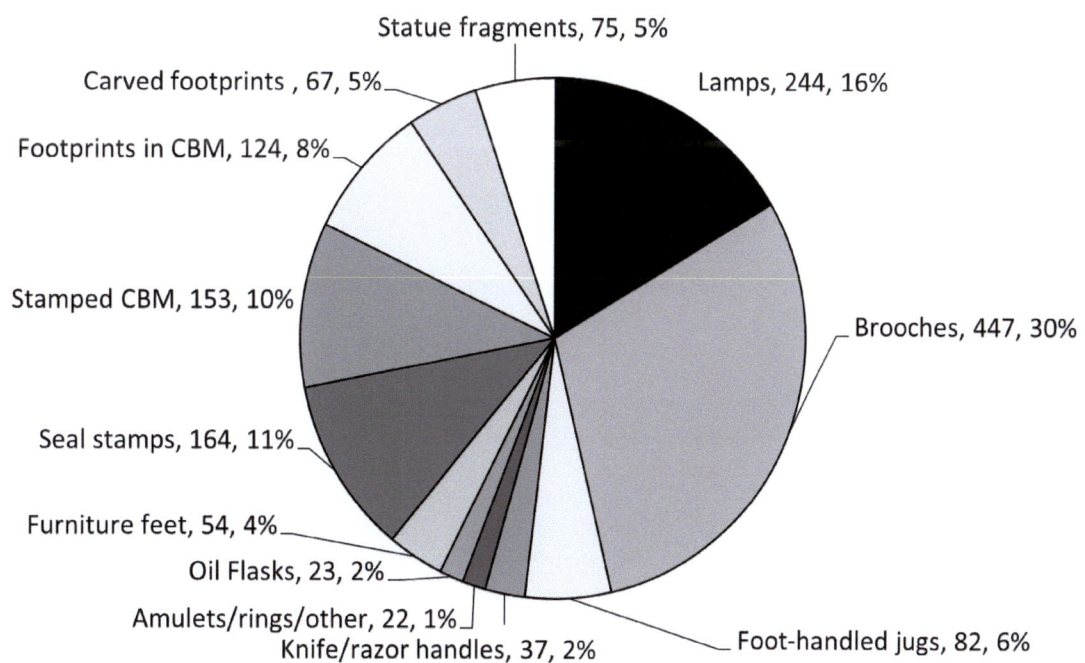

Figure 10.1: Chart to show the artefact type of 1,492 Roman foot-shaped objects.

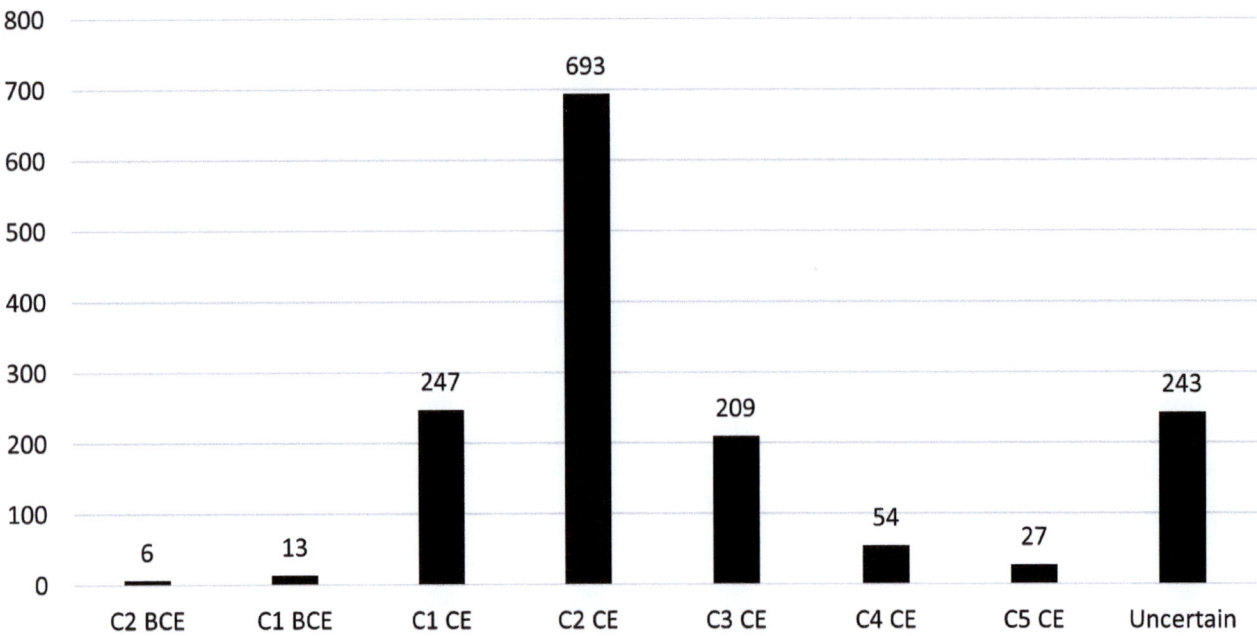

Figure 10.2: Chart to show the date-range of 1,492 Roman foot-shaped artefacts.

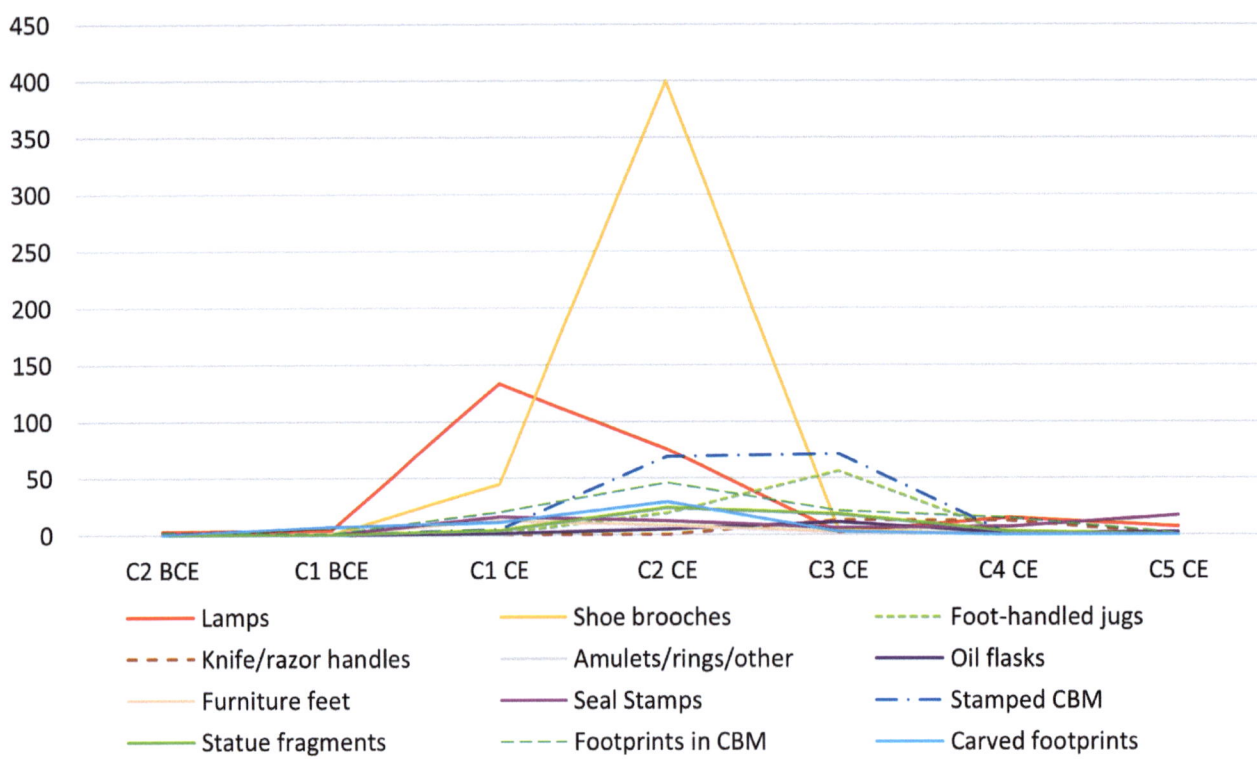

Figure 10.3: Chart to show the known date-range of 1,249 Roman foot-shaped artefacts.

artefacts seem part of a long tradition, although the Roman forms are substantially different from their predecessors, especially those depicting hobnailing, in that the feet and shoes tend to be depicted more realistically, and there is a greater range of symbolism.

10.2 Geographical distribution

Some types of Roman foot- and shoe-shaped artefact were found across the empire, particularly lamps and carved footprints (Figure 10.4). Others, for example, sandal *fibulae*, knife/razor handles, and jugs whose handles terminate in feet, mostly occur in the north-western provinces and along the Danube (Figure 10.5). Indeed, 703 (51%) of the study's 1,492 objects were found in the north-western provinces, with a further 250 (17%) coming from the Danube region. One should, however, bear in mind that metal small finds in particular are much less well published in Spain, Italy and in eastern Europe, and any such papers may be less accessible to some scholars due to language barriers (Eckardt 2022: personal comment).

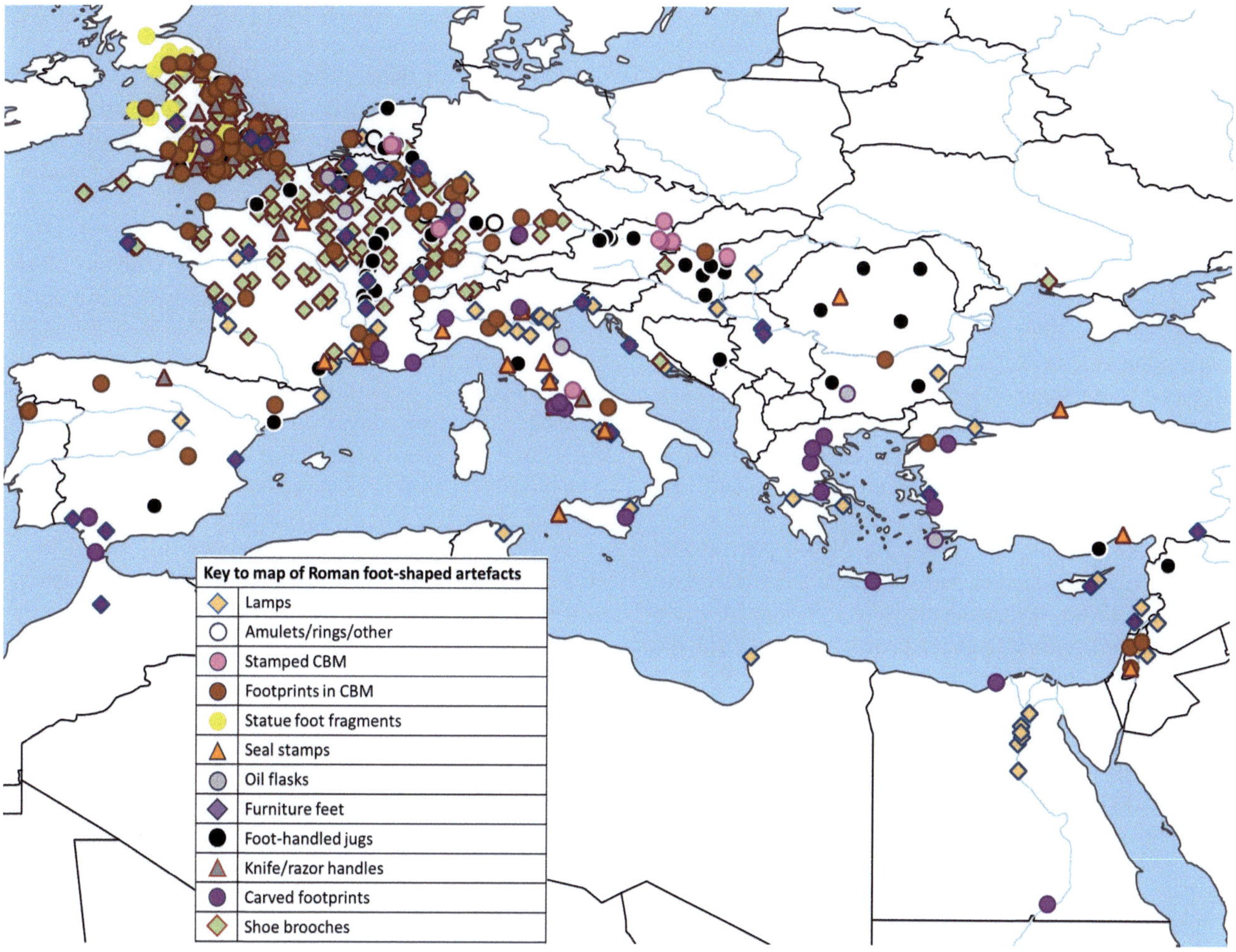

Discussion and Conclusions

Figure 10.4: Distribution map of 1,145 Roman foot-shaped artefacts with a known find location.

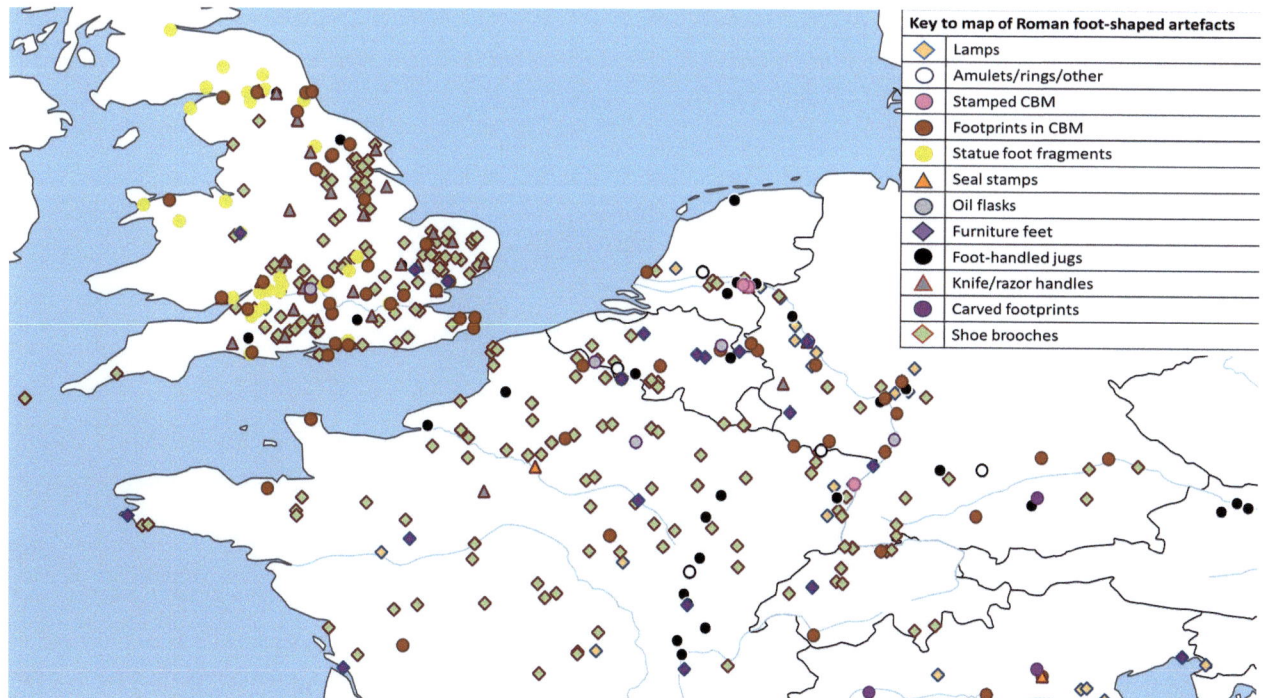

Figure 10.5: Distribution map of Roman foot-shaped artefacts from the north-western provinces.

As with the lack of recorded dates, we should note that 347 (25.3%) of the 1,492 foot-shaped artefacts have no exact find location. If just the 1,143 objects with a known find location are taken into account, almost 70% of the corpus comes from the north-western provinces. This points to a special significance for Roman foot- and shoe-shaped artefacts in this study's target region.

10.3 Distribution of site types and find settings

Apart from rare inscriptions, the key to interpreting the social significance of Roman foot- and shoe-shaped artefacts is applying contextual archaeological theory and analysing the type of site and setting in which they were found (Figure 10.6). This section will only comment on the proportions of the different site types and find settings, while the significances will be discussed below. As explained earlier, the categories are very broad and tend to lump sites together, and some objects could belong in several categories simultaneously. Nevertheless, the site types and find settings do provide evidence for the significance of foot-shaped artefacts. Once again, the data are sometimes not recorded, in this case for 537 (36%) site types and 810 (54%) find settings of the 1,492 objects in the corpus (Figure 10.7). Once these are removed from consideration, we are left with 953 foot-shaped artefacts with a known site type and 681 with a known find setting.

As has already been observed, the distinction between different site types is not always clearly defined. Of this study's site types, the largest and most nebulous category is 'urban', which accounts for 491 (51%) objects with a known site type. The next largest is 'military', accounting for 311 (33%). This could indicate a possible link between the Roman army and the significance of foot-shaped artefacts, which may represent power and authority, or be a religious or apotropaic symbol. However, there is an excavation bias towards military and urban sites (Cool and Baxter 2016: 9). Villa/rural sites account for at least 142 (15%) artefacts with a known site type, although this may be more due to 89 finds from the PAS database.

With regard to the known find settings (Figure 10.8), 84 (12%) are 'domestic' and 154 (23%) from industrial settings, many of them potteries or tile works. Settings labelled 'other', which covers a range of contexts including a classroom, a rubbish dump, a doctor's surgery, two sand quarries, theatres, amphitheatres, and ditches, account for 183 (27%).

One hundred and four of the foot-shaped objects (15%) come from a funerary setting, being found either in a grave or part of a cemetery, and 129 (19%) were found in temples or shrines. In addition, 28 items (2%) came from watery places such as wells, rivers, and bogs, and may have been votive offerings. This means that almost half of the Roman foot-shaped artefacts with a known find setting may have been used in ritual activities. Such settings will be discussed in the following sections.

10.4 The ritual significance of Roman representations of feet and footwear

This section summarizes the ritual significance of foot- and shoe-shaped artefacts deposited in temples, shrines and other sanctuaries, and those given as offerings in watery places. It also gives a résumé of the meaning of foot-shaped objects deposited in funerary settings.

10.4.1 Foot-shaped artefacts found in sanctuaries

Foot- and shoe-shaped artefacts seem to have been considered appropriate offerings at temples and shrines. Of the corpus as a whole, 129 (23% of those with a known find setting) fit these criteria. It is possible that some from an unknown find setting also fall into this category. Like the variation of dating between different object types, some foot-shaped artefacts are more commonly found in temples and shrines than others. One of the largest categories, perhaps unsurprisingly, is carved footprints, where 41 of the 67 (61%) are known to come from shrines or temples. It is worth bearing in mind that these do skew the data. In addition, of those with an unknown find setting,

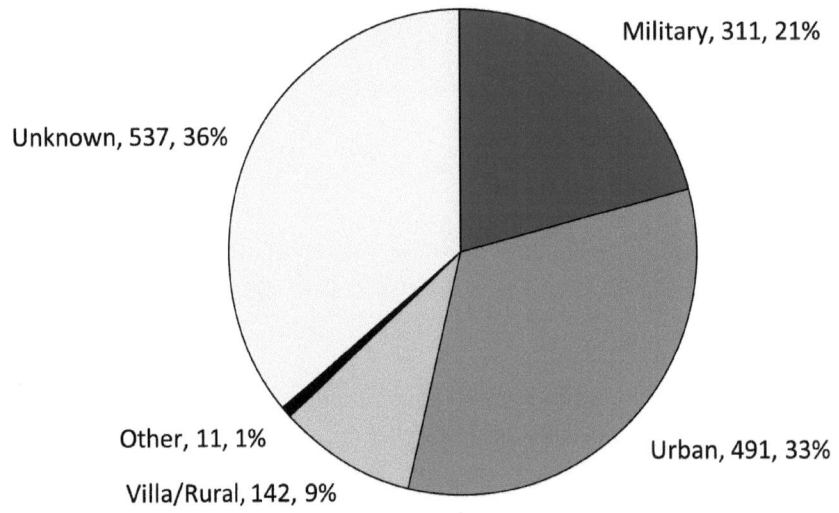

Figure 10.6: Chart to show the site type of 1,492 Roman foot-shaped artefacts.

Discussion and Conclusions

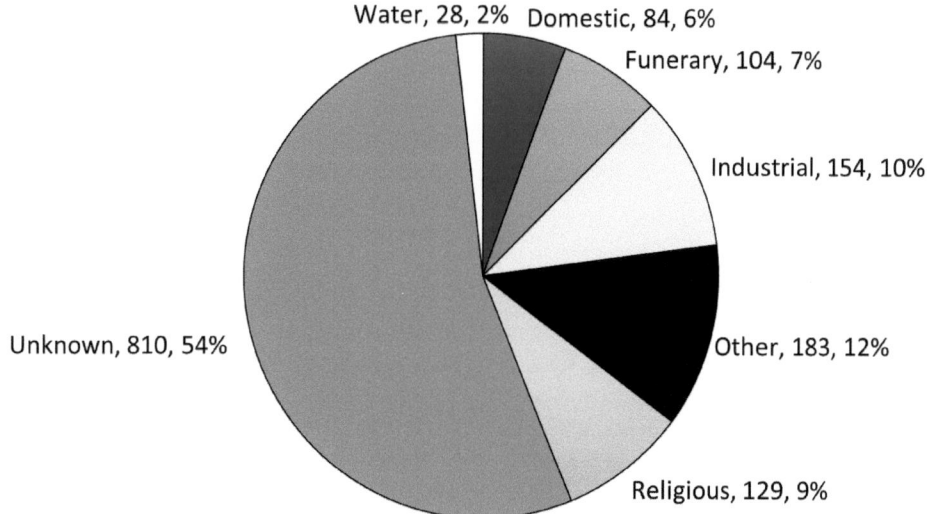

Figure 10.7: Chart to show the find setting of all 1,492 Roman foot-shaped artefacts.

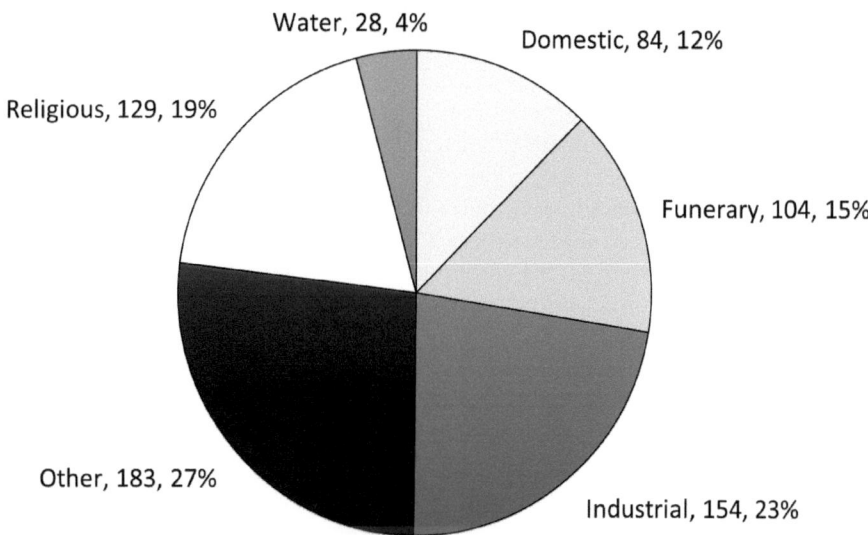

Figure 10.8: Chart to show the known find setting of 682 Roman foot-shaped artefacts.

six are thought to depict the feet of Isis, two Serapis, two Caelestis, and four Dexiva, a deity from Gaul. These footprints are polysemous and may represent the presence of a divinity, or of a pilgrim in the sanctuary. They may also be votives in thanks for healing or a safe journey.

The other largest category is sandal *fibulae*, with 41 found in temples or sanctuaries (26.5% of shoe brooches with a known find setting). As items of personal adornment, they may have been convenient offerings which could simply be unclasped and given. They may also have been pilgrim badges (Johns 1995: 104; Allason-Jones 2015: 79; Eckardt 2013: 221), or carried the same meanings as carved footprints. Indeed, these ideas of feet as a proxy for a being, or as votives for a safe journey, apply across the range of artefacts.

10.4.2 Offerings in watery places

The widespread Roman 'practice of depositing valuables in watery places' (Merrifield 1987: 24) has been discussed throughout this book. One of the first case studies was that of actual shoes deposited in Roman wells, which could be votives, signs of a contract between depositor and divinity (Driel-Murray 1999a: 137), or appropriate markers for the biography of wells (van Driel-Murray 2011a: 337; van Haasteren and Groot 2013: 25). Foot- and shoe-shaped artefacts have also been found deposited in watery places. Of the corpus as a whole, 28 (4% of those with a known find setting) are recorded as being deposited in wells, springs, rivers or bogs. These comprise 18 jugs with handles terminating in feet, which may have been made specifically for ritual purposes (Crummy 2011: 114), including purification. The feet on the handles made them more appropriate as votive offerings. Other items found in watery settings are a knife/razor handle that forms part of the ritual assemblage from the river Tees, and an oil flask known as the 'Hardwick boot'. Additionally, five statue foot-fragments came from a bog near Milsington, Scotland, a Roman well in the crypt of Southwark Cathedral, and the Roman riverside wall of London. Finally, a shoe brooch was found deposited in the Walbrook, London, together with a model *caduceus*, linking it to Mercury, and two further sandal *fibulae* may be fen-edge votives (Eckardt 2013: 224, 226). These artefacts deposited in or near watery places were seen as appropriate votive offerings, possibly because they represent the feet of the donor or the deity concerned.

10.4.3 Funerary feet and footwear

Actual Roman shoes are found in burials, both worn by the deceased and placed. This study has found 1,756 Roman graves containing evidence of footwear, both leather and hobnails, and this sample is not exhaustive. Shoes in Roman graves both provide the dead with footwear for the afterlife, and protect them on their journey to the Underworld (see Chapter 4). Foot- and shoe-shaped artefacts in burials serve a dual purpose, both as grave furniture and as the provision of footwear, albeit symbolic. As we have already seen, not all categories of foot-shaped artefact are found in funerary settings. However, 104 examples in the corpus (15% of those with a known find setting) were. The largest group is 33 lamps in the shape of feet. These would have formed part of the burial rites (Bailey 1963: 12; Eckardt 2000: 16; Philpott 1991: 192), provided light in the darkness of death, and were a proxy for actual footwear (Pirling *et al.* 2006: 409). Sandal *fibulae* were both worn on the body and deposited separately after burial, and there are 24 funerary examples in the corpus. They also symbolise footwear and may have provided protection on the journey to the Underworld. This is also the case for the few oil flasks found in burials, which may also have symbolised luxury. Likewise the sets of furniture feet from tombs, some of which were emblems of power, since they were attached to *curule* chairs and feet were emblems of domination.

Of the 82 jugs with handles ending in feet, 14 of the corpus (17%) were found in funerary settings. They are linked to burial rites involving purification and feasting. Since the feet are mostly bare, it is more likely that these provided the protection of a deity on the journey, rather than symbolising shoes. The same may be said for the six carved footprints from tombs. Two of these depict the feet of Isis and one of Serapis, both deities liked with death, healing and resurrection. A fourth set is dedicated to Silvanus, among whose patronage was the protection of human health (Palmer 1978: 222). Of the other two sets, one is barefoot and probably represents a god, while the other is shod, and may depict the deceased, or his daughter who erected the monument. Foot-fragments from statues associated with burials are all parts of grave markers, and were originally portraits, but may have been retained due to their ritual associations.

In funerary settings, then, foot-shaped artefacts are multi-faceted, symbolising the provision of footwear, and the presence of a being, often divine, bringing protection. Many formed part of the burial rites, and all could demonstrate the status and beliefs of the dead and their nearest and dearest.

10.5 Pars pro toto

We have seen that some Roman representations of feet and footwear can stand as proxy for a being, whether human or divine (Dunbabin 1990: 86). This may be related to the foot being the foundation of a being, the point of contact by which we experience the earth beneath us. The synecdochical function of foot-shaped artefacts has many facets, which this section will summarize.

In some cases, such as human footprints in CBM, and stamp matrices, the foot-shape functions as a kind of signature (van Driel-Murray 1999a: 132), either to claim creatorship or ownership of an object. *Planta pedis* stamps were also used to advertise manufacturers. There is an element of expressing power and authority here (Brodribb 1987: 117). Carved footprints signify a presence, often of a deity, but sometimes of a devotee, and sometimes of both simultaneously (Chiarini 2017: 155). Shoe brooches may perform similar functions, as they may be pilgrim badges (Johns 1995: 104). They may also represent the donor. Footwear deposited in tombs may have comforted those left behind to know that something of theirs would accompany the dead as a reminder. Thus, there is an aspect of memorialisation in foot-shaped artefacts.

This study has argued that many foot-shaped lamps represent the feet of deities, which can be the case for other artefacts. The next section examines the deities commonly symbolised by representations of human feet.

10.5.1 The feet of the gods

This study has found that foot-shaped artefacts are commonly associated with a number of divinities. In this corpus, the deity most frequently represented by feet is Isis, originally an Egyptian goddess, with a close relationship to the Imperial Cult and emperor worship from the time of Vespasian (Takács 2007: 356). She is often depicted wearing thonged sandals, or *soleae*, and accompanied by the symbols of a sistrum, ivy leaves, or a serpent. She is a deity of healing and resurrection (Caseau 2012: 122), which links her to the funerary use of footwear. Her consort, Serapis, who performed similar roles (Nicgorski 2014: 154), is also portrayed by feet, usually bare (Parkin 2018: 183), but sometimes wearing *crepidae,* the style of sandal associated with healers and philosophers. Feet are also a common proxy for Mercury, another deity associated with death through his role as psychopomp (Crummy 2007: 227). He is also patron of travellers (Henig 2015), linking him to the role of footwear as protection for a journey. This study has argued that Bacchus can be depicted by feet, especially as far as foot-shaped lamps decorated with vine leaves or scallop shells are concerned. Like Mercury, Isis and Serapis, Bacchus was a god of reincarnation and the afterlife (Henrichs 2012).

In addition, Christ is linked to feet in later Roman artefacts, especially those bearing Christian symbols, such as fourth-century lamps and stamp matrices. There are a number of references to Christ's feet and sandals in the New Testament, and some early Christian catacombs are decorated with a pair of sandals, a symbol of mission (Arnold 1997: 232). Jesus is also associated with resurrection and everlasting life. We have thus seen a connection between representations of feet and footwear, deities, and life after death.

Although gods are usually depicted barefoot, feet clad in *caligae*, the iconic Roman army boot, may represent Mars. Feet have also been found to be *pars pro toto* for other deities: Nemesis, Caelestis, Vulcan, Diana, Minerva, Apollo, Jupiter and Victory. Their feet could be symbols of devotion, of religious affiliation, of entreaty or thanks to the god for their favour, or for their protection.

10.6 Apotropaic feet

Another major theme that runs through this work is the metaphorical protection afforded by feet and footwear. Actual shoes protect the feet, from dirt, cold and injury (Forrer 1942: 77; van Driel-Murray 1999a: 131) and, in the Roman world, are associated with crushing an enemy, including a supernatural one, underfoot (Dasen 2015: 184). Shoe-shaped artefacts may have been apotropaic, protecting travellers on a journey, which could be the journey of life, or to the Underworld. The representation of deities through their feet adds to the protective effect.

This apotropaic role of feet was the most difficult to prove satisfactorily, however, Iron Age and Roman amulets in the shape of feet and footwear are known. There is also some use of such talismans in Ancient Egypt and Ancient Greece, so this aspect may not be purely Roman. Hobnailing patterns are what distinguishes Roman shoe-shaped amulets from earlier ones, and some symbols used in nailing designs, such as swastikas, were also apotropaic. When the foot-shape, the representation of a deity and nailed symbols are put together, this adds up to very strong apotropaic protection.

10.6.1 The sinister side

In the Roman world, chirality – whether something is left or right – is an important aspect of feet. This study has discussed at length documented Roman beliefs concerning the good luck associated specifically with the right foot and the bad luck brought by the left. As far as the overall numbers are concerned, there is a definite preference for right-footed artefacts (Figure 10.9). However, a closer look at the different categories reveals that, while there are more right-footed (168) than left-footed (46) lamps, the proportions are different for sandal *fibulae* (188 right; 176 left). If the statistics are broken down into our 12 categories, we can see that the occurrence of right-footed objects is more common in some than in others (Figure 10.10).

Why there should be a preference for left feet in some artefacts is unclear. It may be linked to the persistence of local beliefs, as seen in Iron Age amulets, or to some form of resistance. It could also indicate the contractual use of left and right shoes proposed by van Driel-Murray (1999a: 136), although this study has shown that the preference for left shoes in this instance is not particularly marked. It may simply be that, for many people, the left foot was just as significant as the right.

10.7 The importance of hobnailing

Throughout this study, the significance of Roman hobnailing patterns, be they on actual footwear, or on ornamental objects, has been highlighted. That artefacts were produced with depictions of nails which could not be seen under normal circumstances demonstrates a fascination with Roman hobnailing designs, if not their ideological importance.

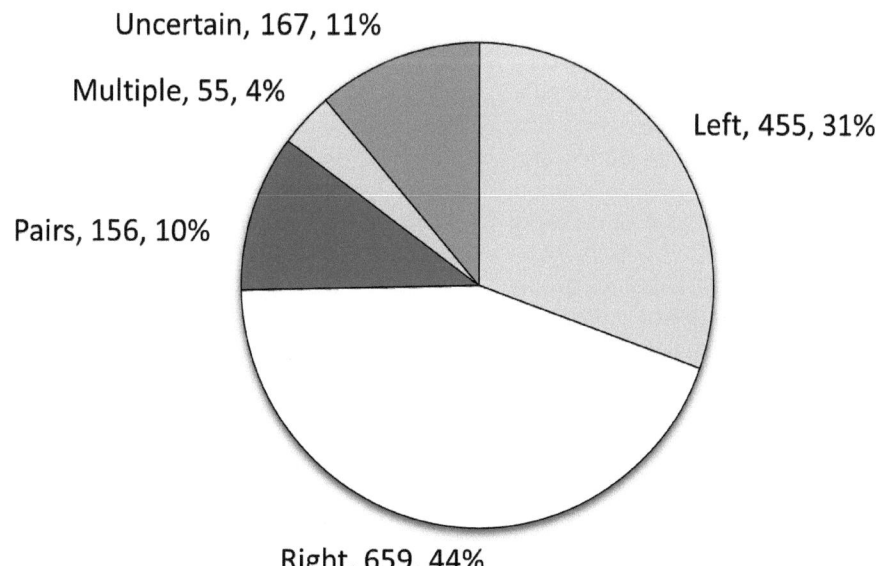

Figure 10.9: Chart to show the overall chirality for 1,492 Roman foot-shaped artefacts.

Roman Feet and Shoes

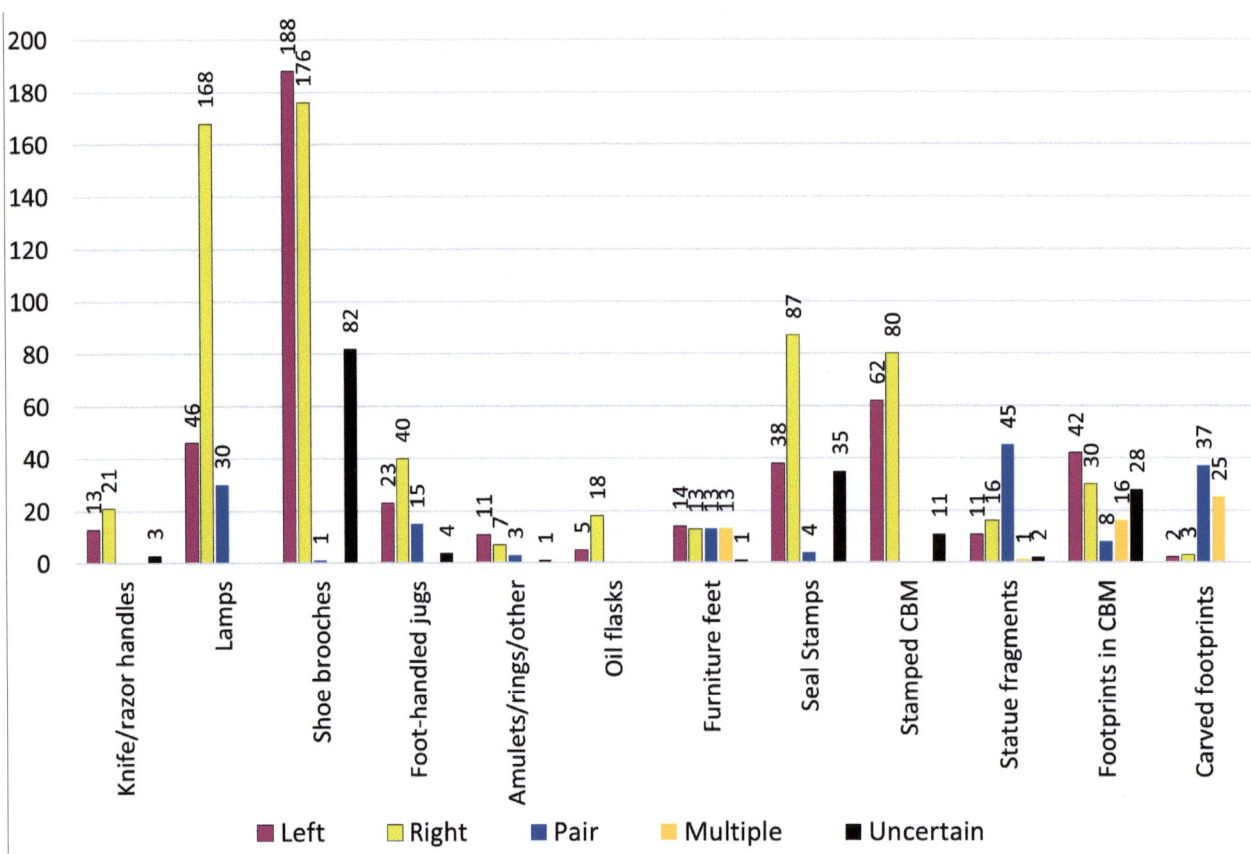

Figure 10.10: Chart to show details of chirality for 1,492 Roman foot-shaped artefacts.

Nailed designs echo and reinforce the themes that run through this research. The patterns could be whimsical or humorous. Hobnailing patterns followed fashions, which are dateable, and also demonstrated cultural capital. The designs became a sort of signature, and a statement of personal identity (van Driel-Murray 1999a: 132). Hobnailing is particularly associated with the army, as are some of the artefacts in the corpus.

The symbols depicted in hobnailing could show that people were under the protection of, or committed to, a particular deity (van Driel-Murray 1999a: 132). Hobnailing patterns played an apotropaic role, even in artefacts where they were not always visible in use. This apotropaic effect may be implicit in some designs, such as circles, swastikas, and diamonds. Like the significance of foot- and shoe-shaped artefacts, hobnailing could be polysemous. These attributes show that hobnailing was socially and cosmologically significant throughout the Roman Empire and explain why many artefacts feature representations of hobnailing.

10.8 How far evidence from ancient texts applied to the north-western provinces

This study set out to examine the extent to which the ancient evidence in texts and art for how feet and footwear were considered in the Roman world was applicable to the north-western provinces. We have already seen from the geographical distribution that almost 70% of the corpus with a known find-location comes from the north-western provinces, so the foot- and shoe-shaped artefacts can be taken as evidence for some beliefs surrounding feet in the Roman era.

Early in this work, Roman opinions and beliefs about footwear were examined in detail (see Chapter 2). It was found that ancient authors thought that appropriate footwear was bound up with the wearer's identity in terms of rank, status, and gender. Many grave markers from the north-western provinces depict soldiers wearing *caligae* with their uniforms, or prominent men sporting *calcei* with their togas. While the appropriateness question may not be applicable to foot- and shoe-shaped artefacts from the north-western provinces, the objects were often used to display aspects of status and, in some cases, gender. Certainly, the copper alloy artefacts, which were more expensive than ceramics, would have shown that their owners had money.

For ancient authors, feet and footwear were also bound up with ideas of power and authority. There is some evidence that the idea of the foot as the seat of power was also current in the north-western provinces. This is particularly the case with furniture feet attached to *curule* chairs. It is also shown by some stamp matrices. That some pieces of Roman CBM produced by the military are stamped with *planta pedis* designs is a particular instance of this aspect of significance. While the soldiers involved may not have hailed originally from the north-western provinces, they were stationed there.

The idea of feet or footprints standing for a whole being, often divine, can be seen in Apuleius *Metamorphoses* (11.17; 11.23; 11.24). The concept of *pars pro toto* is visible in some foot- and shoe-shaped artefacts from the north-western provinces.

This work has discussed Roman ideas of good fortune attached to feet in detail. The bringing of good luck was also attributed to feet by those living in the north-western provinces. However, as summarized above, chirality may not have been as significant a factor for apotropaism in the North West as it appears to have been in Rome, if the texts are to be believed. Nevertheless, concepts to do with the feet, as documented by ancient authors, appear to be applicable in the north-western provinces.

There is, however, another side to the coin. Since some of the artefacts, namely sandal *fibulae*, knife or razor handles ending in a foot, and jugs whose handles terminate in feet, are almost exclusive to the north-western provinces, we may be seeing associated cosmology that is regional rather than Roman. This may be particularly true for the ritual deposition of footwear and foot- and shoe-shaped artefacts. However, these regional artefacts also display the same significances as other, more widespread, foot- and shoe-shaped objects.

10.9 The limitations of this research

This work represents a thorough, in-depth study of Roman representations of feet and footwear. Nevertheless, no survey of this kind of material can ever hope to be complete and, despite every attempt to ensure as thorough research as possible, some information proved unobtainable, meaning that some artefacts were inevitably missed.

One must also take into account the inherent bias of findings. The paucity of some recording means that some of the data are inevitably skewed. Publishing bias should also be considered, since small finds are much less well published in Spain, Italy and eastern Europe (Eckardt 2022: personal comment). The problem of bias is further exacerbated by the types of site excavated, in that there may be a concentration on urban and military sites or funerary settings. However, by taking these biases into account, it was felt that creditable analysis could be carried out on the material.

It is worth remembering at this point that, apart from footwear deposited in graves and wells, and the significance of hobnailing, this study did not set out to deal with actual Roman shoes in much detail, since these have been covered at length by van Driel-Murray and many other scholars. Neither has it researched anatomical foot-shaped votives to do with healing, which have been studied in depth by other scholars, such as Chiarini (2017). There has not been space to investigate the significance of images of sandals on mosaics, especially those found in baths, discussed in detail by Dunbabin (1990), or carved into funerary *stelae*.

10.10 Conclusions

In a uniquely focussed study of Roman representations of feet and footwear, this work set out to research why the Romans chose foot iconography for decorative objects. It found that the ideological significance of representations of feet and footwear in the Roman world is complex and multi-faceted, but can show us much about the identity and beliefs of the people who owned them. We have seen that Roman foot- and shoe-shaped artefacts can simultaneously display a sense of humour, and of fashion, by which the owner could also demonstrate their status. The association of feet with personal identity is found in ancient texts and also across the north-western provinces. Foot-shaped objects were of ritual significance, being deposited in religious, funerary, and watery settings. Since they stood as a proxy for a being, both human and divine, they acted as a kind of signature, and memorialised a presence. The use of depictions of feet and footwear as a signature, a sign of ownership and also creatorship, is linked to the idea of feet as a symbol of power and authority. This facet is seen in the works of ancient authors and in objects from the north-western provinces. The protection provided by actual shoes to actual feet became a metaphor for apotropaic protection, particularly on a journey. As *pars pro toto* for divinities, representations of feet and footprints may have strengthened this apotropaic effect. The knowledge gap filled by this research has shown that, thanks to the complex and polysemous significance of Roman representations of feet and footwear, such objects were special in the Roman world.

Bibliography

Ancient Sources

Acts 13:25, Holy Bible: New International Version.

Aeschylus, *Choephoroe Oresteia: Agamemnon. Libation-Bearers. Eumenides*. Ed. and trans. Sommerstein, A.H. (2009) Loeb Classical Library 146. Cambridge, MA: Harvard University Press: 236–239.

Apuleius *Metamorphoses (The golden ass)* Volume I: Books 1–6. Ed. and trans. Hanson, J.A. (1996), Loeb Classical Library 44, Cambridge, MA: Harvard University Press: 10–11.

Archeologie van Zuid-Holland (2022) *Fibula/mantelspeld*. Inventory number 9379.

Archéologie Alsace (2019) *Lampe à huile en forme de pied portant une sandale*.

Ashmolean Museum (2017) collection online 'Pottery stamp with Greek inscription'. Accession number AN1873.131.

British Museum (2020) *Bronze ring-stamp in the form of a shoe*. Museum number 1872,0604.263

British Museum (2021) *Amulet*. Museum number 1872,0604.859

Cato, *On agriculture* 13.22, trans. Hooper, W.D., Boyd Ash, H. (1934), Loeb Classical Library 283, Cambridge, MA: Harvard University Press: 72–73.

Catullus 61.159–160, trans. Cornish, F.W., Postgate, J.P., Mackail, J.W., revised Goold, G.P. (1913) Loeb Classical Library 6, Cambridge, MA: Harvard University Press: 78–79.

Catullus 98.4, trans. Cornish, F.W., Postgate, J.P., Mackail, J.W., revised Goold, G.P. (1913) Loeb Classical Library 6, Cambridge, MA: Harvard University Press: 170–171.

Cicero *Phillipics* 13.13.28, ed. and trans. Shackleton Bailey, D.R. Revised Ramsey, J and Manuwald, G. (2010), Loeb Classical Library 507, Cambridge, MA: Harvard University Press: 260–261.

Cicero *Pro Rabirio Postumo,* trans. Watts, N.H. (1931), Loeb Classical Library 252, Cambridge, MA: Harvard University Press: 366–416.

Cicero, *De Divinatione* 2.84. trans. Falconer, WA. (1923), Loeb Classical Library 154, Cambridge, MA: Harvard University Press: 466–467.

Deutsche Akademie der Wissenschaften zu Berlin (1862-) Corpus inscriptionum latinarum, Berlin: G. Reimer: Volumes III, IV, V, VI, VII, IX, XI, XIII, XIV.

Collectie Gelderland (2020a) *Tegel van baksteen met voetafdruk en stempel uit de Romeinse tijd*. Object number BB.I.C.10.

Collectie Gelderland (2020b) *IJzeren vouwstoel uit de Romeinse tijd*. Object number CC.279

Colossal statue of Constantine the Great, early 4th century, marble, Capitoline Museums, Rome.

Colossians 3.16, Holy Bible: New International Version.

Dio Cassius *Roman History* 50.24.3 in *Volume V: Books 46–50* trans. Cary, E. and Foster, H.B. (1917), Loeb Classical Library 82. Cambridge, MA: Harvard University Press: 486–487.

Dio Cassius *Roman History* 52.34.8 in *Volume VI: Books 51–55* trans. Cary, E. and Foster, H.B. (1917), Loeb Classical Library 83. Cambridge, MA: Harvard University Press: 168–169.

Diocletian, *Edict on maximum prices* IX, trans. Kropff, A. (2016)

Ephesians 5.18b–19a, Holy Bible: New International Version.

Ezekiel 16:25, Holy Bible: New International Version.

Feugère, M., Bourrieau, Y. and Webley, R. (2021) *Clasp-knife: human leg* (Artefacts: CNF-4036).

Fitzwilliam Museum, Cambridge (2022) *Figurine of Serapis with Cerberus* inv. no. Loan Ant.103.93.

Frontinus, *Stratagems. Aqueducts of Rome*, trans. Bennett, C.E. and McElwain, M.B. (1925) Loeb Classical Library 174. Cambridge, MA: Harvard University Press: 339.

Gallo-Romeins Museum, Tongeren (2020) *Kruidenpotje (balsamarium) in de vorm van een laarsje*. Inventory number GRM 4523.

Garland, H.P. (2007) *Roof tiles Roman 04*, flickr.com.

Harl, F. and Harl, O. (2018a) 'Porträtstele des Publius Flavoleius Cordus', *Ubi Erat Lupa,* no. 7079.

Harl, F. and Harl, O. (2018b) 'Porträtstele des Caius Iulius Clemens und des C Iulius Sabinus', *Ubi Erat Lupa,* no.15749.

Harl, F. and Harl, O. (2019a) 'Fragment der Grabstele einer jungen Frau', *Ubi Erat Lupa,* no. 16496.

Harl, F. and Harl, O. (2019b) 'Weihung für Isis', *Ubi Erat Lupa*, no. 6455.

Harl, F. and Harl, O. (2020) 'Fragmente einer Reiterstatue', *Ubi Erat Lupa,* no. 19987.

Herodotus, *The Persian wars, volume I: books 1–2*, trans. Godley, AD (1920) Loeb Classical Library 117, Cambridge, MA: Harvard University Press: 326–327 and 450–452.

Horace, *Epistles* 2.2.37, trans. Rushton Fairclough, H. (1926) Loeb Classical Library 194, Cambridge, MA: Harvard University Press: 426–427.

Horace, *Satire* 1.3, trans. Rushton Fairclough, H. (1926) Loeb Classical Library 194, Cambridge, MA: Harvard University Press: 270–274.

Horace, *Satire* 2.8.77, trans. Rushton Fairclough, H. (1926) Loeb Classical Library 194, Cambridge, MA: Harvard University Press: 244–245.

Inscriptiones graecae IG XII.1165.

Isidore of Seville, 'Footwear (*de calciamentis*)' in Barney, S., Lewis, W. and Beach, J. (2006) *The etymologies of Isidore of Seville*, Cambridge: Cambridge University Press.

Jerome, *Letter* 52.10, trans. Wright, F.A. (1933), Loeb Classical Library 262. Cambridge, MA: Harvard University Press: 217.

Joconde (2018) museum collections database: 'tuile', Musée archéologique de Strasbourg. Inventory number 11.2015.1.1

Joconde (2019) museum collections database: 'Sandal fibula from Sens'. Inventory number 2017.0.ARC.94

Joconde (2021) museum collections database: 'Pot (à anse)' Inventory numbers 73.1.14 and 96.53.28.

John 1.27 and 13, Holy Bible: New International Version.

Josephus, *The Jewish war* 6.1.8, trans. Thackeray, H. St. J. (1928) Loeb Classical Library 210. Cambridge, MA: Harvard University Press: 202–203.

Juvenal, *Satire* 3.247–248, trans. Braund, S.M. (2004) Loeb Classical Library 91, Cambridge MA: Harvard University Press: 186–187.

Juvenal, *Satire* 16.13–14 and 22–25, trans. Braund, S.M. (2004) Loeb Classical Library 91, Cambridge MA: Harvard University Press: 506–509.

Koninklijk Instituut voor het Kunstpatrimonium KIK-IRPA (2008) *chaise pliante*, object number:10142083.

Landeskunde online (2008) *Römerkastell Saalburg Sonderausstellung: Ton + Technik—Römische Ziegel*.

Livius.org (2020) *Mušov, tile of X Gemina*.

Livy, *History of Rome* 29.19.12, Volume VIII: Books 28–30, trans. Moore, F. (1949), Loeb Classical Library 381, Cambridge, MA: Harvard University Press: 266–267.

Luke 3.15, Holy Bible: New International Version.

Mark 1.7, Holy Bible: New International Version.

Martial, *Epigrams* 2.29.7–8 in *Volume I: Spectacles, Books 1–5*, ed. and trans. Shackleton Bailey, D.R. (1993) Loeb Classical Library 94, Cambridge, MA: Harvard University Press: 148–149.

Matthew 3.1, Holy Bible: New International Version.

Metropolitan Museum of Art, New York (2019) 'Hanging lamp in the form of a sandaled right foot'. Accession Number: 62.10.1.

Ministerio de Cultura y Deporte (2020) *Placa con vestigia*, Ceres online database.

Mishnah Shabbat 6.2.

Musée Archéologique de l'Oise (2016) 'Une fibule découverte au grand théâtre de Vendeuil-Caply'.

Musée d'Archéologie Nationale (MAN) Saint-Germain-en-Laye (2020) *Encrier*. Accession number MAN75452.

Musée de l'Éphèbe (2022) 'Lampe en forme de pied'.

Musées de Strasbourg (2007) 'Tuile de type tegula avec empreinte'. Inventory number MAS 8293 A.

Musée des Antiquités - Bibliotheca Alexandrina (2020) *Offrande à Sérapis en forme de bloc portant une empreinte de pied*. Inventory number BAAM 0498

Museo Archeologico Nazionale di Napoli (2019a) *Fresco of Isiac ceremony from Herculaneum*, inv. no. 8924.

Museo Archeologico Nazionale di Napoli (2019a) *Statue of Aesculapius*, marble, inv. no. 6360.

Museo Archeologico Nazionale di Napoli (2019c) *Statue of Mammius Maximus*, copper alloy, inv. no. 5591.

Museo Archeologico Nazionale di Napoli (2019d) *Farnese Lar, marble,* inv. no. 5975.

Museu Nacional Arqueològic de Tarragona (2020). Inventory number MNAT 2820.

Museum of Gloucester (2020) *Roman tile with an adult hobnail sole print in it*, X.

National Archaeological Museum, Florence (2010) *Magical gem in a gold setting: bust of Serapis on a foot on the Campbell Bonner magical gems database*. Inventory number CBd-4167.

Pliny the Elder, *Natural Histories* 2.24, trans. Rackham, H. (1938) Loeb Classical Library 330, Cambridge, MA: Harvard University Press: 184–185.

Pliny the Elder, *Natural Histories* 13.4, trans. Rackham, H. (1938) Loeb Classical Library 370, Cambridge, MA: Harvard University Press: 110–111.

Pliny the Younger, *Epistles* 9.17.3 in *Letters, Volume II: Books 8–10*, trans. Radice, B (1969) Loeb Classical Library 59, Cambridge, MA: Harvard University Press: 112–113.

Plutarch *Roman Questions* 30 (*Moralia* 271e) in *Moralia* Vol. IV, trans. Babbitt, F.C. (1936), Loeb Classical Library 305, Cambridge, MA, Harvard University Press: 52–53.

Portable Antiquities Scheme (PAS) online database (2020) 'Vessel' YORYM-68EAC1.

Portonaccio Sarcophagus, late 2nd century, marble, Capitoline Museums, Rome. Inv. No. 112327.

Psalms 119, verse 105, Holy Bible: New International Version.

Revelation 1:8; 21:6; 22:13, Holy Bible: New International Version.

Roman Inscriptions of Britain (RIB) 105

RIB 1199

RIB 1299

RIB 1301

RIB 1303

RIB 3162

RIB 321

RIB 418

RIB 429

RIB 492

RIB 497

RIB 523

RIB 524

RIB 558

RIB 562

RIB 563

RIB 567

RIB 568

RIB 645

RIB 943

RIB 952

Roman Imperial Coinage (RIC) 360

RIC II Trajan 666

RIC IIa 812

RIC III 246

RIC IV 289

RIC V 19

RIC VI 96

RIC VIII 494

Rijksmuseum van Oudheden (2019) online collection 'Emailfibula in de vorm van een voetzool'. Inventory number f 1941/12.15

Rijksmuseum van Oudheden (2020) online collection ' Stempel in "planta pedis" vorm en retrograde'. Inventory number e 1944/1.76.

Rijksmuseum van Oudheden (2021) online collection 'Kan'. Inventory number NS 25.

Sailko (2012) *Sigilli in bronzo per imprimere marca di fabbrica su oggetti in terracotta*, Wikimedia Commons.

Scriptores Historiae Augustae: Probus 14 and 20 in *Historia Augusta, Volume III* trans. Magie, D. (1932) Loeb Classical Library 263. Cambridge, MA: Harvard University Press: 364–365; 378–379.

Scriptores Historiae Augustae: The two Maximini 28.7 in *Historia Augusta, Volume II* trans. Magie, D. (1924) Loeb Classical Library 140. Cambridge, MA: Harvard University Press: 368–369.

Statue of Isis, marble, Capitoline Museums inv. No. MC0744.

Strabo, *Geography Volume II*, trans. Jones, H.L. (1923) Loeb Classical Library 50. Cambridge, MA: Harvard University Press: 201–203.

Suetonius, *Augustus* 73, in *Lives of the Caesars, Volume I*, trans. Rolfe, J.C. (1914) Loeb Classical Library 31, Cambridge, MA: Harvard University Press: 260–261.

Suetonius, *Gaius Caligula* 14.2 in *Lives of the Caesars, Volume I*, trans. Rolfe, J.C. (1914) Loeb Classical Library 31, Cambridge, MA: Harvard University Press: 434–435.

Suetonius, *Gaius Caligula* 52, in *Lives of the Caesars, Volume I*, trans. Rolfe, J.C. (1914) Loeb Classical Library 31, Cambridge, MA: Harvard University Press: 494–495.

Suetonius, *Nero* 51, in *Lives of the Caesars, Volume II*, trans. Rolfe, J.C. (1914) Loeb Classical Library 38, Cambridge, MA: Harvard University Press: 174–175.

Suetonius, *Tiberius* 38, in *Lives of the Caesars*, Volume I, trans. Rolfe, J.C. (1914) Loeb Classical Library 31, Cambridge, MA: Harvard University Press: 366–367.

Suetonius, *Vespasian* 7.2, in *Lives of the Caesars, Volume II*, trans. Rolfe, J.C. (1914) Loeb Classical Library 38, Cambridge, MA: Harvard University Press: 282–285.

Tacitus *Histories 4.81.1–3: Books 4–5. Annals: Books 1–3,* trans. Moore, C.H. and Jackson, J. (1931) Loeb Classical Library 249, Cambridge, MA: Harvard University Press: 160–163.

Tertullian *Apology* 39.18, trans. Glover T.R., Rendall, G.H. (1931) Loeb Classical Library 250, Cambridge, MA: Harvard University Press: 181.

Thorvaldsens Museum, Copenhagen (2020) *Amulet with a left foot*. Inventory number H2221.

Tyne and Wear archives and museums (2020) collections, search for 'child; tile'.

Vatican Museums (2019) *Aldobrandini Wedding*, Augustan wall painting, Inv. No. 79631.

Vatican Museums (2021) *Augustus Prima Porta*, Inv. No. 2290.

Vindolanda tablets online (2019)

Vindolanda tablets II online (2019).

Virgil *Aeneid* 4.139, trans. Rushton Fairclough, H. (1916), Revised Goold, G.P., Loeb Classical Library 63, Cambridge, MA: Harvard University Press: 430–431.

Vitruvius, *On Architecture* 3.4.4, trans. Granger, F. (1931) Loeb Classical Library 251, Cambridge, MA: Harvard University Press: 88–95.

York Museums and Gallery Trust online collections (2019) *Shoe-shaped brooch*. Object number YORYM : 1974.112.3

York Museums and Gallery Trust online collections (2020) *Tile tomb*. Object number YORYM : 2010.345.

York Museums and Gallery Trust online collections (2021) *Figurine*. Object number YORYM : 2012.377.

Modern Sources

Achrati, A. (2003) 'Hand and foot symbolisms: from rock art to the Qur'ān', *Arabica* 50(4): 464–500.

Adams, N. (1977) 'The leather', in Rogerson, A. (ed.) 'Excavations at Scole, 1973', *East Anglian Archaeology* 5: 97–224.

Addyman, P. (2015) *British historic towns atlas volume V: York*, Oxford: Historic Towns Trust and York Archaeological Trust.

Agusta-Boularot S., Golosetti, R. and Isoardi, D. (2010) 'La déesse *Dexiua* du Castellar (Cadenet, Vaucluse). Confrontation des témoignages épigraphiques et des données archéologiques à l'occasion des premières fouilles', *Revue archéologique de Narbonnaise* 43: 109–125.

Albert, R. and Fauduet, I. (1976) 'Les fibules d'Argentomagus' (2e partie), *Revue archéologique du Centre de la France* 15.3: 199–240.

Albrecht, N. (2014) *Römerzeitliche Brunnen und Brunnenfunde im rechtsrheinischen Obergermanien und in Rätien*. Doctoral thesis (unpublished) Universität Heidelberg.

Aldhouse-Green, M.J (1976) *A corpus of religious material from the civilian areas of Roman Britain*, Oxford: British Archaeological Reports 24.

Aldhouse-Green, M.J. (1978) *A corpus of small cult-objects from the military areas of Roman Britain*, Oxford: British Archaeological Reports 52.

Allason-Jones, L. (1988) 'Small finds from turrets on Hadrian's Wall', in Coulston, J.C. (ed.) *Military equipment and the identity of Roman soldiers: Proceedings of the fourth Roman military equipment conference*, BAR Int Ser 394: 197–233.

Allason-Jones, L. (1995) 'Sexing small finds', in Rush, P. (ed.) *Theoretical Roman archaeology: second conference proceedings,* Aldershot: Avebury: 22–32.

Allason-Jones, L. (2008) 'The metalwork (excluding brooches and enamelled objects)', in Cool, H.E.M. & Mason D.J.P. (eds.) *Roman Piercebridge: excavations by D.W. Harding & Peter Scott 1969–1981*, Durham: Architectural and Archaeological Society of Durham and Northumberland Research Report 7: D11.1–116.

Allason-Jones, L. (2009) 'The small finds', in Rushworth, A. (ed.) *Housesteads Roman fort—the grandest station* vol. 2, Swindon: English Heritage: 430–487.

Allason-Jones, L. (2011) *Artefacts in Roman Britain: their purpose and use*, Cambridge: Cambridge University Press.

Allason-Jones, L. (2015) 'Zoomorphic brooches in Roman Britain: decoration or religious ideology?', in Marzel, S.-R. and Stiebel, G.D. (eds.) *Dress and ideology: fashioning identity from antiquity to the present*, London: Bloomsbury: 69–86.

Allason-Jones, L. (forthcoming) *Roman sculpture from northern England*, Oxford: Oxford University Press for the British Academy. *Corpus Signorum Imperii Romani* Great Britain 1.11.

Allason-Jones, L. and Jones, D.M. (1994) 'Jet and other materials in Roman artefact studies', *Archaeologia Aeliana Series 5*. Vol 22: 265–272.

Allason-Jones, L. and McKay, B. (1985) *Coventina's Well: a shrine on Hadrian's Wall*, Hexham: Trustees of the Clayton Collection, Chesters Museum.

Allason-Jones, L. and Miket, R. (1984) *The catalogue of small finds from South Shields Roman fort*, Newcastle upon Tyne: Society of Antiquaries Monograph, Series 2.

Allison, P.M. (2006a) 'Mapping for gender. Interpreting artefact distribution inside 1st- and 2nd-century AD forts in Roman Germany', *Archaeological Dialogues*: 13: 1–20.

Allison, P.M. (2006b) *The Insula of the Menander in Pompeii vol. iii: the finds, a contextual study* online companion.

Alram-Stern, E. (1989) *Die römischen Lampen aus Carnuntum*, Vienna: Verlag der Österreichischen Akademie der Wissenschaften.

Ambrose, T. (1977) 'The leather', in Cunliffe, B. (ed.) *Excavations at Portchester Castle* London: Society of Antiquaries of London: Distributed by Thames and Hudson, Report 34: 247–262.

Ambroz, A.K. (1966) *Фибула найдена на юге европейской части СССР*, Moscow: ГЛАВНАЯ РЕДАКЦИЯ ВОСТОЧНОЙ ЛИТЕРАТУРЫ.

Aemilia online (2019) 'Lucerne dal santuario di Cittanova'.

Anderson-Stojanović, V.R. (1987) 'The chronology and function of ceramic unguentaria', *American Journal of Archaeology* 91(1): 105–122.

Andreae, B. (1975) 'Über das Antikenmuseum im Rahmne der Kunstsammlungen der Ruhr-Universität Bochum', *Jahrbuch der Ruhr-Universität Bochum* 1975.x.

Antonine Wall, the, online (2017) *Bar Hill: fort, military way, wall, and temporary camps.*

Appadurai, A. (1986) 'Introduction: commodities and the politics of value', in Appadurai, A. (ed.) *The social life of things: commodities in cultural perspectives*, Cambridge: Cambridge University Press: 3–63.

Applebaum S. (1963) 'Where Saul and Jonathan perished: Bet Shean in Israel. The Roman theatre revealed and a Greek statue discovered', *The Illustrated London News* vol. 381, 16 March: 380–383.

Archaeology Data Service (2018a) *Defended Small Towns of Roman Britain.*

Archaeology Data Service (2018b) *The rural settlement of Roman Britain: an online resource.*

Archeologie Mušov (2020) museum website.

Armand-Calliat, L. (1937) *Le châlonnais gallo-romain: répertoire des découvertes archéologiques faites dans l'arrondissement de Châlon*, Châlon-sur-Saône: Société d'histoire et d'archéologie.

Armour, N., Dodwell, N. and Timberlake, S. (2007) *The Roman cemetery, the Babraham Institute, Cambridgeshire: an archaeological excavation*, Cambridge: Cambridge Archaeological Unit, Report No. 754.

Arnold, E. (1997) *The early Christians in their own words*, Farmington PA: Plough Publishing House.

Arrowsmith, P. and Power, D. (2012) *Roman Nantwich: a salt-making settlement: excavations at Kingsley Fields 2002*, Oxford: Archaeopress.

Artefacts: encyclopédie collaborative en ligne des objets archéologiques (2021) online.

Asser, M. (2008) 'Bush shoe-ing worst Arab insult', *BBC News* Monday, 15 December 2008 online.

Atkinson, M. and Preston, S.J. (2015) 'Heybridge: A Late Iron Age and Roman settlement, excavations at Elms Farm 1993–5', *Internet Archaeology* 40.

Aubin, G. (1981) 'Circonscription des Pays de la Loire', *Gallia* 39.2: 333–362.

Austen, P.S. (1991) *Bewcastle and old Penrith: A Roman outpost fort and a frontier vicus: excavations 1977–78*, Kendal, England: Cumberland and Westmorland Antiquarian and Archaeological Society.

Babelon, E. (1916) *Le trésor d'argenterie de Berthouville*, Paris: Librairie centrale des Beaux-arts.

Babelon, E. and Blanchet, A. (1895) *Catalogue des bronzes antiques de la Bibliothèque nationale*, Paris: E. Leroux.

Bachofen, J. (1912) *Römische Grablampen nebst einigen andern Grabdenkmälern vorzugsweise eigener Sammlung*, Basel: J.J. Bachofen.

Bagshawe, R., Green, C., Gregory, T., Rogerson, A., Wade-Martins, P. and Edwards, D.A. (1977) 'Norfolk, various papers', *East Anglian Archaeology* 5.

Bailey, D.M. (1975) *A catalogue of the lamps in the British Museum Volume 1. Greek, Hellenistic and early Roman pottery lamps*, London: British Museum Publications.

Bailey, D.M. (1980) *A catalogue of the lamps in the British Museum Volume 2. Roman lamps made in Italy*, London: British Museum Publications.

Bailey, D.M. (1988) *A catalogue of the lamps in the British Museum Volume 3. Roman provincial lamps*, London: British Museum Publications.

Bailey, D.M. (1996) *A catalogue of the lamps in the British Museum Volume 4. Lamps of metal and stone, and lampstands*, London: British Museum Publications.

Bailey, D.M. (1963) *Greek and Roman pottery lamps*, London: Trustees of the British Museum.

Baker, P. (2013) *The archaeology of medicine in the Greco-Roman world*, Cambridge: Cambridge University Press.

Balestra, L. and Gerri, L. (2011) 'Bolli su terra sigillata dagli "scavi delle fognature" di Aquileia (1968–1972)', *Quaderni Friulani di Archeologia* XXI: 119–126.

Baratta, G. (2006) 'La produzione della pelle nell'Occidente e nelle province africane', *L'Africa Romana* XVII: 203–221.

Baratta, G. (2014) 'Il signaculum al. di là del testo: la tipologia delle lamine', in: Buonopane, A., Braito, S. and Girardi, C. (eds.) *Instrumenta inscripta V. Signacula ex aere. Aspetti epigrafici, archeologici, giuridici, prosopografici, collezionistici*, Roma: Scienze e Lettere: 101–132.

Barber, B. and Bowsher, D. (2000) *The eastern cemetery of Roman London: excavations 1983–1990*, London: Museum of London Archaeology Service, monograph 4.

Barker, S.J. (2020) 'Reuse of statuary and the recycling habit of late antiquity: an economic perspective', in Duckworth, C.N. and Wilson, A. (eds.) *Recycling and reuse in the Roman economy*, Oxford: Oxford University Press: 105–190.

Barnabei, F. (1922) 'Este—Scoperte archeologiche nella necropoli atestina del nord, riconosciuto nel fondo Rebato', *Notizie degli scavi di antichità* XIX: 3–57.

Barnard, M. (2020) 'Introduction', in Barnard, M. (ed.) *Fashion theory: a reader* (2nd edn.), London: Routledge: 1–10.

Bar-Oz, G. and Tepper, Y. (2010) 'Out on the tiles: animal footprints from the Roman site of Kefar 'Othnay (Legio), Israel', *Near Eastern Archaeology* 73.4: 244–247.

Barthel, W. and Kapf, E. (1907) 'Das Kastell Cannstatt', in Fabricius, E., Hettner, F. and von Sarwey, O. (eds.) *Der obergermanisch-raetische Limes des Römerreiches*, Abteilung B, Band 5, Kastell Nr. 59.

Barthes, R. (1983 [1967]) *The fashion system*, trans. Ward, M. and Howard, R., New York: Hill and Wang.

Barthes, R. (2006 [1993]) *The language of fashion*, trans. Carter, M. and Stafford, A., Oxford and New York: Berg.

Basey, J. (2018) *Roman wells and their contents: the significance of the deposition of deer bones, Roman sculpture and human remains in Britannia, the Upper-Rhine and Raetia*, BA Dissertation, Newcastle University.

Bastelaer, D.A. van (1877) *Le cimetière belgo-romano-franc de Strée*, Mons: H. Manceaux.

Bateson, J.D. (1981) *Enamel-working in Iron Age, Roman, and sub-Roman Britain: the products and techniques*, Oxford: BAR British Series 93.

Bateson, J.D. and Hedges, R.E.M. (1975) 'The scientific analysis of a group of Roman-age enamelled brooches', *Archaeometry* 17.2.

Bayley, J. and Butcher, S. (1988) 'The enamelled brooches', in Wickenden, N.P. (ed.) *Excavations at Great Dunmow*, Chelmsford: East Anglian Archaeology Report 41: microfiche 1D 25–28.

Bayley, J. and Butcher, S. (2004) *Roman brooches in Britain: a technological and typological study based on the Richborough Collection*, London: Society of Antiquaries of London.

BBC News (2003) 'Decoding Iraq's symbols of celebration', Thursday, 10 April.

Becker, W.A. (1838) trans. Metcalfe, F. (1891), *Gallus; or, Roman scenes of the time of Augustus*. London: Longmans, Green.

Bedford Roman Villa Project (2017) *The story so far...* online.

Bémont, C. and Chew, H. (2007) *Catalogue des lampes en terre cuite antiques*, Saint-Germain-en-Laye: Musée d'Archéologie Nationale.

Berganza Auction House (2020) *Ancient Roman sandal ring.*

Bersu, G. and Unverzagt, W. (1961) 'Le *castellum* de Fanum Martis (Famars, Nord)', *Gallia* 19.1: 159–190.

Betts, E. (2016) 'Places of transition and deposition: Phenomenon of water in the sacred landscape of Iron Age central Adriatic Italy', *Accordia Research Papers* 14: 63–83.

Betts, I.M. (1990) 'Roman brick and tile', in Wrathmell, S. and Nicholson, A. (eds.) *Dalton Parlours: Iron Age settlement and Roman villa*, Wakefield: West Yorkshire Archaeology Service: 165–170.

Betts, I.M., Black, E.W. and Gower, J. (1997) 'A corpus of relief-patterned tiles in Roman Britain', *Journal of Roman Pottery Studies* 7.

Biddulph, E. and Booth, P. (2006) *The Roman cemetery at Pepper Hill, Southfleet, Kent*, Oxford: Oxford Wessex Archaeology Joint Venture.

Bienert, B. (2007) *Die römischen Bronzegefäße im Rheinischen Landesmuseum Trier*, Trier: Beihefte Trierer Zeitschrift 21.

Biernacki, A.B. (1976) 'Abdruck einer Schuhsohle auf der keramischen Platte aus Novae', *Archaeologia* 27: 133–136.

Binet, E., Chaidron, C., Canny, D. and Thuet, A. (2010) 'Les débuts de l'urbanisation du quartier 1ère moitié du 1er siècle après J. -C.', *Revue archéologique de Picardie* numéro spécial 27: 23–32.

Birley, A. and Blake, J. (2007) *Vindolanda research report: the excavations of 2005–2006*, Hexham: The Vindolanda Trust.

Birley, B. (2020) 'Our curator's collection' online, *Vindolanda Charitable Trust.*

Birley, P. (2007) 'The sculptured stone', in Birley, A. and Blake, J. (eds.) *Vindolanda research report: the excavations of 2005–2006*, Hexham: The Vindolanda Trust: 138–143.

Birley, R. (1977) *Vindolanda: a Roman frontier post on Hadrian's Wall*, London: Thames and Hudson.

Bishop, D. (2012) *The soles of our feet*, Columbia International University.

Bishop, M.C. and Coulston, J.C. (2006) *Roman military equipment: from the Punic war to the fall of Rome* (2nd edn.), London: Batsford.

Blagg, T. (1980) 'The sculptured stones', in Hill, C., Millett, M., Blagg, T. and Dyson, T. (1980) *The Roman riverside wall and monumental arch in London: excavations at Baynard's Castle, Upper Thames Street, London 1974–6*, London: London and Middlesex Archaeological Society: 125–193.

Blundell, S. (2018) 'One shoe off and one shoe on', in Pickup, S. and Waite, S. (eds.) *Shoes, slippers and sandals: feet and footwear in classical antiquity*, Abingdon: Routledge: 221–228.

Boelicke, U. (2002) *Die Fibeln aus dem Areal der Colonia Ulpia Traiana*, Mainz: Phillipp von Zabern, Xantener Berichte 10.

Boesterd, M.H.P. den (1956) *The bronze vessels in the Rijksmuseum G. M. Kam at Nijmegen*, Nijmegen: Uitgegeven in Opdracht van het Departement van Onderwijs, Kunsten en Wetenschappen.

Boffey, D. (2020) 'French detectorist accused of looting on vast scale after haul discovered at home', *The Guardian* 16 December 2020.

Böhme, A. (1972) 'Die Fibeln der Kastelle Saalburg und Zugmantel', *Saalburg Jahrbuch* 29: 5–112.

Böhme, H.W. (1974) *Germanische Grabfunde des 4. [i.e. vierten] bis 5. [i.e. fünften] Jahrhunderts zwischen unterer Elbe und Loire: Studien zur Chronologie und Bevölkerungsgeschichte* Vols. I and II, Munich: Beck.

Bohstrom, P. (2017) 'Cremated soldier found in cooking pot at vast Roman camp in Israel', *Haaretz* 26.12.2017.

Bond, S.E. (2014) 'Follow me: courtesan sandals, shoemakers, and ephemeral epigraphic landscapes', *History from below*.

Bonnamour, L. (1977) 'Vases en bronze d'époque romaine trouvés dans la Saône', in Boucher, S. (ed.) *Actes du IVe Colloque international sur les bronzes antiques, 17–21 mai 1976*, Lyon: L'Hermès: 19–26.

Bonner, C. (1950) *Studies in magical amulets: chiefly Graeco-Egyptian*, Ann Arbor: University of Michigan Press.

Boon, G. (1972) *Isca, the Roman legionary fortress at Caerleon, Mon.* (3rd edn.), Cardiff: National Museum of Wales.

Booth, P. (1980) *Roman Alcester*, Warwick: Warwickshire Museum.

Booth, P. (1992) *Asthall, Oxfordshire: excavations in a Roman 'small town'*, Oxford: Oxford Archaeological Unit, Thames Valley landscapes monograph 9.

Booth, P. (2010) *The late Roman cemetery at Lankhills, Winchester: excavations 2000–2005*, Oxford: Oxford Archaeology, Oxford archaeology monograph no. 10.

Booth, P. and Cool, H.E.M. (2006) *Small finds from Pepper Hill Roman cemetery, Southfleet, Kent (ARC PHL97 and NBR98)*, CTRL specialist report series.

Bosanquet, R.C. (1925) 'Whitley Castle Roman camp, Northumberland', *Proceedings of the Society of Antiquaries of Newcastle upon Tyne* 4.1: 249–255.

Bossen, L. and Gates, H. (2017) *Bound feet, young hands: tracking the demise of footbinding in village China*, Stanford, CA: Stanford University Press.

Boube-Piccot. C. (1975) *Les bronzes antiques du Maroc II: le mobilier* (2 vols.) Rabat: Direction des monuments historiques et des antiquités.

Bourdieu, P. (1977) *Outline of a theory of practice*, Cambridge: Cambridge University Press.

Bourdieu, P. (1984) *Distinction: a social critique of the judgement of taste*, Cambridge, MA: Harvard University Press.

Bourdieu, P. (1995) 'Haute couture and haute culture', in *Sociology in question*, London: Sage: 132–138.

Božič, D. (2001) 'Über den Verwendungszweck einiger römischer Messerchen', *Instrumentum* 1: 28-30.

Božič, D. and Feugère, M. (2004) 'Les instruments de l'écriture', *Gallia* 61: 21-41.

Brady, K., Brown, L., and Smith, A. (2005) *A Romano-British landscape at Brockley Hill, Stanmore, Middlesex: excavations at Brockley Hill House and the former MoD site*, Oxford: Oxford Archaeological Unit, OA Job No. 2211.

Brassington, M. (1969) 'Roman Wells at Little Chester', *Derbyshire Archaeological Journal*, 89: 115–19.

Breeze, D.J. (2018) *Maryport: a Roman fort and its community*, Oxford: Archaeopress Publishing.

Brekle, H. (2011) 'Typ und Exemplar: Zur Theorie und Vor- und Frühgeschichte der Typographie', Regensburg: Universität Regensburg.

Breuer, J., Roosens, H. and Mertens, J. (1952) 'Le cimetière belgo-romain de Cerfontaine (Namur)', *Archaeologia Belgica* 6.

Brewer, R.J. (1986) *Wales*, Oxford: Oxford University Press for the British Academy. *Corpus Signorum Imperii Romani* Great Britain 1.5.

Brill, A. A. (1938) *The basic writings of Sigmund Freud*, New York: The modern library.

Brodribb, G. (1979) 'A Survey of Tile from the Roman bath house at Beauport Park, Battle, E. Sussex', *Britannia* 10: 139–156.

Brodribb, G. (1987) *Roman brick and tile*, Gloucester: Alan Sutton.

Brooks, R.T. (1977) 'The Roman villa at Hill Farm, Abridge', *Essex Journal* 12: 50–61.

Brown, L.A. and Walker, W.H. (2008) 'Prologue: archaeology, animism and non-human agents', *Journal of archaeological method and theory*, 15(4): 297–299.

Bruce, J.C. (1867) *The Roman wall: a description of the mural barrier of the north of England*, London: Longmans, Green, Reader and Dyer.

Brück, J. (1999) 'Ritual and rationality: some problems of interpretation in European archaeology', *European Journal of Archaeology*, 2(3): 313–344.

Brück, J. (2006) 'Fragmentation, personhood and the social construction of technology in middle and late Bronze Age Britain', *Cambridge Archaeological Journal*, 16(3): 297–315.

Buonopane, A. (2014) 'Schiavi e liberti imperiali nei *signacula ex aere*', in Buonopane, A., Braito, S. and Girardi, C. (eds.) *Instrumenta inscripta V. Signacula ex aere: aspetti epigrafici, archeologici, giuridici, prosopografici, collezionistici*, Roma: Scienze e Lettere: 141–148.

Buora, M. and Lafli, E. (2014) 'Tre signacula dall'Asia Minore', in Buonopane, A., Braito, S. and Girardi, C. (eds.) *Instrumenta inscripta V. Signacula ex aere: aspetti epigrafici, archeologici, giuridici, prosopografici, collezionistici*, Roma: Scienze e Lettere: 417–422.

Burandt, B. (2016) 'Iron footed—hobnail patterns under Roman shoes and their functional meaning', in Hoss, S. and Whitmore, A. (eds.) *Small finds and ancient social practices in the northwest provinces of the Roman Empire*, Oxford: Oxbow Books: 9–15.

Burgers, A. (2001) *The water supplies and related structures of Roman Britain.* Oxford, British Archaeological Reports (British Series) 324.

Burrow, J.G. (2015) 'Ghosting of images in barefoot exemplar prints collection: issues for analyses', *Journal of forensic identification* 65: 884–900.

Busch, A.L. (1965) 'Die Römerzeitlichen Schuh- und Lederfunde der Kastelle Saalburg, Zugmantel und Kleiner Feldberg', *Saalburg Jahrbuch* 22: 158–210.

Bush, T.S. (1907) *Report on the exploration on Little Down Field, Lansdown, May and September, 1907*, Bath: J. B. Keene.

Bussière, J. and Lindros Wohl, B. (2017) *Ancient lamps in the J. Paul Getty Museum*, Los Angeles: J. Paul Getty Museum.

Butcher, S. (1977) 'Enamels from Roman Britain', in Apted, M.R., Gilyard-Beer, R. and Saunders, AD (eds.) *Ancient monuments and their interpretation: essays presented to A.J. Taylor*, London: Phillimore: 41–70.

Butcher, S. (1982) 'The metalwork', in Carlyon, P.M. (ed.) 'A Romano-British site at Kilhallon, Tywardreath: Excavation in 1975', *Cornish Archaeology* 21: 162–163.

Butcher, S. (2004) 'Roman Nornour, Isles of Scilly: a reconsideration', *Hendhyscans Kernow* 39–40: 5–44.

Butcher, S. (2008) 'Part II: The Romano-British brooches and enamelled objects', in Cool, H.E.M. and Mason D.J.P. (eds.). (2008) *Roman Piercebridge: Excavations by D.W. Harding and Peter Scott 1969–1981*, Durham: Architectural and Archaeological Society of Durham and Northumberland Research Report 7: D11.186–216.

Cadenat, P. (1980) 'Les fibules d'Ussubium (Commune du Mas-d'Agenais, Lot-et-Garonne)', *Revue de l'Agenais* 107.1: 5–22.

Callewaert, M. (2014) 'Les fibules en contexte funéraire dans le nord-est de la Gaule durant le Haut-Empire: quelques chiffres', *Signa* 3: 37–46.

Campbell, K. and Compton, J. (2003) *Archaeological excavation at the former council depot, Haslers Lane, Great Dunmow, Essex*, Chelmsford: Essex County Council Field Archaeology Unit.

Canto de Gregorio, A.M. (1985) *La epigrafía Romana de Itálica*, Doctoral Thesis, Madrid: Universidad Complutense.

Canto, A.M. (1984) 'Les plaques votives avec *plantae pedum* d'Italica: Un essai d'interprétation', *Zeitschrift für Papyrologie und Epigraphik* 54: 183–194.

Carlyon, P.M. (1982) 'A Romano-British site at Kilhallon, Tywardreath: Excavation in 1975', *Cornish Archaeology* 21: 155–170.

Carr, G. (2001) "Romanisation' and the body', in Davies, G., Gardner, A. and Lockyear, K. (eds.) *TRAC 2000: Proceedings of the tenth annual Theoretical Roman Archaeology Conference*, Oxford: Oxbow Books: 112–124.

Caseau, B. (2011) 'Religious intolerance and pagan statuary', in Lavan, L. and Mulryan, M. (eds.) *The archaeology of late antique 'paganism'*, Leiden; Boston: Brill: 479–504.

Caseau, B. (2012) 'Magical protection and stamps in Byzantium', in Regulski, I., Duistermaat, K. and Verkinderen, P. (eds.) *Seals and sealing practices in the Near East*, Leuven: Peeters: 115–132.

Casey, P.J., Evans, J. and Davies, J.L. (1993) *Excavations at Segontium (Caernarfon) Roman fort, 1975–1997*, London: Council for British Archaeology, Research Report 90.

Castellano Hernández, Á., Gimeno, H. and Sytlow, A.U. (1999) 'Signacula: Sellos Romanos en bronce del Museo Arqueológico Nacional', *Boletín del Museo Arqueológico Nacional* 17: 59–95.

Castiglione, L. (1968a) 'Inverted footprints: a contribution to the ancient popular religion', *Acta Ethnographica Academiae Scientiarum Hungaricae* 17: 121–137.

Castiglione, L. (1968b) 'Inverted footprints again', *Acta Antiqua Academiae Scientiarum Hungaricae* 16: 187–189.

Castiglione, L. (1970) 'Vestigia', *Acta Archaeologica Academiae Scientiarum Hungaricae* 22: 95–132.

Catenaccio, C. (2012) 'Oedipus Tyrannus: the riddle of the feet', *The Classical Outlook* 89(4): 102–107.

Cattelain, P., Bozet, N. and di Stazio, G. (eds.) (2012) *La parure de Cro-Magnon à Clovis*, Treignes: Editions du Cedarc, Guides Archéologiques du Malgré-Tout.

Caylus, A. (1752) *Recueil d'antiquités égyptiennes, étrusques, grecques et romaines* v.4, Paris: Desaint et Saillant.

Chapman, J. (2000) *Fragmentation in archaeology: people, places, and broken objects in the prehistory of south eastern Europe*, New York: Routledge.

Chiarini, S. (2017) 'The foot as gnórisma', in Draycott, J. and Graham, E.-J. (eds.) *Bodies of evidence: ancient anatomical votives past, present and future*, London; New York: Routledge: 147–164.

Christensen, A.M. (2016) 'Some very preliminary thoughts about footprints on Roman roof tiles', *Nescio Quid* 10 September 2016.

Christodoulou, P. (2011) 'Les reliefs votifs du sanctuaire d'Isis à Dion', *Bibliotheca Isiaca* II: 11–22.

Chrzanovski, L. (ed.) (2003) *Nouveautés lychnologiques*, Hauterive CH: Lychno Services.

Cimarosti, E. (2014) 'Tre *signacula* da raccolte museali nell'Italia nordoccidentale', in Buonopane, A., Braito, S. and Girardi, C. (eds.) *Instrumenta inscripta V. Signacula ex aere: aspetti epigrafici, archeologici, giuridici, prosopografici, collezionistici*, Roma: Scienze e Lettere: 319–324.

Claes, P. and Milliau, E. (1961) 'Liberchies: Bons-Villers', *L'Antiquité Classique* 30(1): 157–158.

Clark, J. and Sheldon, H. (eds.) (2008) *Londinium and beyond: essays on Roman London and its hinterland for Harvey Sheldon*, York: Council for British Archaeology.

Clarke, A. and Fulford, M. (2011) *Silchester: city in transition*, London: Society for the Promotion of Roman Studies.

Clarke, C.P. (1998) 'Excavations to the south of Chignall Roman villa, Essex, 1977–81', *East Anglian Archaeology* 83.

Clarke, G. (1979) *The Roman cemetery at Lankhills* (Winchester studies; 3, pt. 2), Oxford: Clarendon Press.

Clarke, G., Rigby, V. and Shepherd, J. (1982) 'The Roman Villa at Woodchester', *Britannia* 13: 197–228.

Clarke, S. (1997) 'Abandonment, rubbish disposal and 'special' deposits at Newstead', in Meadows, K., Lemke, C., and Heron, J. (eds.) *TRAC 96: Proceedings of the sixth annual theoretical Roman archaeology conference*. Oxford: Oxbow Books: 73–81.

Clarke, S. and Jones, R. (1996) 'The Newstead pits', in Driel-Murray, C. van (ed.) *Military equipment in context: proceedings of the ninth international Roman military equipment conference, held at Leiden, the Netherlands, 15th–17th September 1994*, Oxford: Oxbow Books: 110–124.

Clifford, E.M. (1938) 'Roman altars in Gloucestershire', *Transactions of the Bristol and Gloucestershire Archaeological Society* 60: 297–307.

Cochran, M.D. and Beaudry, M.C. (2006) 'Material culture studies and historical archaeology', in Hicks, D. and Beaudry, M. (eds.) *The Cambridge companion to historical archaeology*, Cambridge: Cambridge University Press: 191–204.

Coeuret, G. (1981) 'Prospection sur le site de Pouillé (Loir et Cher)', *Revue archéologique du Centre de la France* 20.1: 5–18.

Collins, R. (2008) 'Identity in the frontier: theory and multiple community interfacing', in Fenwick, C., Wiggins, M., and Wythe, D. (eds.) *TRAC 2007: Proceedings of the seventeenth annual theoretical Roman archaeology conference*, Oxford: Oxbow Books: 45–52.

Collins, R. (2020) 'The phallus and the frontier', in Ivleva, T. and Collins, R. (eds.) *Un-Roman sex: gender, sexuality, and lovemaking in the Roman provinces and frontiers*, Abingdon: Routledge: 274–309.

Cook, B.F. (1976) 'The classical marbles from the Arundel House site', in Hammerson, M.J. (ed.) 'Excavations on the site of Arundel House in the Strand, W.C.2., in 1972', *Transactions of the London and Middlesex Archaeological Society* 26: 209–251.

Cool, H.E.M. (1998) 'The brooches', in Cool, H.E.M. and Philo, C. (eds.) *Roman Castleford: volume1, the small finds*, Wakefield: West Yorkshire Archaeology Service: 29–57.

Cool, H.E.M. (2005) 'The glass', in Brady, K., Brown, L., and Smith, A. (eds.) *A Romano-British landscape at Brockley Hill, Stanmore, Middlesex: excavations at Brockley Hill House and the former MoD site*, Oxford: Oxford Archaeological Unit, OA Job No. 2211: 51–53.

Cool, H.E.M. (2006a) 'The small finds', in Booth, P. and Cool, H. 'The small finds from Pepper Hill, Southfleet, Kent (ARC PHL97 and NBR98)', *CTRL Specialist Archive Report*: Channel Tunnel Rail Link: 3–56.

Cool, H.E.M. (2006b) *Eating and drinking in Roman Britain*, Cambridge: Cambridge University Press.

Cool, H.E.M. and Baxter, M. (2016a) 'Brooches and Britannia', *Britannia* 47: 71–98.

Cool, H.E.M. and Richardson, J. (2013) 'Exploring ritual deposits in a well at Rothwell Haigh, Leeds', *Britannia* 44: 191–217.

Coombe, P. (2006) 'The Hardwick boot: a Roman bronze balsamarium', in Henig, M. (ed.) *Roman art, religion, and society: new studies from the Roman Art Seminar, Oxford 2005*, Oxford: Archaeopress: 1–27.

Coombe, P. (2015) 'Copper alloy statuary', in Killock, D. (ed.) *An assessment of an archaeological excavation at Tabard Square, 34–70 Long Lane and 31–47 Tabard Street, London SE1, London Borough of Southwark*, Brockley: Pre-Construct Archaeology Limited: 194–198.

Coombe, P., Grew, F., Hayward, K.M.J and Henig, M. (2015) *Roman sculpture from London and the South-east*, Oxford: Oxford University Press for the British Academy. *Corpus Signorum Imperii Romani* Great Britain 1.10.

Cooper, N. (1996) 'Searching for the blank generation: consumer choice in Roman and post-Roman Britain', in Webster, J. and Cooper, N. (eds.) *Roman imperialism: post-colonial perspectives: proceedings of a symposium held at Leicester University in November 1994*, Leicester: School of Archaeological Studies, University of Leicester: 85–98.

Cordischi, L. (1990) 'La dea Caelestis ed il suo culto attraverso le iscrizioni: 1. le iscrizioni latine di Roma e dell'Italia', *Archeologia Classica* 42: 161–200.

Corinium Museum (2019) online collections.

Corrocher, J. (1981) *Vichy antique*, Clermont-Ferrand: Presses universitaires Blaise Pascal.

Corzo-Sánchez, R. (1991) 'Isis en el teatro de Itálica', *Boletín de Bellas Artes* (Sevilla) 19: 123–148.

Cotton, J. (1996) 'A miniature chalk head from the Thames at Battersea and the "Cult of the Head" in Roman London', in Bird, J., Hassall, J. and Sheldon, H. (eds.) *Interpreting Roman London*, Oxford: Oxbow Monograph 58: 85–96.

Couchez, K. (2016) *Daar waar het Romeins schoentje wringt*, Masters Dissertation, University of Gent.

Coulston, J.C. (1997) 'The stone sculptures', in Wilson, R.J.A. and Jarrett, M.G. (eds.) *Roman Maryport and its setting: essays in memory of Michael G. Jarrett*, Penrith: Cumberland and Westmorland Antiquarian and Archaeological Society on behalf of the Trustees of the Senhouse Roman Museum, Maryport: 112–131.

Coulston, J.C. and Phillips, E.J. (1988) *Hadrian's Wall west of the North Tyne and Carlisle*, Oxford: Oxford University Press for the British Academy. *Corpus Signorum Imperii Romani* Great Britain 1.6.

Couppé, J., Dupas, M.-J. and Pal'ta, E. (1977) 'Les fibules du Musée de Quentovic', *Cahiers de Quentovic* 2–1977, fasc. 3–4.

Cousins, E.H. (2020) *The sanctuary at Bath in the Roman Empire*, Cambridge: Cambridge University Press.

Coutil, L. (1901) 'Les fouilles de Pitres (Eure)', *Bulletin Monumental* 65: 434–456.

Cracknell, S. (1994) 'Discussion', in Cracknell, S. and Mahany, C. (eds.) *Roman Alcester: southern extramural area 1964–1966 excavations, vol. 1 part 2: finds and discussion*, York: Council for British Archaeology: 149–159.

Cram, L. (1998) 'Human and animal foot impressed tiles', in Cool, H.E.M. and Philo, C. (eds.) *Roman Castleford: volume1, the small finds*, Wakefield: West Yorkshire Archaeology Service: 232–238.

Cram, L. and Fulford, M. (1979) 'Silchester tile making: the faunal environment', in McWhirr, A. (1979) *Roman brick and tile: studies in manufacture, distribution and use in the Western Empire*, Oxford: BAR. International Series 68: 201–210.

Crane, D. and Bovone, L. (2006) 'Approaches to material culture: the sociology of fashion and clothing', *Poetics* 34: 319–333.

Crease, S.M.E. (2015) *Re-thinking ritual traditions: interpreting structured deposition in watery contexts in late pre-Roman Iron Age and Roman Britain*, Doctoral thesis, University College London.

Creemers G. (2006) 'Hoeselt: Romeins bronzen laarsje', in Creemers G. and Vanderhoeven A. (eds.) *Archeologische kroniek van Limburg 2001*, Limburg Het Oude Land van Loon 85: 34–39.

Criniti, N. (2012) 'La produzione fittile veleiate: sintesi documentaria', *Ager Veleias* 7.04: 1–11.

Cripps, W. J. (1901) 'On a Roman altar and other sculptured stones found at Cirencester in April, 1899', *Proceedings of the Society of Antiquaries of London*, Series 2, 18: 177–184.

Croom, A. (2010) *Roman clothing and fashion* (3rd edn.), Stroud: Amberley.

Croom, A. (2018) 'A 'shoe' brooch from the Roman fort at South Shields', in Pickup, S. and Waite, S. (eds.) *Shoes, slippers and sandals: feet and footwear in classical antiquity*, Abingdon: Routledge: 301–309.

Crosby, V. and Hembrey, N. (2013) 'An evaluation in the fields south of Silbury Hill in 2010: Romano-British settlement, later alluviation and water meadows', *The Wiltshire archaeological and natural history magazine* 106: 101–166.

Crouvezier, F. (2019) 'Strasbourg: une nécropole romaine découverte en marge du chantier du tram', *Pokaa*.

Croxford, B. (2003) 'Iconoclasm in Roman Britain?', *Britannia* 34: 81–95.

Croxford, B. (2016) 'Metal sculpture from Roman Britain: scraps but not always scrap', in Myrup Kristensen, T. and Stirling, L. (eds.) *The afterlife of Greek and Roman sculpture: late antique responses and practices*, Michigan: University of Michigan Press: 27–46.

Crummy, N. (1983) *The Roman small finds from excavations in Colchester, 1971–9*, Colchester: Colchester Archaeological Trust, Colchester archaeological report 2.

Crummy, N. (2006) 'A jug handle from Silchester', *Lucerna, Roman Finds Group Newsletter* 32: 4–6.

Crummy, N. (2007) 'Brooches and the cult of Mercury', *Britannia* 38: 225–230.

Crummy, N. (2011) 'The small finds: well 5735', in Clarke, A. and Fulford, M. (eds.) *Silchester: city in transition*, London: Society for the Promotion of Roman Studies: 113–116.

Crummy, N. (2015) 'The copper alloy jug', in Atkinson, M. and Preston, S.J. (eds.) 'Heybridge: a late Iron Age and Roman settlement, excavations at Elms Farm 1993–5', *Internet Archaeology* 40.

Crummy, N., Crossan, P., Crummy, P. and Crossan, C. (1993) *Excavations of Roman and later cemeteries, churches and monastic sites in Colchester, 1971–88*, Colchester, Essex: Colchester Archaeological Trust, Colchester archaeological report 9.

Crummy, N. and Holmes, S. (2003) ' Hunter-god handle from Yorkshire', *Lucerna, Roman Finds Group Newsletter* 26: 5-6.

Cunliffe, B. (1977) *Excavations at Portchester Castle*, London: Society of Antiquaries of London: Distributed by Thames and Hudson, Report (Society of Antiquaries of London. Research Committee) no.34.

Cunliffe, B. (1999) *Fishbourne Roman palace* (revised and updated edition), Stroud: Tempus.

Cunliffe, B. (2013) *The Roman villa at Brading, Isle of Wight: the excavations of 2008–10*, Oxford: University of Oxford School of Archaeology, Monograph 77.

Cunliffe, B. and Fulford, M. (1982) *Bath and the rest of Wessex*, Oxford: Oxford University Press for the British Academy. *Corpus Signorum Imperii Romani* Great Britain 1.2.

Curle, J. (1911) *A Roman frontier post and its people*, Glasgow: James Maclehose and Sons.

Curle, J. (1932) 'An inventory of objects of Roman and provincial Roman origin found on sites in Scotland not definitely associated with Roman constructions', *Proceedings of the Society of Antiquaries of Scotland* 66: 277–397.

Dananai, A. (2012) 'Les fibules romaines en Gaule Belgique: étude d'une micro-région, le Douaisis', *Du néolithique aux temps modernes: 40 ans d'archéologie territoriale : mélanges offerts à Pierre Demolon*, Revue Du Nord Hors-Série 17: 207–259.

Daremberg, C. and Saglio, E. (1877) *Dictionnaire des antiquités Grecques et Romaines,* Paris: Hachette.

Darvill, T. and McWhirr, A. (1984) 'Brick and tile production in Roman Britain: models of economic organisation', *World Archaeology* 15(3): 239–261.

Dasen, V. (2015) 'Probaskania: amulets and magic in antiquity', in Boschung, D. and Bremmer, J.N. (eds.) *The materiality of magic*, Paderborn: Wilhelm Fink: 177–204.

Dasen, V. (2018) 'Amulets, the body and personal agency', in Parker, A. and McKie, S. (eds.) *Material approaches to Roman magic: occult objects and supernatural substances*, Oxford: Oxbow Books: 127–135.

Daveau, I. and Yvinec, J-H. (2002) 'L'occupation gallo-romaine du site de Fontenay-en-Parisis "La Lampe" (Val-d'Oise): établissement agricole spécialisé ou lieu de culte?', *Revue archéologique du Centre de la France* 41: 129–172.

Davies, G. (2012) 'Art, funerary, Roman', in Hornblower, S., Spawforth, A. and Eidinow, E. (eds.) *The Oxford classical dictionary* (4th ed.), Oxford: Oxford University Press.

Davies, P. (2013) 'An evaluation in the fields south of Silbury Hill in 2010: Romano-British settlement, later alluviation and water meadows', *Wiltshire Archaeological and Natural History Magazine* 106: 101–166.

Davies, S., Allen, M. and Bellamy, P. (2002) *Excavations at Alington Avenue, Fordington, Dorchester, Dorset, 1984–87*, Dorchester: Dorset Natural History and Archaeological Society, monograph series no. 15.

Davis, G. (2018) 'Rubbing and rolling, burning and burying: the magical use of amber in Roman London', in Parker, A. and McKie, S. (eds.) *Material approaches to Roman magic: occult objects and supernatural substances*, Oxford: Oxbow Books: 69–83.

Davis, R. (2000) *The book of pontiffs (Liber pontificalis): the ancient biographies of the first ninety Roman bishops to AD 715* (rev.) Liverpool: Liverpool University Press.

De Laet, S.J, van Doorselaer, A., Spitaels, P. and Thoen, H. (1972) *La Nécropole gallo-romaine de Blicquy (Hainaut, Belgique)*, Brugge: de Tempel, Dissertationes archaeologicae Gandenses 14.

Deetz, J. (1996) *In small things forgotten : an archaeology of early American life* (2nd edn.), New York: Random House.

Dehn, W., Hussong, L. and Koethe, H. (1937) 'Fundchronik: Arbeitsgebiet des Landesmuseums Trier', *Germania* 21.3: 195–197.

Delattre, R. (1898) 'Les cimetières romains superposés de Carthage (1896)', *Revue Archéologique*, 33: 82–101.

Delestre, X. (1979) 'Contribution à l'étude des lampes antiques en forme de pied', *Revue archéologique du Centre de la France*, 18.3–4: 175–176.

Deonna, W. (1927) 'L'ornementation des lampes romaines', *Revue Archéologique* 5e Série, T. 26: 233–263.

Deschler-Erb, E. (2006) 'Die Funde aus Bronze und Blei', in Schucany, C. (ed.) *Die römische Villa von Biberist-Spitalhof/SO (Grabungen 1982, 1983, 1986–1889). Untersuchungen im Wirtschaftsteil und Überlegungen zum Umland* Band 2, Remshalden: Bernhard Albert Greiner: 417–458.

Deschler-Erb, E. (2010) 'Römische Kleinfunde und Münzen aus Schleitheim-Juliomagus', *Beiträge zur Schaffhauser Archäologie* 4, Schaffhausen: Baudepartement des Kantons Schaffhausen, Kantonsarchäologie 2010.

Devillers, S. (2000) 'Les fibules du sanctuaire de la forêt d'Halatte (commune d'Ognon, Oise)', *Revue Archéologique de Picardie 18*: 267–276.

Dieudonné-Glad, N., Feugère, M. and Önal, M. (2013) *Zeugma V: Les objets*, Lyon: Maison de l'Orient et de la Méditerranée.

Dobosi, L. (2016) 'Animal and human footprints on Roman tiles from Brigetio', *Dissertationes Archaeologicae* Ser. 3. No. 4, Budapest: Eötvös Loránd University: 117–134.

Dollfus, A. (1975) 'Catalogue des fibules de bronze gallo-romaines de Haute-Normandie', in *Mémoires présentés par divers savants à l'Académie des inscriptions et belles-lettres de l'Institut de France*, première série, sujets divers d'érudition, tome 16,1: 9–261.

Donderer, M. (2004) 'Zur Interpretation des Weißenburger Schatzfundes', *Germania* 82.1: 235–246.

Douglas, A., Gerrard, J.F. and Sudds, B. (2011) *A Roman settlement and bath house at Shadwell: Excavations at Tobacco Dock and Babe Ruth restaurant, the Highway, London*, London: Pre-Construct Archaeology, Monograph (Pre-Construct Archaeology Limited) no. 12.

Douglas, C.R. (2015) *A comparative study of Roman-period leather from Northern Britain*, MPhil. Thesis, University of Glasgow.

Dow, S. and Upson, F. (1944) 'The foot of Sarapis', *Hesperia: the Journal of the American School of Classical Studies at Athens* 13(1): 58–77.

Driel-Murray, C. van (1987) 'Roman footwear: a mirror of fashion and society', in Friendship-Taylor, D., Swann, J. and Thomas, S. (eds.), *Recent research in archaeological footwear*, Association of Archaeological Illustrators and Surveyors Technical Paper no. 8: 32–42.

Driel-Murray, C. van (1993) *The early wooden forts: preliminary reports on the leather, textiles, environmental evidence and dendro-chronology*, Hexham: Roman Army Museum Publications for the Vindolanda Trust, Vindolanda research reports: new ser., v.3.

Driel-Murray, C. van (1995) 'Gender in question', in Rush, P. (ed.) *Theoretical Roman archaeology: second conference proceedings*, Aldershot: Avebury: 3–21.

Driel-Murray, C. van (1997a) 'Die Schuhe aus Schiff I und ein lederner Schildüberzug', in Haalebos, J. 'Ein römisches Getreideschiff in Woerden', *Jahrbuch des Römisch-Germanischen Zentralmuseums Mainz*, 43: 490–498.

Driel-Murray, C. van (1997b) 'Women in forts?', *Jahresbericht Gesellschaft Pro Vindonissa 1997*, Brugg: Vindonissa Museum: 55–61.

Driel-Murray, C. van (1999a), 'And did those feet in ancient time...Feet and shoes as a material projection of the self', in Baker, P., Forcey, C., Jundi, S. and Witcher, R. (eds.) *TRAC 98. Proceedings of the eighth annual theoretical Roman archaeology conference*, Oxford: Oxbow Books: 131–140.

Driel-Murray, C. van (1999b) 'Dead mens' shoes', in Schlüter, W. and Wiegels, R. (eds.) *Rom, Germanien und die Ausgrabungen von Kalkriese*. Osnabrück: Universitätsverlag Rasch: 189–169.

Driel-Murray, C. van (1999c) 'A set of Roman clothing from les Martres-de-Veyre, France', *Archaeological Textiles Newsletter* 28: 11–14.

Driel-Murray, C. van (2001a) 'Vindolanda and the dating of Roman footwear', *Britannia* 32: 185–197.

Driel-Murray, C. van (2001b) 'A brazen boot', *Archaeological Leather Group Newsletter* 13: 1–3.

Driel-Murray, C. van (2002a) 'Regarding the stars', in Carruthers, M., van Driel-Murray, C., Gardner, A., Lucas, J., Revell, L. and Swift, E. (eds.), *TRAC 2001: Proceedings of the eleventh annual theoretical Roman archaeology conference, Glasgow 2001*, Oxford: Oxbow Books: 96–103.

Driel-Murray, C. van (2002b) 'The leather trades in Roman Yorkshire and beyond', in Wilson, P.R. and Price, J. (eds.) *Aspects of industry in Roman Yorkshire and the North*, Oxford: Oxbow Books: 109–23.

van Driel-Murray, C. (2009a) 'Tanning and leather', in Oleson, J. (ed.), *The Oxford handbook of engineering and technology in the classical world*, Oxford, Oxford University Press.

Driel-Murray, C. van (2009b) 'Leerresten uit Geldermalsen-Hondsgemet: voddenhandel?', in Renswoude, J. van and Kerckhove J. van (eds.) Opgravingen in Geldermalsen-Hondsgemet: een inheemse nederzetting uit de Late IJzertijd en Romeinse tijd Amsterdam: Archeologisch Centrum Vrije Universiteit, Hendrik Brunsting Stichting: 854–856.

Driel-Murray, C. van (2009c) 'Ethnic recruitment and military mobility', in Morillo, A., Hanel, N. and Martín, E. (eds.) *Limes XX: XX Congreso Internacional de Estudios sobre la Frontera Romana: León (España), Septiembre, 2006*, Madrid: Polifemo: 813–822.

Driel-Murray, C. van (2011a), 'Footwear in the North-western provinces of the Roman Empire', in Goubitz, O., Groenman-van Waateringe, W. and van Driel-Murray, C. (eds.) *Stepping through time: archaeological footwear from prehistoric times until 1800* (3rd ed.), Zwolle: SPA Uitgevers: 337–376.

Driel-Murray, C. van (2011b) 'Leather and footwear', in Richardson, J. (ed.) *Rothwell Haigh, Rothwell, Leeds, West Yorkshire: Excavation Report*, Leeds: Archaeology Advisory Service report 2170: 47–54.

Driel-Murray, C. van (2016) 'Fashionable footwear: craftsmen and consumers in the north-west Provinces of the Roman Empire', in Wilson, A. and Flohr, M. (eds.) *Urban craftsmen and traders in the Roman world*, Oxford: Oxford University Press: 132–152.

Driel-Murray, C. van (2018) Conversation with Elizabeth Shaw, 14 April.

Driel-Murray, C. van and Gechter, M. (1983) 'Funde aus der Fabrica der Legio I Minervia am Bonner Berg', *Rheinische Ausgrabungen* 23: 1–83.

Drummond-Murray, J. and Thompson, P. with Cowan, C. (2002) *Settlement in Roman Southwark: archaeological excavations (1991–8) for the London Underground Limited Jubilee Line extension project*, London: Museum of London Archaeology Service.

Drury, P.J. (1978) *Excavations at Little Waltham 1970–7*, London: Council for British Archaeology Research Report 26.

Dudley, D. (1967) 'Excavations on Nornour in the Isles of Scilly 1962–1966', *Archaeological Journal* 124: 1–64.

Dumont, A. (2002) *Les passages à gué de la Grande Saône: Approche archéologique et historique d'un espace fluvial (de Verdun-sur-le-Doubs à Lyon)*, ARTEHIS Éditions.

Dunbabin, K.M.O. (1990) '*Ipsa deae vestigia* ... Footprints divine and human on Graeco-Roman monuments', *Journal of Roman Archaeology* Vol. 3: 85–109.

Dungworth, D. (1998) 'Mystifying Roman nails: *clavus annalis, defixiones* and *minkisi*', in Forcey, C., Hawthorne, J., and Witcher, R. (eds.) *TRAC 97: Proceedings of the seventh annual theoretical Roman archaeology conference, Nottingham 1997*, Oxford: Oxbow Books: 148–159.

Eckardt, H. (2000) 'Illuminating Roman Britain' in Fincham, G., Harrison, G. Holland, R. and Revell, L. (eds.) *TRAC 99: Proceedings of the ninth annual theoretical Roman archaeology conference*, Oxford: Oxbow Books: 8–21.

Eckardt, H. (2002) *Illuminating Roman Britain*, Montagnac: M. Mergoil, Monographies Instrumentum 23.

Eckardt, H. (2004) 'Remembering and forgetting in the Roman provinces', in Croxford, B., Eckardt, H., Meade, J., and Weekes, J. (eds.) *TRAC 2003: Proceedings of the thirteenth annual theoretical Roman Archaeology Conference*, Oxford: Oxbow Books: 36–50.

Eckardt, H. (2005) 'The social distribution of Roman artefacts: the case of nail-cleaners and brooches in Britain', *Journal of Roman Archaeology* 18: 139–160.

Eckardt, H. (2013) 'Shoe brooches in Roman Britain', in Eckardt, H. and Rippon, S. (eds.) *Living and working in the Roman world*, Journal of Roman Archaeology Supplementary Series 95: 217–234.

Eckardt, H. (2014) *Objects and identities: Roman Britain and the north-western provinces*, Oxford: Oxford University Press.

Eckardt, H. and Walton, P.J. (2021) *Bridge over troubled waters: the Roman finds from the River Tees at Piercebridge in context*, London: Society for the Promotion of Roman Studies, Britannia Monograph Series 34.

Eckardt, H., Brewer, P., Hay, S. and Poppy, S. (2009) 'Roman barrows and their landscape context: a GIS case study at Bartlow, Cambridgeshire', *Britannia* 40: 65–98.

Edmondson, J. (2008) 'Public dress and social control in late republican and early imperial Rome', in Edmondson, J. and Keith, A. (eds.) *Roman dress and the fabrics of Roman culture*, Toronto: University of Toronto Press: 21–46.

Edmondson, J. and Keith, A. (2008) 'Introduction: from costume history to dress studies', in Edmondson, J. and Keith, A. (eds.) *Roman dress and the fabrics of Roman culture*, Toronto: University of Toronto Press: 1–17.

Eggers, H.J. (1966) 'Römische Bronzegefässe in Britannien', *Jahrbuch des Römisch-Germanischen Zentralmuseums Mainz* 13: 67–164.

Egging-Dinwiddy, K. (2007) *A late Roman cemetery at Little Keep, Dorchester, Dorset*, Salisbury: Wessex Archaeology.

Elbern, V.H. (1979) 'Four bread stamps', in Weitzmann, K. (ed.) *Age of spirituality: Late Antique and early Christian art, third to seventh century*, New York: The Metropolitan Museum of Art: 627–628.

Ellis, P. (1984) *Catsgore, 1979: further excavation of the Romano-British village*, Gloucester: Alan Sutton for the Western Archaeological Trust, Excavation monograph no. 7.

Ellis, P. (ed.) (2000) *The Roman baths and macellum at Wroxeter*, London: English Heritage Archaeological Report 9.

Ellis, S. (1995) 'Lighting in late Roman houses', in Cottam, S., Dungworth, D., Scott, S., and Taylor, J. (eds.) *TRAC 94: Proceedings of the fourth annual theoretical Roman archaeology conference, Durham 1994*, Oxford: Oxbow Books: 65–71.

Emele, J. (1825) *Beschreibungen römischer und deutscher Altertümer in dem Gebiet der Provinz Rheinhessen*, Mainz: Stenz.

Encyclopaedia Britannica (2020) 'Cross'.

Espérandieu, E. (1900) *Musée Calvet. Inscriptions antiques, par le capitaine Émile Espérandieu*, Avignon: Seguin.

Ettlinger, E. (1973) *Die römischen Fibeln in der Schweiz*, Bern: Francke.

Evans, C. and Lucy, S. (2008) *Mucking excavations, Essex. archive and publication project—Prehistoric and Roman—overview and assessment*, Cambridge: Cambridge Archaeological Unit.

Evans, E. (2000) *The Caerleon canabae*, London: Society for the Promotion of Roman Studies, Britannia Monograph Series 16.

Evans, E., Maynard, D., Evans, D., Fox, S., Wilkinson, J and Zienkiewicz, J.D. (1997), 'Caerleon Lodge Hill cemetery: the Abbeyfield site 1992', *Britannia* 28: 169–243.

Evans, J. (2001) 'Material approaches to the identification of different Romano-British site types', in James, S. and Millett, M. (eds.) *Britons and Romans: advancing an archaeological agenda*, York: Council for British Archaeology: 26–35

Exner, K. (1941) 'Die provinzialrömischen Emailfibeln der Rheinlande', *Bericht der Römisch-Germanischen Kommission* Bd. 29: 31–121.

Fabretti, A. (1876) 'Sigillo in bronzo', *Atti della Società di Archeologia e Belle Arti per la provincia di Torino* I: 202–203.

Fagan, G.G. (1999) *Bathing in public in the Roman world*, Ann Arbor: University of Michigan Press.

Faider-Feytmans, G. (1979) *Les bronzes romains de Belgique* vol. II, Mainz am Rhein: Verlag P. von Zaubern.

Farwell, D., Molleson, T., and Atkinson, S. (1993). *Excavations at Poundbury. Vol. 2, The cemeteries*, Dorchester: Dorset Natural History and Archaeological Society, monograph series no. 11.

Fauduet, I. (1999) *Fibules préromaines, romaines et mérovingiennes du Musée du Louvre*, Paris: Presses de l'École Normale Supérieure.

Fauduet, I. and Pommeret, C. (1985) 'Les fibules du sanctuaire des Bolards à Nuits-Saint-Georges (Côte-d'Or)', *Revue archéologique de l'Est et du Centre-Est*, tome XXXVI, fasc. 1–2: 61–116.

Fernandez-Chicarro de Dios, C. (1950) 'Lapidas votivas con huellas de pies y exvotos reproduciendo parejas de pies, del Museo arqueológico provincial de Sevilla', *Revista de archivos bibliotecas y museos* LVI.3: 617–635.

Ferris, I. (2003) 'An empire in pieces. Roman archaeology and the fragment', in Carr, G., Swift, E., and Weekes, J. (eds.) *TRAC 2002: Proceedings of the twelfth annual Theoretical Roman Archaeology Conference, Canterbury 2002*, Oxford: Oxbow Books: 14–28.

Feugère, M. (1985) *Les fibules en Gaule méridionale, de la conquête à la fin du Ve siècle après Jésus-Christ*, Paris: Editions du Centre national de la recherche scientifique.

Feugère, M. (1998) 'Amulettes en forme de pied', *Instrumentum, bulletin du groupe de travail européen*, 8 décembre: 23.

Feugère, M. (2003) 'Penknives from Newstead: writing accessories', *Lucerna, Roman Finds Group Newsletter* 26: 9-12.

Feugère, M. (2010) '*Comendo tibi amicitiam*. Nouvelles fibules romaines à inscription ponctuée', in Ebnöther, C. and Schatzmann R. (eds.) *Oleum non perdidit. Festschrift für Stefanie Martin-Kilcher zu ihrem 65. Geburtstag*, Bern: Archéologie Suisse, Antiqua 47: 315–321.

Feugère, M. (2015) 'Fibules, identités et déplacements individuels ou collectifs dans l'Antiquité', *Journal of Roman Archaeology* 28.2: 699–704.

Feugère, M. and Lambert, P.Y. (2010) 'Une belle gauloise...à propos d'une fibule inscrite de Laon', *Etudes celtiques*, Droz, XXXVII: 147–152.

Feugère, M. and Mauné. S. (2005) 'Les signacula de bronze en Gaule Narbonnaise', *Revue archéologique de Narbonnaise* 38–39: 437–455.

Fittock, M. (2015) 'Broken deities: the pipe-clay figurines from Roman London', *Britannia* 46: 111–134.

Fitz, J. (1998) *Religions and cults in Pannonia : exhibition at Székesfehérvár, Csók István Gallery: 15 May–30 September 1996*, Székesfehérvár: István Király Múzeum.

Fiumi, E. (1977) *Volterra: das etruskische Museum und die Monumente der Antike*, Pisa: Pacini.

Fleming, R. (2021) *The material fall of Roman Britain, 300–525 CE*, Philadelphia: University of Pennsylvania Press.

Fontijn, D. (2002) *Sacrificial landscapes: cultural, biographies of persons, objects and 'natural' places in the Bronze Age of the southern Netherlands*, Leiden: Leiden University Press.

Foreman, A. (2015) 'Why footbinding persisted in China for a millennium', *Smithsonian Magazine*.

le Forestier, C. (2013) 'Les chaussures gallo-romaines en Île-de-France, approche archéo-anthropologique', *Revue archéologique d'Île-de-France* 6: 161–184.

Formigé, J. (1944) 'Le sanctuaire de Sanxay (Vienne)', *Gallia* 2: 43–120.

Forrer, R. (1907) *Reallexikon der prähistorischen, klassischen und frühchristlichen Altertümer*, Berlin and Stuttgart: W. Spemann.

Forrer, R. (1927) *Strasbourg-Argentorate: préhistorique, gallo-romain et mérovingien*, Strasbourg: Librairie Istra.

Forrer, R. (1942) *Archäologisches zur Geschichte des Schuhes aller Zeiten; dem Bally-Schuhmuseum gewidmet*, Schoenenwerd: Verlag des Bally-Schuhmuseums.

Forster, R.H. and Knowles, W.H. (1913) 'Corstopitum: report on the excavations in 1912', *Archaeologia Aeliana* ser. 3.9: 230–80.

Fowler, C. (2010) 'From identity and material culture to personhood and materiality', in *The Oxford handbook of material culture studies*, Oxford: Oxford University Press: 352–358.

Franken, N. (1996) 'Die antiken Bronzen im Römisch-Germanischen Museum Köln. Fragmente von Statuen. Figürlicher Schmuck von architektonischen Monumenten und Inschriften. Hausaustattung, Möbel, Kultgeräte, Votive und verschiedene Geräte', *Kölner Jahrbuch* 29: 7–203.

Franken, N. (1998) 'Römische und spätantike Bronzen im Akademischen Kunstmuseum der Universität Bonn', *Bonner Jahrbuch* 198: 49–99.

Fremersdorf, F. (1926) 'Ein Fund römischer Ledersachen in Köln', *Germania* 10.1: 44–56.

Frézouls, E. (1977) 'Circonscription de Champagne-Ardenne', *Gallia* 35, 2: 389–418.

Friedenberg, D. (1994) 'The evolution and uses of Jewish Byzantine stamp seals', *The Journal of the Walters Art Gallery* 52/53: 1–21.

Fulford, M. (1989) 'A Roman shipwreck off Nornour, Isles of Scilly?', *Britannia* 20: 245–249.

Fulford, M. (2001) 'Links with the past: pervasive 'ritual' behaviour in Roman Britain', *Britannia 32*: 199–218.

Fulford, M. and Machin, S. (2021) 'Building Britannia: Pre-Flavian private and public construction across southern Britain', *Britannia* 52: 207-225.

Furger, A. (1989) *Kurztexte und Hintergrundinformationen. Römermuseum und Römerhaus Augst*, Augst: Römermuseum, Augster Museumshefte 10.

Gage, J. (1836) 'XI. A letter from John Gage, Esq. F.R.S., Director, to Hudson Gurney, Esq., F.R.S., Vice-President, communicating the recent discovery of Roman sepulchral relics in one of the greater Barrows at Bartlow, in the parish of Ashdon, in Essex', *Archaeologia* XXVI: 300–317.

Galavaris, G. (2006) 'The power of the foot. The foot as talisman', in Kazakou, M. and Fioretou, A. (eds.) *Εξορκίζοντας το κακο: πιστη και δεισιδαιμονιες στο βυζαντιο*, Athens: Ταμείο Αρχαιολογικών Πόρων και Απαλλοτριώσεων: 41–52.

Galerie Sangiorgi, Jandolo and Tavazzi, Rome (1909) *Catalogue de la vente après décès de Mr. Joachim Ferroni*, Rome: Imprimerie de l'Unione Cooperativa Editrice.

Gansser-Burckhardt, A. (1942), 'Das Leder und seine Verarbeitung im römischen Legionslager Vindonissa', *Veröffentlichungen der Gesellschaft Pro Vindonissa* Bd. 1, Basel: Birkhäuser.

Garbsch, J. (1994) 'Römischer Gewandschmuck in Bayern', in Reichert, L. (ed.) *125 Jahre Bayerische Handelsbank in München, 1869–1994*, München: Bayerische Handelsbank: 237–262.

Gardner, A. (2013) 'Thinking about Roman imperialism: postcolonialism, globalisation and beyond?', *Britannia* 44: 1–25.

Garrow, D. (2012) 'Odd deposits and average practice. a critical history of the concept of structured deposition', *Archaeological Dialogues* 19(02): 85–144.

Gascou, J. (1990) 'Les inscriptions', *Gallia* 47: 194–201.

Gaspar, N. (2007) *Die keltischen und gallo-römischen Fibeln vom Titelberg*, Luxembourg: Musée national d'histoire et d'art, Dossiers d'archéologie du Musée national d'histoire et d'art XI.

Gaultier, M., Guillon, M., Corde, D. and Trébuchet, E. (2009) 'Les chaussures dans les sépultures antiques: dépôts et habillement', in Bizot, M. and Signoli, M. (eds.) *Rencontre autour des sépultures habillées*, Actes des journées d'étude organisées par le Groupement d'Anthropologie et d'Archéologie funéraire et le Service Régional de l'Archéologie de Provence-Alpes-Côte d'Azur, Carry-le-Rouet, 13–14 décembre 2008: 76–93.

Gell, A. (1998) *Art and agency: an anthropological theory*, Oxford: Clarendon Press.

Gennep, A. van (1909) *The rites of passage*, trans. Vizedom, M. and Caffée. L. (1960) Chicago: Chicago University Press.

Germain, M. (1925) 'Musée de Bourg', *Revue des musées et collections archéologiques* 4: 119–121.

Germany, M. (2003) 'Excavations at Great Holts Farm, Boreham, Essex 1992–4', *East Anglian Archaeology* 105.

Gerrard, J.F. (2007) 'The temple of Sulis Minerva at Bath', *The Antiquaries Journal* 87: 148–164.

Gerrard, J.F. (2009) 'The Drapers' Gardens hoard: a preliminary account', *Britannia*, 40: 163–184.

Gerrard, J.F. (2011) 'Wells and belief systems at the end of Roman Britain: A case study from Roman London', in Lavan, L. and Mulryan, M. (eds.) *The archaeology of late antique "paganism"*, Leiden: Brill, Late antique archaeology 7: 551–572.

Gerrard, J.F. (2013) *The ruin of Roman Britain: an archaeological perspective*, Cambridge: Cambridge University Press.

Gerrard, J.F. (2015a) 'Synthesis, chronology, and 'late Roman' cemeteries in Britain', *American Journal of Archaeology*, 119.4: 565–572.

Gerrard, J.F. (2015b) 'The fate of statues', in Killock, D. (ed.) *Temples and suburbs: excavations at Tabard Square, Southwark*, Brockley: Pre-Construct Archaeology Limited: 198.

Gerrard, J.F. (forthcoming) 'The social lives of wells in Roman Britain and beyond', in Lundock, J. and Sivilich, M (eds.) *Aspects of water in the Roman world*, Gainesville: University of Florida Press.

Gerrard, J.F. and Major, H. (2009) 'Roman Small Finds', in Killock, D. (ed.) *An assessment of an archaeological excavation at Tabard Square, 34–70 Long Lane and 31–47 Tabard Street, London SE1, London Borough of Southwark*, Brockley: Pre-Construct Archaeology Limited: 240–279.

Gherchanoc, F. and Huet, V. (2015) 'Le corps et ses parures dans l'Antiquité grecque et romaine: bilan historiographique' in *L'histoire du corps dans l'Antiquité*: bilan historiographique. Journée de printemps de la SOPHAU du 25 mai 2013, Dialogues d'histoire ancienne, Supplément 14: 127–149.

Giddens, A. (2013) *The constitution of society: outline of the theory of structuration*, Hoboken: Wiley.

Godwin, E.W. (1856) 'Roman villa at Colerne, Wiltshire', *The Archaeological Journal* 13: 328–332.

Goethert, K. (1997) *Romische Lampen und Leuchter*, Trier, Rheinisches Landesmuseum Trier.

Goette, H.R. (1988) 'Mulleus, Embas, Calceus. Ikonografische Studien zu römischem Schuhwerk', *Jahrbuch des Deutschen Archäologischen Instituts* 103: 401–464.

Goh, I. (2017) 'Members only? The non-aggression of phalluses in Lucilian satire', *Arethusa* 50(1): 35–64.

Goldman, N. (2001) 'Roman footwear', in Bonfante, L. and Sebesta, J.L. (eds.) *The world of Roman costume*, Madison, WI: University of Wisconsin Press: 101–132.

Gómez-Pantoja, J. (2000) 'Legio X *Gemina*', in Le Bohec, Y. and Wolff, C. (eds.) *Les légions de Rome sous le Haut-Empire*, Lyon: Coll. du Centre d'Études Romaines et Gallo-Romaines: 169–190.

Goodburn, R. (1972) *The Roman villa, Chedworth*, London: National Trust.

Goodburn, R. (1984) 'The non-ferrous metal objects', in Frere, S. (ed.) *Verulamium excavations volume III*, London: Society of Antiquaries of London: 19–68.

Goodchild, R. and Kirk, J.R. (1954) 'The Romano-Celtic temple at Woodeaton', *Oxoniensia* 19: 15–37.

Goorle, A. van. (1778) *Cabinet de pierres antiques gravées*, Paris: Lamy.

Göpfrich, J. (1986) 'Römische Lederfunde aus Mainz', *Saalburg Jahrbuch 42*: 5–67.

Gorny and Mosch (2016) *Katalog zur Auktion 239 'Kunst der Antike'*, Munich: Gorny and Mosch.

Gosden, C. and Marshall, Y. (1999) 'The cultural biography of objects', *World Archaeology* 31.2: 169–178.

Gouyet, G. (1976) 'Les fibules du vicus gallo-romain de Taverny', *Jeunesse préhistorique et géologique de France* 6: 81–89.

Graham, E.-J. (2020) *Reassembling religion in Roman Italy*, Abingdon: Routledge.

Grandjouan, C. (1961) *Terracottas and plastic lamps of the Roman period*, Princeton, N.J.: American School of Classical Studies at Athens.

Gravett, S.L., Bohmbach, K.G., Greifenhagen F.V. and Polaski, D.C. (2008) *An introduction to the Hebrew Bible: a thematic approach*, London: Westminster John Knox Press.

Green, C. (2007) *Roman religion and the cult of Diana at Aricia*, Cambridge: Cambridge University Press.

Greene, E.M. (2014) 'If the shoe fits: Style and function of children's shoes from Vindolanda', in Collins, R. and McIntosh, F. (eds.) *Life in the limes: studies of the people and objects of the Roman frontiers*, Oxford: Oxbow Books: 29–36.

Greene, E.M. (2018a) 'Metal fittings on the Vindolanda shoes', in Pickup, S. and Waite, S., (eds.) *Shoes, slippers sandals: feet and footwear in antiquity*, London and New York: Routledge: 310–324.

Greene, E.M. (2018b) Conversation with Elizabeth Shaw, 9 October.

Greenough, J.B., D'Ooge, B.L. and Daniell, M.G. (1899) *Caesar's Gallic War*, Boston: Ginn & Co.

Gregory, T. (1977) 'The enclosure at Ashill', *East Anglian Archaeology* 5: 9–30.

Grimal, P. and Kershaw, S. (1991) *The Penguin dictionary of classical mythology*, London: Penguin Books.

Groenman-van Waateringe, W. (1967) *Romeins lederwerk uit Valkenburg Z.H.* Groningen: Wolters, Nederlanse Oudheden II.

Groenman-van Waateringe, W. (1974) 'Römische Lederfunde aus Vindonissa und Valkenburg Z. H.: ein Vergleich', *Jahresbericht Gesellschaft Pro Vindonissa 1974*: 62–84.

Groot, M. (2009) 'Searching for patterns among special animal deposits in the Dutch river area during the Roman period', *Journal of Archaeology in the Low Countries* 1–2: 49–81.

Groot. M. (2012) 'Dealing with deposits in the Dutch river area: animals in settlement rituals in the Roman period', in Pluskowski, A. (ed.) *The ritual killing and burial of animals: European perspectives*, Oxford: Oxbow Books: 137–151.

Gros P. (1984) 'L'*augusteum* de Nîmes', *Revue archéologique de Narbonnaise* 17: 123–134.

Grünbart, M. (2006) 'Byzantine Metal Stamps in a North American Private Collection', *Dumbarton Oaks Papers* 60: 13-24.

Guarducci, M. (1943) 'Le impronte del 'Quo vadis' e monumenti affini, figurati ed epigrafici', *Rendiconti della Pontificia Accademia Romana di Archaeologia* 19, 1942–1943: 305–344.

Guerra, E. (2009) 'Le fibule d'epoca Romana nel Locarnese: tradizione e Romanità', *Jahrbuch Archäologie Schweiz* 92: 165–200.

Guéry, R. and Hallier, G. (1990) 'Tombes et architecture', *Gallia* 47: 148–185.

Guiraud, H. (1989) 'Bagues et anneaux à l'époque romaine en Gaule', *Gallia* 46: 173–211.

Gurney, D. (ed.) (1986) *Settlement, religion and industry on the Fen-Edge; three Romano-British sites in Norfolk*, Dereham: Norfolk Archaeological Unit, East Anglian Archaeology 31.

Haasteren, M. van and Groot, M. (2013) 'The biography of wells: a functional and ritual life history', *Journal of Archaeology in the Low Countries* 4.2: 25–51.

Hammerson, M. (1978) 'Excavations under Southwark Cathedral', *London Archaeologist* 03.08: 206–212.

Hampel, J. (1893) 'A nemzeti múzeum régiségtárának gyarapodása', *Archaeologiai Értesítő* 13: 448–453.

Hanson, J.A. (1959) *Roman theater-temples*, Princeton NJ: Princeton University Press.

Harden, D.B. (1987) *Glass of the Caesars*, Milan: Olivetti.

Harding, A. (2016) 'Introduction: biographies of things', in Albery, H., Lohmann, P. and Zurhake, L. (eds.) *Continuities and changes of meaning*, Distant Worlds Journal 1: 5–10.

Harlow, M. and Nosch, M. L. (2014) 'Weaving the threads: methodologies in textile and dress research for the Greek and Roman world—the state of the art and the case for cross-disciplinarity', in Harlow, M. and Nosch, M. L. (eds.) *Greek and Roman textiles and dress: an interdisciplinary anthology*, Oxford: Oxbow Books: 1–33.

Harris, O.J.T. and Cipolla, C.N. (2017) *Archaeological theory in the new millennium: introducing current perspectives*, London; New York: Routledge, Taylor and Francis Group.

Harris, W. (1980) 'Roman terracotta lamps: the organization of an industry', *Journal of Roman Studies* 70: 126–145.

Haselgrove, C. (1997) 'Iron Age brooch deposition and chronology', in Gwilt, A. and Haselgrove, C. (eds.) *Reconstructing Iron Age societies: new approaches to the British Iron Age*, Oxford: Oxbow Books: 51–72.

Hassall, M. (1979) 'Military tile-stamps from Britain', in McWhirr, A. (ed.) *Roman brick and tile: studies in manufacture, distribution and use in the Western Empire*, Oxford: B.A.R. International Series 68: 261–266.

Hattatt, R. (1982) *Ancient and Romano-British brooches*, Sherborne, Dorset: Dorset publishing.

Hattatt, R. (1985) *Iron Age and Roman brooches: a second selection of brooches from the author's collection*, Oxford: Oxbow Books.

Hattatt, R. (1987) *Brooches of antiquity: a third selection of brooches from the author's collection*, Oxford: Oxbow Books.

Hattatt, R. (1989) *A visual catalogue of Richard Hattatt's ancient brooches*, Oxford: Oxbow Books.

Haverfield, F. (1898) 'Roman shoe found at Birdoswald', *The Classical Review*, vol. 12, no. 2: 142.

Haverfield, F. (1900) 'Catalogue of the Roman inscribed and sculptured stones in the Grosvenor Museum, Chester', *Journal of the Chester Archaeological Society* 7: 5–100.

Haverfield, F. (1906) 'Romano-British Somerset: part 3, other locations', in Page, W. (ed.) *A history of the county of Somerset* vol. 1: 207–372.

Haverfield, F. (1911) 'An inaugural address delivered before the first annual general meeting of the society, 11th May, 1911', *The Journal of Roman Studies* 1: xi–xx.

Haverfield, F. (1914) 'An account of the Roman remains in Corbridge parish', in Craster, H.H.E. (ed.) *A history of Northumberland* vol. 10, Newcastle upon Tyne: Reid and company: 457–522.

Haverfield, F. (1917) 'Roman Cirencester', *Archaeologia: or miscellaneous tracts relating to antiquity* volume LXIX, London: T. Bensley: 161–209.

Haverfield, F. (1919) 'The Tullie House fibulae', *Transactions of the Cumberland and Westmorland Antiquarian and Archaeological Society* 19: 1–19.

Haverfield, F. (1923) *The Romanization of Roman Britain*, Oxford: Clarendon Press.

Haynes, I.P. (2013a) *Blood of the provinces: the Roman auxilia and the making of provincial society from Augustus to the Severans*, Oxford: Oxford University Press.

Haynes, I.P. (2013b) 'Advancing the systematic study of ritual deposition in the Greco-Roman World', in Lindström, G., Schäfer, A. and Witteyer, M. (eds.) *Rituelle Deponierungen in Heligtümern der hellenistisch-römischen Welt: Internationale Tagung Mainz, 28.–30. April 2008*, Mainz: Generaldirektion Kulturelles Erbe Rheinland-Pfalz: 7–19.

Haynes, I.P. (2020a) Personal email to Elizabeth Shaw, 9 September.

Haynes, I.P. (2020b) 'Site discussion', in Haynes, I.P. and Wilmott, T. (2020) *A cult centre on Rome's north west frontier: excavations at Maryport, Cumbria 1870–2015*, Cumbria: Cumberland and Westmorland Antiquarian and Archaeological Society, Research Series 12: 197-222.

Haynes, I.P. (2021) Personal comment to Elizabeth Shaw, 10 May.

Haynes, I.P. and Wilmott, T. (2012) 'The Maryport altars: an archaeological myth dispelled', *Historia* 57.1: 25–37.

Haynes, I.P. and Wilmott, T. (2020) *A cult centre on Rome's north west frontier: excavations at Maryport, Cumbria 1870–2015*, Cumbria: Cumberland and Westmorland Antiquarian and Archaeological Society, Research Series 12.

Heeren, S. (2014) 'Brooches and burials: variability in expressions of identity in cemeteries of the Batavian civitas', *Journal of Roman Archaeology*, 27: 443–455.

Heeren, S. and Feist, L. van der (2017) *Prehistorische, Romeinse en Middeleeuwse fibulae uit de Lage Landen*, Amersfoort: Stijn Heeren and Lourens van der Feijst.

Henrichs, A. (2012) 'Dionysus', in Hornblower, S., Spawforth, A. and Eidinow, E. (eds.) *The Oxford classical dictionary* (4th ed.), Oxford: Oxford University Press.

Henig, M. (1977) 'Death and the maiden: funerary symbolism in daily life', in Toynbee, J. M. C., Munby, J. and Henig, M. (eds.) *Roman life and art in Britain: a celebration in honour of the eightieth birthday of Jocelyn Toynbee*, Oxford: British Archaeological Reports 41: 347–366.

Henig, M. (1984) *Religion in Roman Britain*, London: Batsford.

Henig, M. (1993) 'Votive objects: images and inscriptions' in Woodward, A. and Leach, P. (eds.) *The Uley shrines: excavation of a ritual complex on West Hill, Uley, Gloucestershire 1977–9*, English Heritage Archaeology Report 17: 89–112.

Henig, M. (2015) 'Figural bronzes', in Atkinson, M. and Preston, S.J. (eds.) 'Heybridge: a Late Iron Age and Roman settlement, excavations at Elms Farm 1993–5', *Internet Archaeology* 40.

Henig, M., Webster, G. and Blagg, T. (1993) *Roman sculpture from the Cotswold region*, Oxford: Oxford University Press for the British Academy. *Corpus Signorum Imperii Romani* Great Britain 1.7.

Henig, M., Webster, G. and Blagg, T. (2004) *Roman sculpture from the North West Midlands*, Oxford: Oxford University Press for the British Academy. *Corpus Signorum Imperii Romani* Great Britain 1.9.

Henkel, F. (1913) *Die Römischen Fingerringe der Rheinlande und der benachbarten Gebiete*, Berlin: Georg Reimer.

Hermann Historica Auctions (2019) *Ziegel mit Legionsstempel und Schuhabdruck*.

Héron de Villefosse, A. (1900) 'Séance du 19 Décembre', *Bulletin de la société nationale des antiquaires de France*: 317–323.

Hill, C., Millett, M., Blagg, T. and Dyson, T. (1980) *The Roman riverside wall and monumental arch in London: excavations at Baynard's Castle, Upper Thames Street, London 1974–6*, London: London and Middlesex Archaeological Society.

Hill, D.K. (1946) 'Material on the cult of Sarapis', *Hesperia: the journal of the American School of Classical Studies at Athens* 15(1): 60–72.

Hill, J. (1995) *Ritual and rubbish in the Iron Age of Wessex: A study on the formation of a specific archaeological record*, Oxford: Tempus Reparatum, BAR British series 242.

Hill, J. and Rowsome, P. (2011) *Roman London and the Walbrook stream crossing: excavations at 1 Poultry and vicinity, City of London*, London: Museum of London Archaeology, Monograph 37.

Historic England (2021) *Lexden Tumulus Iron Age barrow*.

Historic Environment Scotland (2021a) *Clickimin broch*.

Historic Environment Scotland (2021b) *Kilmartin Glen: Dunadd Fort*.

Hodder, I. (1987) 'The contextual analysis of symbolic meanings', in Hodder, I. (ed.) *The archaeology of contextual meanings*, Cambridge: Cambridge University Press: 1–10.

Hodder, I. (1992) *Theory and practice in archaeology*, London: Routledge.

Hodder, I. (2005) 'Architecture and meaning: the example of Neolithic houses and tombs', in Parker Pearson, M. and Richards, C. (eds.) *Architecture and order* (2nd edn.), London: Routledge: 67–78.

Hodder, I. (2007) 'The "social" in archaeological theory: an historical and contemporary perspective', in Meskell, L. and Preucel, R. (eds.) *A companion to social archaeology*, Oxford: Blackwell: 23–42.

Hodder, I. (2011a) 'Human-thing entanglement: towards an integrated archaeological perspective', *Journal of the Royal Anthropological Institute* 17.1: 154–177.

Hodder, I. (2011b) 'Wheels of time: some aspects of entanglement theory and the secondary products revolution', *Journal of World Prehistory* 24.2: 175–187.

Hodder, I. (2016) *Studies in human-thing entanglement*.

Hoek, A. van den, Feissel, D. and Hermann Jr., J.J. (2015) 'More lucky wearers: the magic of portable inscriptions', in Boschung, D. and Bremmer, J.N. (eds.) *The materiality of magic*, Paderborn: Wilhelm Fink, Morphomata 20: 309–356.

Hoët-van Cauwenberghe, C. (2013) 'Supports d'écriture et gestion de production au quotidien dans le nord de la Gaule (Nerviens, Atrébates): estampilles et graffiti sur briques et sur tuiles', *Gallia* 70.2: 295–313.

Holtorf, C. (1998) 'The life-histories of megaliths in Mecklenburg-Vorpommern (Germany)', *World Archaeology* 30.1: 23–38.

Hoorn, G. van (1936) *Gids door de verzameling van Nederlandsche en Romeinsche oudheden van het Provinciaal Utrechtsch Genootschap van Kunsten en Wetenschappen in het Centraal-Museum te Utrecht*, Utrecht: Boekhoff.

Höpken, C. and Liesen, B. (2013) 'Römische Gräber im Kölner Süden II: Von der Nekropole um St. Severin bis zum Zugweg', *Kölner Jahrbuch* 46: 369–571.

Hoskins, J. (1998) *Biographical objects: how things tell the stories of people's lives*, London: Routledge.

Hoskins, J. (2006) 'Agency, biography and objects', in Tilley, C., Keane, W., Küchler, S., Rowlands, M., and Spyer, P. (eds.) *Handbook of material culture*, London: Sage: 74–84.

Hoss, S. (2014) 'Metaal', in Driessen, M. and Besselsen, E. (eds.) *Voorburg-Arentsburg: Een Romeinse havenstad tussen Rijn en Maas* vol. II, Amsterdam: University of Amsterdam: 613-674.

Hoss, S. (2015) 'Frontier finds—military fashions', in Breeze, D.J., Jones, R.H, Ioana A. Oltean, I.A. and Hanson, W.S. (eds.) *Understanding Roman frontiers: a celebration for Professor Bill Hanson*, Edinburgh: John Donald: 135–153.

Hoss, S. (2016) 'Of brooches and men' in Hoss, S. and Whitmore, A. (eds.) *Small finds and ancient social practices in the northwest provinces of the Roman Empire*, Oxford: Oxbow Books: 35–53.

Hoss, S. (2020) 'De metaalvondsten uit het Thermenkomplex van Heerlen (zonder munten of fibulae)', in Jeneson, K. and Vos, W.K. (eds.) *Roman bathing in Coriovallum*, Amersfoort: Rijksdienst voor het Cultureel Erfgoed, Nederlandse Archeologische Rapporten 65, Appendix XIII.

Houben, P. and Fiedler, F. (1839) *Denkmäler von Castra Vetera und Colonia Traiana im Ph. Houben's Antiquarium zu Xanten*, Xanten: Gebrüder Becker.

Houlbrook, C. and Armitage, N. (2015) *The materiality of magic: an artefactual investigation into ritual practices and popular belief*, Oxford; Philadelphia: Oxbow Books.

Howell, I. (2005) *Prehistoric landscape to Roman villa: excavations at Beddington, Surrey, 1981–7*, London: Museum of London Archaeology Service, MoLAS monograph 26.

Howsam, N. and Bridgen, A. (2018) 'A comparative study of standing fleshed foot and walking and jumping bare footprint measurements', *Science and Justice—Journal of the Forensic Science Society* 58.5: 346–354.

Hull, M.R. (1958) *Roman Colchester*, London: Society of Antiquaries of London.

Hull, M.R. (1968) 'The Nor'nour brooches', in Dudley, D. (ed.) 'Excavations on Nor'nour in the Isles of Scilly 1962–1966', *Archaeological Journal* 124: 28–64.

Hull, M.R. and Hawkes, C.F.C (1987) *Corpus of ancient brooches in Britain: pre-Roman bow brooches*, Oxford: BAR British series 168.

Hunter, F. (2017) *Legless Romans*, National Museum of Scotland blog.

Hurrell, H. (1904) 'Roman Objects from Hauxton Mill', *Proceedings of the Cambridge Antiquarian Society 10 (4)*: 496.

Huskinson, J. (1994) *Roman sculpture from eastern England*, Oxford: Oxford University Press for the British Academy. *Corpus Signorum Imperii Romani* Great Britain 1.8.

Ingold, T. (2004) 'Culture on the ground: the world perceived through the feet', *Journal of Material Culture* 9.3: 315–340.

Ingold, T. (2010a) 'Footprints through the weather-world: walking, breathing, knowing', *Journal of the Royal Anthropological Institute*, vol 16, Supplement s1: S121–S139.

Ingold, T. (2010b) 'Bringing things back to life: creative entanglements in a world of materials', NCRM Working Paper, Realities/Morgan Centre, University of Manchester..

Inrap (2020) online. *Ligne à grande vitesse Tours–Bordeaux: cuve à chaux*.

Istvánovits, E. and Gábor, P. (2011) 'Az alföldi Barbaricum mécsesei', *A nyíregyházi Jósa András Múzeum évkönyvei* 53: 83–111.

Iványi, D. (1935) *Die pannonischen Lampen. Eine typologisch-chronologische Übersicht*, Budapest: Dissertationes Pannonicae Serie II 2.

Jackson R.P.J. and Potter T.W. (1996) *Excavations at Stonea, Cambridgeshire, 1980–85*, London: British Museum Press.

Jacobi, L. (1897) *Das Römerkastell Saalburg bei Homburg vor der Höhe: nach den Ergebnissen der Ausgrabungen und mit Benutzung der hinterlassenen Aufzeichnungen des königl. Konservators Obersten A. von Cohausen*, Homburg vor der Höhe: Im selbstverlage des Verfassers.

Janek, T. (2014) *Roman building terracottas between Vindobona and Brigetio and along the Danubian Limes (1.–4. Century AD)*, Doctoral thesis, Prague: Charles University.

Jeanne, L., Paez-Rezende, L., Bocquet-Lienard, A., Duclos, C., Savary, X., Coutard, S., Lemonnier, M., Dodeman, C. and Macqueron, P-L. (2014) 'La production de terres cuites architecturales à l'époque romaine dans le nord du territoire des Unelles (Manche) Les ateliers du Pas du Vivray à Teurthéville-Bocage et du Douetty à Brillevast', *Revue archéologique de l'Ouest* 31: 315–368.

Jeneson, K. and Vos, W.K. (eds.) (2020) *Roman bathing in Coriovallum*, Amersfoort: Rijksdienst voor het Cultureel Erfgoed, Nederlandse Archeologische Rapporten 65.

Jennings, K. (2000) 'The excavation of nine Romano-British burials at Andover, Hampshire in 1984 and 1987', *Proceedings of the Hampshire Field Club and Archaeological Society* 55: 114–13.

Jessup, R.F. (1954) 'Excavation of a Roman Barrow at Holborough, Snodland', *Archaeologia Cantiana* 68: 1–61.

Johns, C. (1995) 'Mounted men and sitting ducks: the iconography of Romano-British plate brooches', in Raftery, B. (ed.) *Sites and sights of the Iron Age: essays of fieldwork and museum research presented to I.M. Stead*, Oxford: Oxbow Books: 103–9.

Johns, C. (2012) *The jewellery of Roman Britain: Celtic and classical traditions*, London: Routledge.

Johnson, M. (1999) *Archaeological theory: an introduction*, Oxford: Blackwell.

Joy, J. (2009) 'Reinvigorating object biography: reproducing the drama of object lives', *World Archaeology* 41.4: 540–556.

Jundi, S. and Hill, J. D. (1998) 'Brooches and identities in first century AD Britain: more than meets the eye?' in Forcey, C, Hawthorne, J., and Witcher, R. (eds.) (1998) *TRAC 97: Proceedings of the seventh annual theoretical Roman archaeology conference*, Oxford: Oxbow Books: 125–137.

Károly, G. (1890) 'Ókori Kocsik Helyreállítása', *Archaeologiai Értesitő* 10: 97–126.

Kaufmann-Heinimann, A. (1998) *Götter und Lararien aus Augusta Raurica. Herstellung, Fundzusammenhänge und sakrale Funktion figürlicher Bronzen in einer römischen Stadt*, Augst: Augst Roman Museum, Forschungen in Augst 26.

Keily, J. (2000) *The Roman leather finds from No 1 Poultry*, London: Museum of London Archaeology.

Keily, J. and Mould, Q. (2017) 'Leatherworking in south-eastern Britain in the Roman period', in D. Bird (ed.) *Agriculture and industry in south-eastern Roman Britain*, Oxford: Oxbow books: 236–254.

Keppie, L.J.F. and Arnold, B.J. (1984) *Scotland*, Oxford: Oxford University Press for the British Academy. *Corpus Signorum Imperii Romani* Great Britain 1.4.

Killock, D. (2009) *An assessment of an archaeological excavation at Tabard Square, 34–70 Long Lane and 31–47 Tabard Street, London SE1, London Borough of Southwark*, Brockley: Pre-Construct Archaeology Limited.

Kirsch, A. (2002) *Antike Lampen im Landesmuseum Mainz*, Mainz: P. von Zabern.

Klein, J. (1889) 'Die kleineren inschriftlichen Denkmäler des Bonner Provinzialmuseums', *Bonner Jahrbuch* 88, Bonn: Verein von Alterthumsfreunde im Rheinlande: 96–116.

Knötzele, P. (2007) 'Römische Schuhe: Luxus an den Füßen', *Schriften des Limesmuseums Aalen* Nr. 59., Stuttgart: Theiss.

Kohle, M. (2013) 'Schuhgefäße der Bronze- und Eisenzeit—Überlegungen zur Funktion und Bedeutung', *Ethnographisch-Archäologische Zeitschrift* 54: 49–70.

Kohlert-Németh, M. (1990) *Römische Bronzen II aus Nida-Heddernheim. Fundsachen aus dem Hausrat: Auswahlkatalog*, Frankfurt am Main, Museum für Vor- und Frühgeschichte.

Kopytoff, I. (1986) 'The cultural biography of things: commoditization as process', in Appadurai, A. (ed.) *The social life of things: commodities in cultural perspectives*, Cambridge: Cambridge University Press: 64–91.

Köstner, B. (2016) 'Wearing socks in sandals: the height of Roman fashion?', in Hoss, S. and Whitmore, A. (eds.) *Small finds and ancient social practices in the northwest provinces of the Roman Empire*, Oxford: Oxbow Books: 16–27.

Kötzsche, L. (1979) 'Four bread stamps', in Weitzmann, K. (ed.) *Age of spirituality: Late Antique and early Christian art, third to seventh century*, New York: The Metropolitan Museum of Art: 627–628.

Koutoussaki, L. (2007) 'Antike plastische Tonlampen in der Archäologischen Sammlung der Universität Zürich', *Archäologische Sammlung Zürch* 33: 19–27.

Los Angeles County Museum of Art LACMA (2021) online collection.

Lacroix, P. and Duchesne, A. (1852) *Histoire de la chaussure, depuis l'antiquité la plus reculée jusqu'à nos jours*, Paris: Seré.

Laing, J. (1999) *Art and society in Roman Britain*, Stroud: Sutton Publishing.

Lambot, B. (1975) 'Les fibules du Musée Vivenel', *Cahiers archéologiques de Picardie* 2.2: 15–28.

Lambot, B. (1983) 'Les fibules gallo-romaines du sud du département des Ardennes', *Bulletin de la Société archéologique champenoise* 76, 4: 15–49.

Lambot, B. (1989) 'Le sanctuaire gaulois et gallo-romain de Nanteuil-sur-Aisne/Népellier (Ardennes)', *Bulletin de la Société archéologique champenoise* 76.4: 15–49.

Larese, A. (2003) 'Le lucerne Romane fittili e bronzee del Museo Archeologico Romano di Adria', in Chrzanovski, L. (ed.) *Nouveautés Lychnologiques*, Hauterive CH: Lychno Services: 123–146.

Larsson-Lovén, L. (2014) 'Roman art: what can it tell us about dress and textiles?', in Harlow, M. and Nosch, M. L. (eds.) *Greek and Roman Textiles and Dress: An Interdisciplinary Anthology*, Oxford: Oxbow Books: 260–278.

Lau, O. (1967) *Schuster und Schusterhandwerk in der griechisch-römischen Literatur und Kunst*, Doctoral thesis, Universität Bonn.

Lavan, L. and Mulryan, M. (2011) *The archaeology of late antique "paganism"*, Leiden; Boston: Brill.

Lavender, N.J. (1993) 'A 'principia' at Boreham, near Chelmsford, Essex: excavations 1990', *Essex Archaeology and History* 24: 1–21.

Laver, P.G. (1927) 'The excavation of a tumulus at Lexden, Colchester', *Archaeologia* 26: 241–54.

Lawrence, A. and Deschler-Erb, S. (2018) *Religion in Vindonissa: Kultorte und Kulte im und um das Legionslager*, Brugg: Gesellschaft Pro Vindonissa XXIV.

Lawrence, P. (2008) 'Unit 3: Empires of the mind', in A326 *Block 1: What are empires?* Milton Keynes: The Open University.

Lawrence, S., Smith, A.T. and Allen, L. (2009) *Between villa and town: excavations of a Roman roadside settlement and shrine at Higham Ferrers, Northamptonshire*, Oxford: Oxford Archaeological Unit Limited.

Lebel, P. (1961) *Catalogue des collections archéologiques de Besançon. V, Les bronzes figurés*, Paris: Les Belles Lettres.

Leech, R., Besly, E., Everton, R. and Fowler, E. (1981) 'The excavation of a Romano-British farmstead and cemetery on Bradley Hill, Somerton, Somerset', *Britannia* 12: 177–252.

Lehner, H (1930) 'Bericht über die Tätigkeit des Provinzialmuseums in Bonn', *Bonner Jahrbuch* Bd. 135, Bonn: Bonner Universitätsbuchdruckerei Gebr. Scheur.

Leibundgut, A. (1976) *Die Römischen Bronzen der Schweiz II: Avenches*, Mainz: Philipp von Zabern.

Lejeune, M. (1985) 'Recueil des inscriptions gauloises, vol. I: textes gallo-grecs', *Gallia* 45e supplement.

Lemoine, Y., Satre, S., Zink, M. and Lavagne, H. (2013) *Nouvel Espérandieu: recueil général des sculptures sur pierre de la Gaule Tome IV, Fréjus*, Paris: Académie des inscriptions et belles-lettres.

Lentacker, A., Bakels, C., Verbeeck, M. and Oesender, K. (1992) 'The archaeology, fauna and flora of a Roman well at Erps-Kwerps (Brabant, Belgium)', *Helinium* 32: 110–131.

Lepage, L. (1978) 'Les fibules du Châtelet de Gourzon, Haute-Marne, d'après les publications du XIXe siècle', *Bulletin de la Société archéologique champenoise* 71.4: 51–64.

Lerat, L. (1954) *Catalogue des collections archéologiques de Besançon. I, les lampes antiques*, Paris: Les Belles Lettres.

Lerat, L. (1979) *Les fibules d'Alésia dans les musées d'Alise-Sainte-Reine*, Semur-en-Auxois: Université de Dijon, Bibl. Pro Alésia, VII.

Lerat, L. and Blind, F. (1956) *Catalogue des collections archéologiques de Besançon II: les fibules gallo-romaines*, Paris: Les Belles Lettres, Annales Littéraires de l'Université de Besançon, 2e Série, Tome III, Fasc. 1.

Levine, D. B. (2005) 'EPATON BAMA ('her lovely footstep'): the erotics of feet in Ancient Greece', in Cairns, D. (ed.) *Body language in the Greek and Roman worlds*, Swansea: Classical Press of Wales: 55–72.

Lévy, I. (1913) '*Sarapis*', extrait de la revue de l'histoire des religions, Paris: Ernest Leroux.

Lewis, C. T. and Short, C. (1879) *A Latin dictionary*, Oxford. Clarendon Press.

Licetus, F. (1652) *De lucernis antiquorum reconditis libri sex*, Venice: Nicolai Schiratti.

Liddel, P. and Low, P. (2019) 'Four unpublished inscriptions (and one neglected collector) from the World Museum, Liverpool', in Noreña, C.F. and Papazarkadas, N. (eds.) *From document to history*, Leiden: Brill: 408–430.

Lindenschmit, L. (1889) *Das römisch-germanische Central-Museum: in bildlichen Darstellungen aus seinen Sammlungen*, Mainz: Zabern.

Lindenschmit, L. and Lindenschmit, L. (1900) *Die Alterthümer unserer heidnischen Vorzeit*, Mainz: Zabern.

Liversidge, J. (1955) *Furniture in Roman Britain*, London: A. Tiranti.

Liversidge, J. (1958) 'Roman discoveries from Hauxton', *Proceedings of the Cambridge Antiquarian Society* 51: 7–17.

Llandudno Museum (2015) online *The Roman room*.

Lloyd, G.E.R. (1973) 'Right and left in Greek philosophy', in Needham, R.(ed.) *Right and left; essays on dual symbolic classification*, Chicago: University of Chicago Press: 167–187.

Lloyd-Morgan, G. (1994) 'Copper alloy objects excluding brooches', in Cracknell, S. and Mahany, C. (eds.) *Roman Alcester: southern extramural area 1964–1966 excavations, vol. 1 part 2: finds and discussion*, York: Council for British Archaeology: 177–194.

Lloyd-Morgan, G. (2000) 'Other objects of copper alloy', in Evans, E. (ed.) *The Caerleon canabae*, London: Society for the Promotion of Roman Studies, Britannia Monograph Series 16: 344–385.

Lockyear, K. (2000) 'Site finds in Roman Britain: a comparison of techniques', *Oxford Journal of Archaeology* 19(4): 397–423.

Loeschcke, S. (1919) *Lampen aus Vindonissa*, Zurich: Beer et Cie.

Louis, R. (1943) 'Les fouilles des Fontaines-Salées en 1942', *Gallia* 1.2: 27–70.

Lourdaux, S. (1999) 'Amulettes en forme de pied de LT A', *Instrumentum* 9: 25.

Lucas, G. (2017) 'The paradigm concept in archaeology', *World Archaeology* 9:2: 260–270.

Luke, M. and Preece, T. (2011) 'Farm and forge: late Iron Age/Romano-British farmsteads at Marsh Leys, Kempston, Bedfordshire', *East Anglian Archaeology* 138.

Lullies, R. Lourdaux, S. (1999) 'Amulettes en forme de pied de LT A', *Instrumentum* 9: 25.

Lutz, M. (1971) 'Le domaine gallo-romain de Saint-Ulrich (Moselle)', *Gallia*, tome 29, fascicule 1: 17–44.

Lysons, S. (1797) *An account of Roman antiquities discovered at Woodchester in the county of Gloucestershire*, London: Strahan.

Lysons, S. (1813) *Reliquiæ Britannico-Romanæ: containing figures of Roman antiquities discovered in the various parts of England*, London: T. Bensley.

MacConnoran, P. (1982) 'Leather footwear', in Wilmott, T. (ed.) 'Excavations at Queens Street, City of London, 1953 and 1960; and Roman timber-lined wells in London', *Transactions of the London and Middlesex Archaeological Society* 33: 55–61.

MacConnoran, P. (1986) 'Footwear', in Miller, L; Schofield, J. and Rhodes, M. (eds.) *The Roman quay at St. Magnus' House, London,* London and Middlesex Archaeological Society Special Paper No.8: 218–226.

MacDonald, G. (1906) *The Roman forts on the Bar Hill, Dumbartonshire.* Glasgow: James Maclehose and sons.

MacGregor, A. (1978*) Roman finds from Skeldergate and Bishophill*, London: Published for the York Archaeological Trust by the Council for British Archaeology, Archaeology of York 17.2.

Mackreth, D.F. (1968) 'The brooches', in Brodribb, A.C.C., Hands, A.R. and Walker, D.R. (eds.) *Excavations at Shakenoak Farm, near Wilcote, Oxfordshire* v.4, Oxford: A.R. Hands, Exeter College.

Mackreth, D.F. (1971) 'The Roman brooches', in Down, A. and Rule, M. (eds.) *Chichester excavations* v.6, Chichester: Chichester Civic Society Excavations Committee: 182–194.

Mackreth, D.F. (1973) *Roman brooches*, Salisbury: Salisbury and South Wiltshire Museum.

Mackreth, D.F. (1982) 'The brooches', in McWhirr, AD, Viner, L. and Wells, C. (eds.) *Cirencester excavations II: Romano-British cemeteries at Cirencester*, Cirencester: Cirencester Excavation Committee: Microfiche 2/5 A13–B07.

Mackreth, D.F. (1994) 'Copper alloy and iron brooches', in Cracknell, S. and Mahany, C. (eds.) *Roman Alcester: southern extramural area 1964–1966 excavations, vol. 1 part 2: finds and discussion,* York: Council for British Archaeology: 162–177.

Mackreth, D.F. (2000) 'The Romano-British brooches', in Ellis, P. (ed.) *The Roman baths and macellum at Wroxeter*, London: English Heritage Archaeological Report 9: 144–159.

Mackreth, D.F. (2011) *Brooches in late Iron Age and Roman Britain*, Oxford: Oxbow Books.

Major, H. (1993) 'The Roman brick and tile', in Lavender, N.J. 'A 'principia' at Boreham: excavations 1990', *Essex Archaeology and History* 24: 9–13.

Major, H. and Tyrrell, R. (2015) 'The Roman tile', in Atkinson, M. and Preston, S.J. (eds.) 'Heybridge: a late Iron Age and Roman settlement, excavations at Elms Farm 1993–5', *Internet Archaeology* 40.

Malafouris, L. (2013) *How things shape the mind: a theory of material engagement*, Cambridge, MA: MIT Press.

Malton Museum (2019) online *Roman collection.*

Manning, W.H. (1989) *Report on the excavations at Usk 1965–1976: the fortress excavations, 1972–1974 and minor excavations on the fortress and Flavian fort*, Cardiff: University of Wales Press.

Manzoni, A. (1976) 'Hanging lamp in the form of a sandalled right foot', *Journal of numismatic fine arts* 5.4.

Marado, L.M. and Ribeiro, J. (2018) 'Biological profile estimation based on footprints and shoeprints from Bracara *Augusta Figlinae* (brick workshops), *Heritage* 2018.1: 33–44.

Marmol. E. del (1862) 'Fouilles au cimetière des Iliats et dans quelques localités voisines', *Annales de la Société Archéologique de Namur* 7 1861–1862.

Marquardt, J. and Mommsen, T. (1888) *Römisches Staatsrecht* 3.2, Leipzig: Hirzel.

Martigny, J.A. (1865) *Dictionnaire des antiquités chrétiennes*, Paris: Hachette.

Mastrocinque, A. (2007) 'Sylloge Gemmarum Gnosticarum II', *Bollettino di Numismatica, Monografia 8.2.III*, Rome: Istituto Poligrafico e Zecca dello Stato.

Matthews, C.L. and Hutchings, J.B. (1972) 'A Roman well at Dunstable', *Bedfordshire Archaeological Journal* 7: 21–34.

Mattingly, D.J. (2002) 'Vulgar and weak 'Romanization', or time for a paradigm shift?', *Journal of Roman Archaeology* 15: 536–540.

Mattingly, H.B., Bruun, P.M., Sutherland, C.H.V. and Carson, R.A.G. (1923–1994) *The Roman imperial coinage*, London: Spink.

Maxe-Werly, A.C.N. (1871) 'Note sur des objets antiques découverts à Gondrecourt (Meuse) et à Grand (Vosges)', *Mémoires de la Société nationale des antiquaires de France* 48: 167–168.

May, T. (1904) *Warrington's Roman remains*, Warrington: Mackie.

Mazis, M. (2020) *Imprint on a Roman roof tile*, X April 21, 2020.

Mazur, A. (1998) 'Les fibules romaines d'Avenches I', *Bulletin Pro Aventico* 40: 5–104.

Mazur, A. (2010) 'Les fibules romaines d'Avenches II', *Bulletin Pro Aventico* 52: 5–104.

McCallum, M., Beckmann, M., Nardelli, S. and Munro, M. (2019) 'The excavations at the so-called Villa of Titus (Castel Sant'Angelo, Rieti)', *Journal of Fasti On-Line* 435.

McCarthy, M.R. (2000) *Roman and medieval Carlisle: the southern lanes: excavations 1981–2*, Carlisle: Carlisle Archaeology.

McComish J.M. (2012) *An analysis of Roman ceramic building material from York and its immediate environs*, M.A. dissertation, University of York.

McDonald, K. (2016) *Four footprints, two languages, one tile*.

McIntosh, F. (2011) 'Regional brooch-types in Roman Britain: evidence from northern England', *Archaeologia Aeliana*, 5th series, vol. 40: 155–182.

McNiven, I.J. (2018) 'Torres Strait canoes as social and predatory object-beings', in Harrison-Buck, E. and Hendon, J.A. (eds.) *Relational identities and other-than-human agency in archaeology*, Boulder: University Press of Colorado: 167–196.

McWhirr, A. (ed.) (1979) *Roman brick and tile: studies in manufacture, distribution and use in the Western Empire*, Oxford: B.A.R. International Series 68.

McWhirr, A. (1984) *The production and distribution of brick and tile in Roman Britain*, Doctoral thesis, University of Leicester.

McWhirr, A. and Viner, D. (1978) The production and distribution of tiles in Roman Britain with particular reference to the Cirencester region', *Britannia* 9: 359–377.

McWhirr, A., Viner, L. and Wells, C. (1982) *Cirencester excavations II: Romano-British cemeteries at Cirencester*, Cirencester: Cirencester Excavation Committee.

Meates, G. (1979) *The Roman villa at Lullingstone, Kent*, Chichester: Kent Archaeological Society; distributed by Phillimore, Monograph series of the Kent Archaeological Society no. 1.3.

Meddens, B. (2000) 'The animal bone', in Ellis, P. (ed.) *The Roman baths and macellum at Wroxeter*, London: English Heritage archaeological report 9: 315–336.

Mele, N. V. (1981) *Catalogo delle lucerne in bronzo: Museo nazionale archeologico di Napoli*, Rome: Istituto poligrafico e Zecca dello stato.

Menzel, H. (1953) 'Lampen im römischen Totenkult', in Klumbach (ed.) *Festschrift des Römisch-Germanischen Zentralmuseums zu Mainz III*, Mainz: Verlag des Römisch-Germanischen Zentralmuseums: 131-138.

Menzel, H. (1966) *Die römischen Bronzen aus Deutschland II Trier*, Mainz: Verlag des Römisch-Germanischen Zentralmuseums.

Menzel, H. (1969) *Antike Lampen im Römisch-Germanischen Zentralmuseum zu Mainz*, Mainz: Römisch-Germanisches Zentralmuseum Mainz, Katalog Nr. 15.

Mercklin, E. von (1940) 'Römische Klappmessergriffe', in *Serta Hoffilleriana: commentationes gratulatorias Victori Hoffiller sexagenario* vols. I and II, Zagreb: Zaklada Tiskare Nerodnih: 339–352.

Merrifield, R. (1987) *The archaeology of ritual and magic*, London: Guild Publishing.

Merrifield, R. (1995) 'Roman metalwork from the Walbrook—rubbish, ritual or redundancy?', *London and Middlesex Archaeological Society* 46: 27–44.

Meskell, L. (2004) *Object worlds in ancient Egypt: material biographies in past and present*, London: Berg.

Meylemans, E., Vanholme, N. and Perdaen, Y. (2013) 'Schellebelle 172 AD. Leven langs de Schelde', *Ex Situ* 3.

Middleton, A. (1997) 'Tiles in Roman Britain', in Freestone, I. and Gaimster, D.R.M. (eds.) *Pottery in the making: world ceramic traditions*, London: British Museum for the Trustees of the British Museum.

Miller, D. (1987) *Material culture and mass consumption*, Oxford: Blackwell.

Miller, D. (2008) *The comfort of things*, Cambridge: Polity.

Miller, D. (2010) *Stuff*, Cambridge: Polity.

Millet, P. and Díaz, J. (2013) 'Los sellos in planta pedis de las ánforas olearias béticas Dressel 23 (primera mitad siglo V d.C.)', *Archivo Español de Arqueología* 85: 193–219.

Millett, M. (1994) 'Treasure: interpreting Roman hoards', in Cottam, S., Dungworth, D., Scott, S. and Taylor, J. (eds.) *TRAC 94: Proceedings of the fourth annual theoretical Roman archaeology conference*, Oxford: Oxbow Books: 99–106.

Millett, M. (2001) 'Approaches to urban societies', in James, S. and Millett, M. (eds.) *Britons and Romans: Advancing an archaeological agenda*, York: Council for British Archaeology: 60-76.

Millett, M. and Ferraby, R. (2021) 'Roman Aldborough', *Current Archaeology Live 2021*.

Millett, M. and Graham, D. (1986) *Excavations on the Romano-British small town at Neatham, Hampshire 1969–1979*, Winchester: Hampshire Field Club and Archaeological Society Monograph 3.

Milne, G. and Museum of London (1992) *From Roman basilica to medieval market: archaeology in action in the City of London*, London: HMSO.

Milne, G. and Wardle, A. (1993) 'Early Roman development at Leadenhall Court, London and related research', *Transactions of the London and Middlesex Archaeological Society* 44: 23–169.

Milton Keynes Heritage Association (date unknown) online 'Death and burial at Blue Bridge'.

Möhring, A. (1989) 'Sonderformen Römischer Lampen im Römisch-Germanischen Museum Köln', *Kölner Jahrbuch für Vor- und Frühgeschichte* 22: 803–873.

Moisin, P.H. (1954) 'Givry', *Archéologie* 1954.1, L'antiquité classique 23.1: 181–182.

Mols, S.T.A.M. (1994a) 'Furniture attachments shaped like human feet', in Ronke, J. (ed.) *Akten der 10. Internationalen Tagung über antike Bronzen, Freiburg 18.–22. Juli 1988*, Stuttgart: Theiss, Forschungen und Berichte zur Vor- und Frühgeschichte in Baden-Württemberg 45: 293–296.

Mols, S.T.A.M. (1994b) *Houten meubels in Herculaneum vorm, techniek en funktie*, Doctoral thesis, Nijmegen: Katholieke Universiteit.

Morgan, D.L. (2014) 'Pragmatism as a paradigm for social research', *Qualitative Inquiry* 20.8: 1045–1053.

Morillo Cerdán, Á. and Salido Domínguez, J. (2013) 'Material constructivo latericio procedente del campamento de la Legio VII *Gemina* en León. La intervención arqueológica de Puerta Obispo', *Lucentum* 32: 147–170.

Morin-Jean (1911) 'Les fibules de la Gaule romaine. Essai de typologie et de chronologie' in *Sixième Congrès préhistorique de France*, Le Mans: de Monnoyer: 803–835.

Morris, J. (2008) 'Associated bone groups; one archaeologist's rubbish is another's ritual deposition', in Davis, O., Sharples, N. and Waddington, K. (eds.) *Changing perspectives on the first millennium BC*, Oxford: Oxbow Books: 83–98.

Mosser, M. and Adler-Wölfl, K. (2015) 'Die Legionsziegelei von Vindobona im 17. Wiener Gemeindebezirk', *Fundort Wien. Berichte zur Archäologie* 18/2015, Vienna: Forschungsgesellschaft Wiener Stadtarchäologie: 50–93.

Mould, Q. (1990) 'The leather objects', in Wrathmell, S. and Nicholson, A. (eds.) *Dalton Parlours: Iron Age settlement and Roman villa*, Wakefield: West Yorkshire Archaeology Service.

Mould, Q. (1997) 'Leather', in Wilmott, T. (ed.) *Birdoswald: excavations of a Roman fort on Hadrian's Wall and its successor settlements 1987–92*, London: English Heritage Archaeological Report 14: 326–340.

Mould, Q. (2005) 'The leather', in Brady, K., Brown, L., and Smith, A. (eds.) *A Romano-British landscape at Brockley Hill, Stanmore, Middlesex: excavations at Brockley Hill House and the former MoD site*, Oxford: Oxford Archaeological Unit, OA Job No. 2211: 53–55.

Mould, Q. (2012) 'The Roman shoes from Drapers' Gardens', to be published by Pre-Construct Archaeology Limited.

Mould, Q. (2013) 'Leather shoes', in Pickstone, A. and Drummond-Murray, J. (eds.) 'A late Roman well or cistern and ritual deposition at Bretton Way, Peterborough', *Proceedings of the Cambridge Antiquarian Society,* 102: 53–54.

Mould, Q. (2018) 'Another piece in the jigsaw: the leather from a Roman well at Tollgate Farm, Staffordshire, UK', in Ivleva, T., Driessen, M. and de Bruin, J. (eds.) *Embracing the provinces: society and material culture of the Roman frontier regions*, Oxford: Oxbow Books: 159–168.

Musée d'archéologie nationale, Saint-Germain-en-Laye, *Chaussures,* Display board [Date observed 9/9/2016].

Mráv, Z. (2013) 'Eiserne Klappstühle aus Kaiserzeitlichen Bestattungen der einheimischen Elite in Pannonien', *Archaeologiai Értesítő* 138: 105–144.

Mráv, Z. (2016) 'Nagybronz Szoborleletek Pannoniában: Rövid áttekintés', *Communicationes Archaeologicae Hungariae 2015–2016*: 173–208.

Murdoch, T.V. (1991) *Treasures and trinkets: jewellery in London from pre-Roman times to the 1930s*, London: Museum of London: 141.

Musée du Pays Châtillonnais-Trésor de Vix (2019) *Le monde gallo-romain.*

Museo Arqueológico Nacional, Madrid (2021) online collection.

Museum of London (2019) collections online.

Mustață, S. (2017) *The Roman metal vessels from Dacia Porolissensis*, Cluj-Napoca: Mega Publishing House.

Nagy, T. (1945) 'A gellérthegyi bronzkorsó', *Budapest Régiségei* 14: 525–533.

Neal, D.S., Wardle, A. and Hunn, J. (eds.) (1990) *Excavation of the Iron Age, Roman and medieval settlement at Gorhambury, St Albans*, Swindon: English Heritage Report 14.

Nenova-Merdjanova, R. (1998) 'The bronze jugs decorated with a human foot from the Roman provinces Moesia and Thracia', *Archaeologia Bulgarica* 2.3: 68–76.

Niccolini, F. and Niccolini, F. (1890) *Le case ed i monumenti di Pompei disegnati e descritti* volume 3, Naples: Richter and Co.

Nicgorski, A, (2014) 'The fate of Serapis: a paradigm for transformations in the culture and art of late Roman Egypt', in Brody, L. and Hoffman, G. (eds.) *Roman in the provinces: art on the periphery of Empire*, Chestnut Hill, MA: McMullen Museum of Art, Boston and University of Chicago Press: 153–166.

Nickel, C. (2011) *Martberg: Heiligtum und Oppidum der Treverer II: die Fibeln vom Martberg*, Koblenz: Hans-Helmut Wegner, Berichte zur Archäologie an Mittelrhein und Mosel 18.

Nierhaus, R. (1959) *Das römische Brand- und Körpergräberfeld "Auf der Steig" in Stuttgart-Bad Cannstatt: die Ausgrabungen im Jahre 1955*, Stuttgart: Verlag Silberburg.

Nilsson, M.P. (1950) *Lampen und Kerzen im Kult der Antike*, Lund: Gleerup.

Oliver, M. (1993) 'Excavation of an Iron Age and Romano-British settlement site at Oakridge, Basingstoke, Hampshire, 1965–6', *Proceedings of the Hampshire Field Club and Archaeological Society*, 48: 55–94.

Olsen, B. (2010) *In defense of things: archaeology and the ontology of objects*, California: AltaMira Press.

Olson, K. (2008) 'The appearance of the young Roman girl', in Edmondson, J. and Keith, A. (eds.) *Roman dress and the fabrics of Roman culture*, Toronto: University of Toronto Press: 139–15.

Olson, K. (2012) *Dress and the Roman woman: self-presentation and society*, Abingdon: Taylor and Francis.

Olson, K. (2017) *Masculinity and dress in Roman antiquity*, Oxford: Taylor and Francis.

O'Neil, H.E. and Toynbee, J.M.C. (1958) 'Sculptures from a Romano-British well in Gloucestershire', *Journal of Roman studies* 48(1–2): 49–55.

Ortalli, J and Maioli, R.G. (2021) *Gli scavi di Piazza Ferrari e la domus 'del Chirurgo'*, Soprintendenza Archeologia

Osborne, R. (2004) 'Hoards, votives, offerings: the archaeology of the dedicated object', *World Archaeology* 36.1: 1–10.

Ostia Antiqua virtual museum (2015) *Objects of ivory or bone.*

Ostoia, V. (1969) *The Middle Ages: treasures from the cloisters and the Metropolitan Museum of Art*, Los Angeles: Los Angeles County Museum of Art.

Ovid *Metamorphoses* 2.412–3 trans. Miller, F.J. (1916) Revised Goold, G.P., Loeb Classical Library 42, Cambridge, MA: Harvard University Press: 88–89.

Oxford University Press (1992) *The Oxford English dictionary online.*

Padley, T. (1991) 'The Roman shoes', in Padley, T., Caruana, I. and Winterbottom, S., *The wooden, leather and bone objects from Castle Street, Carlisle: Excavations 1981-2*, Kendal: Cumberland and Westmorland Antiquarian and Archaeological Society, Research series no. 5, fasc. 3: 228–239.

Padova Cultura (2019) online 'Via Annia'.

Page, W. (1906) *The Victoria history of the county of Somerset*, London: A. Constable.

Palma di Cesnola, A. (1884) *Salaminia (Cyprus): the history, treasures, and antiquities of Salamis in the island of Cyprus*, London: Trübner and Company.

Palmer, R.E.A. (1978) 'Silvanus, Sylvester, and the chair of St. Peter', *Proceedings of the American Philosophical Society* 122(4): 222–247.

Palumbo, A. (2001) 'Manufatti di cultura transalpina e attestazioni de 'militaria'', in Sannazaro, M. (ed.) *Ricerche archeologiche nei cortili dell'Università Cattolica: la necropoli tardoantica*, Milano: Vita e pensiero: 125–140.

Paresys, C., le Goff, I., Delor-Ahü, A., Louis, A. and Fort, B. (2016) 'Espaces funéraires et mobiliers en Champagne-Ardenne durant l'Antiquité tardive', SAE et SAC *L'Antiquité tardive dans l'Est de la Gaule, II. Sépultures, nécropoles et pratiques funéraires en Gaule de l'Est - Actualité de la recherche, 2010*, Châlons-en-Champagne, France: 11–34.

Parker, A. (2016) 'Staring at death: the jet gorgoneia of Roman Britain', in Hoss, S. and Whitmore, A. (eds.) *Small finds and ancient social practices in the northwest provinces of the Roman Empire*, Oxford: Oxbow Books: 98–113.

Parker, A. and McKie, S. (eds.) (2018) *Material approaches to Roman magic: occult objects and supernatural substances*, Oxford: Oxbow Books.

Parker, A.J. and Rogers, J. (1982) 'Animal marks and other casual impressions', in Heighway, C.M. and Parker, A.J. (eds.) 'The Roman tilery at St Oswald's Priory, Gloucester', *Britannia* 13: 76.

Parkin, A. (2018) 'A colossal porphyry foot in Newcastle', in Pickup, S. and Waite, S., (eds.) *Shoes, slippers sandals: feet and footwear in antiquity*, London and New York: Routledge: 174–192.

Parkin, A. (2019) personal e-mail to E. Shaw, 10th September.

Partridge, P. (1981) *Skeleton Green: a late Iron Age and Romano-British site*, London: Society for the Promotion of Roman Studies.

Patek, E. (1942) *A pannoniai fibulatipusok elterjedése és eredete/Verbreitung und Herkunft der römischen Fibeltypen in Pannonien*, Budapest: Institut für Münzkunde und Archäologie der Péter Pázmány-Universität, Dissertationes pannonicae series 2.19.

Pearce, J. (2013) 'Beyond the grave: excavating the dead in the late Roman provinces', in Lavan, L. and Mulryan, M. (eds.) *Field methods and post-excavation techniques in late antique archaeology*, Leiden, Netherlands: Brill: 441–482.

Pearce, J., Millett, M. and Struck, M. (2001) *Burial, society and context in the Roman world*, Oxford: Oxbow Books.

Perdrizet, P. (1921) *Les terres cuites grecques d'Égypte de la collection Fouquet*, Nancy: Berger-Levrault.

Perego, E. (2010) 'Magic and ritual in Iron Age Veneto, Italy', *Papers from the Institute of Archaeology* 20: 67–96.

Petrie, W.M.F. (1905) *Roman Ehnasya: (Herakleopolis Magna)*, London: the Egypt Exploration Fund.

Pfeiffer, S. (2008) 'The god Serapis, his cult and the beginnings of the ruler cult in Ptolemaic Egypt', in McKechnie, P. and Guillaume, P. (eds.): *Ptolemy II Philadelphus and his world*, Leiden and Boston: Brill, Mnemosyne: supplements 300: 387–408.

Pharr, C. (1952) *The Theodosian code and novels and the Sirmondian constitutions*, Princeton: Princeton University Press.

Phillipe, J. (1999) 'Les fibules de Seine-et-Marne du 1er siècle av. J.-C. au 5e siècle ap. J.-C.', *Mémoires archéologiques de Seine-et-Marne* 1.

Phillips, E.J. (1977) *Corbridge. Hadrian's Wall east of the North Tyne*, Oxford: Oxford University Press for the British Academy. *Corpus Signorum Imperii Romani* Great Britain 1.1.

Philpott, R. (1991) *Burial practices in Roman Britain: a survey of grave treatment and furnishing, AD 43–410*, Oxford: Tempus Reparatum, BAR British series 219.

Pickstone, A. and Drummond-Murray, J. (2013) 'A late Roman well or cistern and ritual deposition at Bretton Way, Peterborough', *Proceedings of the Cambridge Antiquarian Society,* 102: 37–66.

Pickup, S. and Waite, S. (2018) *Shoes, slippers sandals: feet and footwear in antiquity*, London and New York: Routledge.

Pietruk, F. (2005) *Les fibules romaines des musées de Metz*, Metz: Communauté d'agglomération Metz métropole.

Pilloy, J. (1864) 'Fouilles faites à Lizy ou *Champ des Lusiaux*', *Bulletin de la Société Académique de Laon XIV*: 207–220.

Pirling, R. (1993) 'Ein Trierer Spruchbecher mit ungewöhlicher Inschrift aus Krefeld-Gellep', *Germania* 71: 387–404.

Pirling, R. and Siepen, M. (2000) *Das römisch-fränkische Gräberfeld von Krefeld-Gellep 1982–1988*, Stuttgart: Steiner.

Pirling, R. and Siepen, M. (2006) *Die Funde aus den römischen Gräbern von Krefeld-Gellep: Katalog der Gräber 6348–6361*, Stuttgart: Steiner, Germanische Denkmäler der Völkerwanderungszeit Serie B, Die fränkischen Altertümer des Rheinlandes Bd. 20.

Piron, D. (1970) 'Les fibules gallo-romaines du Château-Musée de Blois (Loir-et-Cher)', *Revue archéologique du Centre de la France*, tome 9, fascicule 2: 110–122.

Planck, D. (1975) *Arae Flaviae I: Neue Untersuchungen zur Geschichte des römischen Rottweil*, Stuttgart: Müller und Gräff Kommissionsverlag.

Pluton, S., Adrian, Y.M., Kliesch, F. and Cottard, A. (2008) 'La nécropole gallo-romaine du «Clos au Duc» à Évreux (Eure): des sépultures du Ier siècle apr. J.-C.', *Revue archéologique de l'Ouest* 25: 209–260.

Poggi, V. (1876) *Sigilli antichi Romani*, Torino: E. Loescher.

Polak, M. (2000) *South Gaulish terra sigillata with potters' stamps from Vechten*, Nijmegen: Rei Cretariae Romanae Fautorum Acta Supplementum 9.

Pollhammer, E. (2019) 'Schuhwerk und die Darstellungen in der römischen Altagskultur', in Beutler, F., Farka, C., Gugl, C., Humer, F., Kremer, G. and Pollhammer, E. (eds.) *Der Adler Roms: Carnuntum und die Armee der Cäsaren*, Mainz: Nünnerich-Asmus: 250–254.

Pontiroli, G. (1980) *Lucerne antiche dei musei di Cremona*, Milan: Cisalpino-Goliardica.

Poole, C. (2018) 'Ceramic building material'. in Simmonds, A. and Lawrence, S. (eds.) *Footprints from the past: the south-eastern extramural settlement of Roman Alchester and rural occupation in its hinterland: the archaeology of East West Rail Phase 1*, Oxford: Oxford Archaeology Monograph 28:152–171.

Popović, L.B., Mano-Zisi, D., Veličković, M. and Jelićić, B. (1969) *Antička bronza u Jugoslaviji*, Beograd: Narodni Musej.

Portable Antiquities Scheme of the Netherlands (PAN) database (2020).

Pozo-Rodríguez, S.F. (2001) 'Un nuevo documento para el Corpus de la vajilla metálica de la Baetica: jarro broncíneo Romano de boca tri-lobulada procedente de la comarca de Priego (Córdoba)', *Antiquitas* 13: 175–181.

Pozo-Rodríguez, S.F. (2004) 'Bronces Romanos de Arastipi (Villanueva de Cauche-Antequera, Málaga). Notas sobre la vajilla y el mobiliario doméstico Romano', *Mainake* XXVI.

Preucel, R.W. (2006) *Archaeological semiotics*, Malden, MA: Blackwell.

Pringle, H. (2019) 'What's in a Footprint?', *The last word on nothing*, 21 February, 2011.

Pritchard, F. (1993) 'Leather shoes', in Milne, G. and Wardle, A. (eds.) 'Early Roman development at Leadenhall Court, London and related research', *Transactions of the London and Middlesex Archaeological Society* 44: 78–80.

Prowse, T. and Small, A. (2009) 'Excavations in the Roman cemetery at Vagnari, 2008: Preliminary report', *Journal of Fasti Online*, Rome: Associazione Internazionale di Archeologia Classica.

Puccio, L. (2010) 'Pieds et empreintes de pieds dans les cultes isiaques', *Mélanges de la Casa de Velázquez*, 40–2: 137–155.

Pudney, C. (2011) 'Pinning down identity: the negotiation of personhood and the materialisation of identity in the Late Iron Age and early Roman Severn Estuary', in Mladenović, D. and Russell, B. (eds.) *TRAC 2010: Proceedings of the twentieth annual theoretical Roman archaeology conference*, Oxford: Oxbow Books: 115–131.

Puttock, S. (2002) *Ritual significance of personal ornament in Roman Britain*, Oxford: British Archaeological Reports, British Series 327.

Raddato, C. (2011) *Statue of the Emperor Hadrian*, flickr.com.

Raddato, C. (2016) *Exhibition: fragile luxury—Cologne a glass-making centre in Antiquity*, flickr.com.

Radišič, T. (2008) 'Kult Serapisa u rimskim provincijama Gornjoj Meziji i Donjoj Panoniji na teritoriji današnje Srbije', *Petničke Sveske* 64: 362–372.

Radnóti, A. (1938) *Die römischen Bronzegefäße von Pannonien*, Dissertationes Pannonica ser. 2.6.

Radovanović, D. T. (2018) 'Lamp with the representation of the griffin: the Christianisation of pagan motifs during late antiquity', Зборник радова Филозофског факултета у Приштини 48: 219–234.

Rageth, J. (1977) 'Die Grabfunde von Sta. Maria in Calanca GR, 1968', *Zeitschrift für schweizerische Archäologie und Kunstgeschichte* 34.1: 1–20.

Rashleigh, P. (1803) 'Account of antiquities discovered at Southfleet, in Kent', *Archaeologia* 14: 221-223.

Reece, R. (1995) 'Site-finds in Roman Britain', *Britannia* Vol. 26: 179–206.

Reece, R. (2011) 'The coins', in Nowakowski, J.A. and Quinnell, H. (eds.) *Trevelgue Head, Cornwall: the importance of C K C Andrew's 1939 excavations for prehistoric and Roman Cornwall*, Truro: Cornwall Council: 245–56.

Rees, H., Crummy, N., Ottaway, P.J. Dunn, G. and (2008) *Artefacts and society in Roman and medieval Winchester*, Winchester: Winchester Museums.

Reinach, S. and Musée des Antiquités Nationales (1921) *Catalogue illustré du Musée des antiquités nationales au Saint-Germain-en-Laye,* Paris: Musées nationaux.

Reinhold, M. (1971) 'Usurpation of status and status symbols in the Roman Empire', *Historia: Zeitschrift für Alte Geschichte* 20, (2/3): 275–302.

Renfrew, C. and Bahn, P. (2020) *Archaeology: theories, methods and practice* (8th edn.), London: Thames and Hudson.

Revell, L. (2016) 'Footsteps in stone: variability within a global culture', in Alcock, S.E., Egri, M. and Frakes, J.F.D. (eds.) *Beyond boundaries: connecting visual cultures in the provinces of ancient Rome*, Los Angeles: Getty Publications:206–222.

Rever, F. (1827) *Mémoire sur les ruines du Vieil-Évreux*, Évreux: Ancelle.

Reygel P. (2012) 'De opgraving op het Vrijthof te Tongeren', *Signa 1*, Brussels: Presses Universitaires de Bruxelles: 119–123.

Reynolds-Brown, K. (1979) 'Lamp in shape of foot', in Weitzmann, K. (ed.) *Age of spirituality: late antique and early Christian Art, third to seventh century*, New York: Metropolitan Museum of Art: 337–338.

Rhodes, M. (1980) 'Leather footwear', in Jones, D. M. and Rhodes, M. (eds.), *Excavations at Billingsgate Buildings, Lower Thames Street, London, 1974*, London: London and Middlesex Archaeological Society Special Paper 4: 99–128.

Ricci, S. (1898) *Epigrafia Latina: trattato elementare con esercizi pratici e facsimili illustrativi*, Milano: Ulrico Hoepli.

Richards, C. and Thomas, J. (1984) 'Ritual activity and structured deposition in later Neolithic Wessex', *Neolithic studies*: 189–218.

Richardson, J. (2011) *Rothwell Haigh, Rothwell, Leeds, West Yorkshire: excavation report*, West Yorkshire Archaeological Services.

Richlin, A. (2014) *Arguments with silence: writing the history of Roman women*, Ann Arbor, MI: University of Michigan Press.

Richmond, I.A. (1943) 'Roman legionaries at Corbridge, their supply base, temples and religious cults', *Archaeologia Aeliana* Series 4 Vol. 21: 127–224.

Richmond, I.A., Gillam, J.P. and Birley, E. (1951) 'The temple of Mithras at Carrawburgh', *Archaeologia Aeliana* Series 4. Vol 29: 1–92.

Ridder, AD (1913) *Les bronzes antiques du Louvre,* Paris: E. Leroux.

Ridgeway, V., Leary, K., and Sudds, B. (2013) *Roman burials in Southwark: excavations at 52–56 Lant Street and 56 Southwark Bridge Road, London, SE1*, London: Pre-Construct Archaeology, Monograph (Pre-Construct Archaeology Limited) no. 11.

Rieckhoff, S. (1975) 'Münzen und Fibeln aus dem Vicus des Kastells Hüfingen (Schwarzwald-Baar-Kreis)', *Saalburg Jahrbuch* 32: 5–104.

Rigato, D. (2014) 'I *signacula ex aere* del Museo Nazionale di Ravenna: un quadro introduttivo', in Buonopane, A., Braito, S. and Girardi, C. (eds.) *Instrumenta inscripta V. Signacula ex aere: aspetti epigrafici, archeologici, giuridici, prosopografici, collezionistici*, Roma: Scienze e Lettere: 203–216.

Riha, E. (1979) *Die römischen Fibeln aus Augst und Kaiseraugst*, Augst: Amt für Museen und Archäologie des Kantons Basel-Landschaft, Forschung in Augst 3.

Riha, E. (1994) *Die römischen Fibeln aus Augst und Kaiseraugst: Die Neufunde seit 1975*, Augst: Römermuseum, Forschung in Augst 18.

Rinaldi Tufi, S. (1983) *Yorkshire*, Oxford: Oxford University Press for the British Academy. *Corpus Signorum Imperii Romani* Great Britain 1.3.

Robertson, A., Scott, M., and Keppie, L. (1975) *Bar Hill: a Roman fort and its finds* (British archaeological reports 16), Oxford: British Archaeological Reports.

Rocamora, A. (2015) 'Pierre Bourdieu: the field of fashion', in Rocamora, A. and Smelik, A. (eds.) *Thinking through fashion: a guide to key theorists*, London: Bloomsbury: 233–250.

Rodgers M.M. (1988) 'Dynamic biomechanics of the normal foot and ankle during walking and running', *Physical Therapy* 68(12): 1822–1830.

Rodwell, K.A. (1988) *The prehistoric and Roman settlement at Kelvedon, Essex*, CBA Research Report 63: Council for British Archaeology.

Rogerson, A. (1977) 'Excavations at Scole, 1973', *East Anglian Archaeology*, 5: 97–223.

Rolland, H. (1965) *Bronzes antiques de Haute Provence (Basses-Alpes, Vaucluse)*, Paris: Centre national de la recherche scientifique, Gallia: fouilles et monuments archéologiques in France métropolitaine, Supplément 18.

Rohrbacher, D. (2016) *The play of allusion in the Historia Augusta*, Madison, Wisconsin: University of Wisconsin Press.

Rolley C. (1972) 'Circonscription de Bourgogne', *Gallia* 30.2: 443–467.

Roman Britain News (2020) 'Lamp from Chippenham Museum', X January 4, 2020.

Rorive, S. (2019) Personal email to Elizabeth Shaw, 27 August.

Rosenthal, R. and Sivan, R. (1978) 'Ancient lamps in the Schloessinger collection', *Qedem* 8: 3–179.

Roskams, S., Neal, C., Richardson, J. and Leary, R. (2013) 'A late Roman well at Heslington East, York: ritual or routine practices?', *Internet Archaeology* 34.

Ross, A. (1968) 'Shafts, pits, wells—sanctuaries of the Belgic Britons?', in Piggott, S., Coles, J.M. and Simpson, D.D.A. (eds.) *Studies in ancient Europe: essays presented to Stuart Piggott*, Leicester: Leicester University Press: 255–85.

Ross, A. (1974) *Pagan Celtic Britain: studies in iconography and tradition*, London: Cardinal.

Ross, A. and Feacham, R. (1976) 'Ritual rubbish? The Newstead pits', in Megaw, J. (ed.) *To illustrate the monuments: essays on archaeology presented to Stuart Piggott on the occasion of his sixty-fifth birthday*, London: Thames and Hudson: 230–237.

Rossi, W.A. (1977) *The sex life of the foot and shoe*, London: Routledge and Kegan Paul.

Rothe, U. (2009) *Dress and cultural identity in the Rhine-Moselle region of the Roman Empire*, Oxford: Archaeopress, British Archaeological Reports (S2038).

Rouquette, D. (1969) 'Une curieuse lampe en terre sigillée de Mèze (Hérault)', *Revue archéologique du Centre de la France*, 8.3: 239–243.

Rouquette, D. (1972) 'Une nouvelle lampe en terre cuite en forme de pied', *Revue archéologique du Centre de la France* 11.1–2: 172–174.

Rousseau, A. (2004) 'Les Fontaines-Salées, mémoires de sel Saint-Père', *Archéologie en Bourgogne* 1: 1–8.

Royal Commission on Historical Monuments, England (1962) *An inventory of the historical monuments in city of York, volume 1, Eburacum, Roman York*, London: Her Majesty's Stationery Office.

Royal-Athena Galleries (2016) *Art of the ancient world 2017* vol. XXVIII, London and New York: J.M. Eisenberg.

Royal-Athena Galleries (2017) *Art of the ancient world 2018* vol. XXIX, London and New York: J.M. Eisenberg.

Rüpke, J. (2016) *On Roman religion: lived religion and the individual in ancient Rome*, Ithaca, NY: Cornell University Press.

Ruprechtsberger, E.M. (1985) 'Eine Bronzekanne aus Windischgarsten', *Jahrbuch des Oberösterreichischen Musealvereines* 130a: 61-70.

Rushforth, G. (1915) 'Funeral lights in Roman sepulchral monuments', *Journal of Roman Studies* 5: 149–164.

Rushworth, A. (ed.) *Housesteads Roman fort—the grandest station*, Swindon: English Heritage.

Russell, M (2019) 'Farewell two arms: a Roman bronze body part from Halnaker, West Sussex', *Sussex Archaeological Collections* 157: 125–132.

Rusu, A. (1979) 'Bronzuri figurate Romane în Muzeul Județean din Deva', *Sargetia* 14: 173–183.

Saarländischer Museumsverband (2020) *Römermuseum Schwarzenacker*.

Said, E. (1979) *Orientalism*, New York: Vintage Books.

Salemink, R. (2010) *Membra disiecta. Fragmenten van bronzen Romeinse keizers standbeelden in Germania Inferior: een inventarisatie*, Masters Dissertation, Universiteit van Amsterdam.

Salisbury and South Wiltshire Museum (2019) online collections.

Sanie, Ş., Sanie, S. and Cojocaru, M. (1980) 'Tezaurul de la Muncelul de Sus şi unele probleme ale circulaţiei monetare Romane în Moldova', *Cercetări Istorice* 11: 249–268.

Sannazaro, M. (ed.) (2001) *Ricerche archeologiche nei cortili dell'Università Cattolica: la necropoli tardoantica*, Milano: Vita e pensiero.

Sanquer, R. (1977) 'Circonscription de Bretagne', *Gallia* 35.2: 335–367.

Santoro l'Hoir, F. (1983) 'Three sandalled footlamps: their apotropaic potentiality in the cult of Sarapis', *Archäologischer Anzeiger* 1983 Heft 2: 225–237.

Sauer, E.W. (2003) *The archaeology of religious hatred in the Roman and early medieval world*, Stroud: Tempus.

Sauer, E.W. (2011) 'Religious rituals at springs in the late antique and early medieval world', in Lavan, L. and Mulryan, M. (eds.) *The archaeology of late antique 'paganism'*, Leiden: Brill, Late antique archaeology 7: 505–550.

Saussure, F. de (1916) *Cours de linguistique générale*, Paris: Payot; Charles Bally, Albert Sechehaye, and Albert Riedlinger.

Savin, P. (2019) *Roman tile stamp of the Classis Britannica showing hob nails from a Roman sandal*, X July 18, 2019

Schachter, A. (2012) 'Sphinx', in Hornblower, S., Spawforth, A., and Eidinow, E. (eds.) *The Oxford classical dictionary* (4th ed.), Oxford: Oxford University Press.

Schoppa, H. (1960) 'Neue Beobachtungen zum römischen Hofheim, Maintaunuskreis', *Germania* 38.1–2: 184–189.

Schuster, J. (2011) 'Brooches', in Biddulph, E., Seager Smith, R. and Schuster, J. (eds.) *Settling the Ebbsfleet Valley: High Speed 1 excavations at Springhead and Northfleet, Kent: the late Iron Age, Roman, Saxon, and Medieval landscape, volume 2: Late Iron Age to Roman finds reports*, Salisbury: Oxford Wessex Archaeology: 190–231.

Seaford, R. (2012) 'Masks', in Hornblower, S., Spawforth, A., and Eidinow, E. (eds.) *The Oxford classical dictionary* (4th ed.), Oxford: Oxford University Press.

Sedlmayer, H. (1999) *Die römischen Bronzegefässe in Noricum*, Monographies Instrumentum 10.

Selesnow, W. (1988) *Lampen aus Ton und Bronze* (Bildwerke der Sammlung Kaufmann. Band 2), Melsungen: Verlag Gutenberg.

Sellye, I. (1939) *Császárkori emailmunkák Pannoniából: Les bronzes émaillés de la Pannonie romaine*, Budapest: Institut de numismatique et d'archéologie de l'Université Pierre Pázmány.

Shanks, M. and Tilley, C.Y. (1988) *Social theory and archaeology*, Albuquerque: University of New Mexico Press.

Shaw, E.J. (2017) *Shoes and status in Roman art and archaeology*, MA Dissertation, the Open University.

Sieveking, J. (1930) *Bronzen, Terrakotten, Vasen der Sammlung Loeb*, Munich: Buchholz.

Silius Italicus, *Punica* 7.172, trans. Duff, J.D. (1934) Loeb Classical Library 277, Cambridge, MA: Harvard University Press: 348–349.

Simmel, G. (1957) 'Fashion', *The American journal of sociology* 62.6: 541–558.

Simmonds, A. and Lawrence, S. (2018) *Footprints from the past: the south-eastern extramural settlement of Roman Alchester and rural occupation in its hinterland: the archaeology of East West rail phase 1*, Oxford: Oxford Archaeology Monograph 28.

Simonett, C. (1941) *Tessiner Gräberfelder: Ausgrabungen des Archäologischen Arbeitsdienstes in Solduno, Locarno-Muralto, Minusio und Stabio, 1936 und 1937*, Basel: Birkhäuser, Monographien zur Ur- und Frühgeschichte der Schweiz 3.

Simpson, F.G. and Simpson, G. (1976) *Watermills and military works on Hadrian's Wall: excavations in Northumberland 1907–1913*, Kendal: T. Wilson.

Smith, A., Allen, M., Brindle, T. and Fulford, M. (2016) *The rural settlement of Roman Britain Vol 1*, London: The Society for the Promotion of Roman Studies, Britannia Monograph Series 29.

Smith, A.C. (2018) 'The left foot aryballos wearing a network sandal', in Pickup, S. and Waite, S. (eds.) *Shoes, slippers and sandals: feet and footwear in classical antiquity*, Abingdon: Routledge: 195–215.

Smith, C.R. (1857) *Catalogue of the Museum of London antiquities*, London: T. Richards.

Smith, C.R. (1859) *Illustrations of Roman London*, London: T. Richards.

Smith, J.B. (1995) 'Interim report on the votive material from Romano-Celtic temple sites in Oxfordshire', *Oxoniensia* LX: 177–203.

Smith, T.P. (undated) 'Building materials', *ONE94 (no. 1 Poultry)* MOLAS.

Snape, M.E. (1993) *Roman brooches from North Britain: a classification and a catalogue of brooches from sites on the Stanegate*, Oxford: British Archaeological Reports 235.

Society of Antiquaries of London (1806) *Archaeologia: or miscellaneous tracts relating to antiquity* volume XV, London: T. Bensley.

Society of Antiquaries of London (2005) *Catalogue of drawings and museum objects* 'Britannia Romana 116.2', York: Archaeology Data Service.

Sofaer, J. (2006) *The body as material culture: a theoretical osteoarchaeology*, Cambridge: Cambridge University Press, Topics in contemporary archaeology no. 4.

Sopwith, T. (1833) *An account of the mining districts of Alston Moor, Weardale and Teesdale, in Cumberland and Durham*, Alnwick: W. Davison.

Sørensen, M.L.S. (2015) 'Paradigm lost—on the state of typology in archaeological theory', in Kristiansen, K., Šmejda, L. and Turek, J. (eds.) *Paradigm found: archaeological theory—present, past and future. Essays in honour of Evžen Neustupný*, Oxford: Oxbow Books: 84–94.

Sourvinou-Inwood, C. (2012) 'Artemis', in Hornblower, S., Spawforth, A., and Eidinow, E. (eds.) *The Oxford classical dictionary* (4th ed.), Oxford: Oxford University Press.

Spagnolis, M. and de Carolis, E. (1983) *Museo nazionale Romano: I bronzi vol. IV. 1, Le lucerne*, Rome: De Luca.

Spagnolis, M. and de Carolis, E. (1997) *Le lucerne di bronzo del Museo Civico Archeologico di Bologna*, Bologna: Commune di Bologna.

Spânu, D., Dima, M. and Frînculeasa, A. (2016) 'The Mălăieștii de Jos (Prahova County) silver craftsman's hoard from the end of the 3rd century AD', *Dacia. Revue d'archéologie et d'histoire ancienne* 60: 237–273.

Stansbie, D. et al. (2007) 'A Roman cemetery at Sampford Road, Thaxted', *Essex Archaeology and History* 38: 66–88.

Stead, I. (1980) *Rudston Roman villa*, Leeds: Yorkshire Archaeological Society.

Stead, I., Flouest, J., Rigby, V., Pacitto, S., Stead, S. and Pacitto, A.L. (2006) *Iron Age and Roman burials in Champagne*, Oxford: Oxbow Books.

Steiger, R. (1980) 'Zwei Fusslampen aus Augst', *Jahresberichte aus Augst und Kaiseraugst* 1: 59–87.

Stek, T.D. (2009) *Cult places and cultural change in Republican Italy*, Amsterdam: Amsterdam University Press.

Stoll, O. (2007) 'The religions of the armies', in Erdkamp, P. (ed.) *A companion to the Roman army*, Oxford: Blackwell: 451–476.

Strauel, J.-P. (2004) 'Nouvelles prospections sur la villa de Grussenheim', *Annuaire de la Société d'Histoire de la Hardt et du Ried* 17: 15–16.

Strong, J. (2007) *Relics of the Buddha*, Delhi: Motilal Banarsidass.

Stupperich, R. (2016) *Licht! Lampen von der Antike bis zur Neuzeit. Begleitheft zur Ausstellung*, Heidelberg: heiBOOKS.

Sumner, G. (2009) *Roman military dress*, Stroud: History Press.

Swann, J. (1986) 'Tiles with human foot impressions', in Gurney, D. (ed.) *Settlement, religion and industry on the fen-edge; three Romano-British sites in Norfolk*, Dereham: Norfolk Archaeological Unit, East Anglian Archaeology 31.

Swann, J. (1996) 'Concealed shoes in buildings', *Costume* 30: 56–69.

Symonds, M. with Haynes, I.P. and Wilmott, T. (2014) 'Maryport's mysterious monuments', *Current Archaeology* 289: 17–21.

Szabó, K. (1981) 'Emberi lábfejjel díszített fülű bronzkorsók Pannoniából', *Archaeologiai Értesitő* 108: 52–64.

Tache, M. (2015) *Fibules antiques celtiques, romaines, mérovingiennes*, Saint-Germain-en-Laye: Carmanos-Commios.

Takács, S.A. (2007) 'Divine and human feet: records of pilgrims honouring Isis', in Elsner, J. and Rutherford, I. (eds.) *Pilgrimage in Graeco-Roman and early Christian antiquity: seeing the gods*, Oxford: Oxford University Press: 353–372

Tassinari, S. (1973) 'Pots avec une anse dont l'attache inférieure figure un pied humain', in Duval, P.-M. (ed.) *Recherches d'archéologie celtique et gallo-romaine*, Genève: Droz, Collection de la Bibliothèque des Hautes Études 4.III.5: 127–40.

Tassinari, S. (1975) *La vaisselle de bronze, romaine et provinciale, au Musée des Antiquités Nationales*, Gallia Supplément 29.

Terra Sigillata Museum Rheinzabern (2006) online *Ausstellung: eine Zeitreise*.

Thomas, F.W.K. (1879) 'Dunadd, Glassary, Argyleshire: the place of inauguration of the Dalriadic Kings', *Proceedings of the Society Antiquaries, Scotland* 13: 28–47.

Thomas, N. (1991) *Entangled objects: exchange, material culture, and colonialism in the Pacific*, Cambridge, Mass: Harvard University Press.

Thomas, S. (2016) 'From treasured items to trash? The use of brooches in Roman Cornwall in the creation of identity and social memory', in Mandich, M.J., Derrick, T.J., Gonzalez Sanchez, S., Savani, G., and Zampieri, E. (eds.) *TRAC 2015: Proceedings of the twenty-fifth annual theoretical Roman archaeology conference, Leicester 2015*, Oxford: Oxbow Books: 111–124.

Thompson, F. (1965) *Roman Cheshire*, Chester: Cheshire Community Council, History of Cheshire 2.

Thompson, F.H. (1969) 'Excavations at Linenhall Street', Chester, 1961–2, *Journal of the Chester Archaeological Society* 56: 1–21.

Thornton, J. (1984) 'The leather', in Ellis, P. (ed.) *Catsgore, 1979: Further excavation of the Romano-British village*, Gloucester: Alan Sutton for the Western Archaeological Trust, Excavation monograph no. 7: 35–36.

Tilley, C. (1990) *Reading material culture: structuralism, hermeneutics, and post-structuralism*, Oxford: Blackwell.

Tilley, C. (1999) *Metaphor and material culture*, Oxford: Blackwell.

Tilley, C. (2001) 'Ethnography and material culture', in. Atkinson, P., Coffey, A., Delamont, S., Lofland, L.H. and Lofland, J. (eds.) *Handbook of ethnography*, London: Sage: 258–272.

Timby, J. *et al.* (1998) *Excavations at Kingscote and Wycomb, Gloucestershire: A Roman estate centre and small town in the Cotswolds with notes on related settlements*, Cirencester: Cotswold Archaeological Trust.

Topál, J. (2003) *Roman cemeteries of Aquincum, Pannonia: the western cemetery, Bécsi Road II*, Budapest: Aquincum Nostrum.

Toynbee, J.M.C., Munby, J. and Henig, M. (1977) *Roman life and art in Britain: a celebration in honour of the eightieth birthday of Jocelyn Toynbee*, Oxford: BAR 41.

Turk, F.A. (1982) 'The animal bones', in Carlyon, P.M. (ed.) 'A Romano-British site at Kilhallon, Tywardreath: Excavation in 1975', *Cornish Archaeology* 21: 165.

Turner, R. (1990) 'A Romano-British Cemetery at Lanchester, Durham', *Archaeologia Aeliana* 5.18: 63–77.

Vanvinckenroye, W. (1984) *De Romeinse zuidwest-begraafplaats van Tongeren: opgravingen 1972–1981*, Tongeren: het Provinciaal Gallo-Romeins Museum te Tongeren 29.

Vatin, C. (1969) 'Ex-votos de bois gallo-romains à Chamalières', *Revue Archéologique* 1:103–114.

Veldmeijer, A. J. (2013) *Leatherwork from Qasr Ibrim (Egypt). Part I: footwear from the Ottoman period*, Leiden: Sidestone Press.

Veličković, M. (1972) *Rimska sitna bronzana plastika u Narodnom muzeju/Petits bronzes figurés romains au Musée national*, Belgrade: Narodni muzej.

Vermeulen, W.G.J.R. (1932) *Een Romeinsch grafveld op den Hunnerberg te Nijmegen (uit den tijd van Tiberius–Nero)*, Amsterdam: H. J. Paris.

Vernon, W., Simmonite, N., Reel, S. and Reidy, S. (2017) 'An investigation into the cause of the inner dark areas and outer lighter areas (ghosting) seen in dynamically-created two-dimensional bare footprints', *Science and Justice—Journal of the Forensic Science Society* 57.4: 276–282.

Vidman, L. (1969) *Sylloge inscriptionum religionis Isiacae et Sarapiacae*, Berlin; Boston: De Gruyter.

Vierneisel, K. (ed.) (1979) Römisches im Antikenmuseum (2nd edn.) Berlin: J. Schönwald KG, Staatliche Museen Preußischer Kulturbesitz.

Vikan, G. and Nesbitt, J. (1980) *Security in Byzantium: locking, sealing, weighing*, Washington: Dumbarton Oaks Center for Byzantine Studies.

Viner, L. and Leech, R. (1982) 'Bath Gate Cemetery, 1969–1976', in McWhirr, A., Viner, L. and Wells, C. (eds.) *Cirencester excavations II: Romano-British cemeteries at Cirencester*, Cirencester: Cirencester Excavation Committee: 69–111.

Volken, M. (2014) *Archaeological footwear: development of shoe patterns and styles from prehistory till the 1600's*, Zwolle: SPA Uitgevers.

Wait, G. A. (1985) *Ritual and religion in Iron Age Britain*, Oxford: B.A.R. British series 149.

Waldhauer, O. (1914) *Die antiken Tonlampen*, St. Petersburg: Kaiserliche Ermitage.

Walke, N. (1962) 'Eine römische Fußlampe aus Wehringen', in Werner, J. (ed.) *Aus Bayerns Frühzeit; Friedrich Wagner zum 75. Geburtstag*, Munich: C.H. Beck: 215–218.

Wallace-Hadrill, A. (2008) *Rome's cultural revolution*, Cambridge: Cambridge University Press.

Walters, H.B. (1899) *Catalogue of the bronzes, Greek, Roman, and Etruscan, in the department of Greek and Roman antiquities, British Museum*, London: Printed by order of the Trustees.

Walters, H.B. (1914) *Catalogue of the Greek and Roman lamps in the British Museum*, London: Printed by order of the Trustees.

Walton, P.J. (2008) 'Finds from the River Tees at Piercebridge', in Cool, H.E.M. and Mason D.J.P. (eds). *Roman Piercebridge: excavations by D.W. Harding and Peter Scott 1969–1981*, Durham: Architectural and Archaeological Society of Durham & Northumberland Research Report 7: 286–293.

Walton, P.J. (2021) 'Objects of personal adornment', in Eckardt, H. and Walton, P.J. (eds.) *Bridge over troubled waters: the Roman finds from the River Tees at Piercebridge in context*, London: Society for the Promotion of Roman Studies, Britannia Monograph Series 34: 53–72.

Walton, P.J. (2021) 'Toilet, surgical or pharmaceutical equipment', in Eckardt, H. and Walton, P.J. (eds.) *Bridge over troubled waters: the Roman finds from the River Tees at Piercebridge in context*, London: Society for the Promotion of Roman Studies, Britannia Monograph Series 34: 73–81.

Warry, P. (2006) *Tegulae: manufacture, typology and use in Roman Britain*, Oxford: Archaeopress, BAR British Series 417.

Watts, D. (1993) 'An assessment of the evidence for Christianity at the Butt Road site', in Crummy, N., Crossan, P., Crummy, P. and Crossan, C. (1993) *Excavations of Roman and later cemeteries, churches and monastic sites in Colchester, 1971–88*, Colchester, Essex: Colchester Archaeological Trust, Colchester archaeological report 9: 192–202.

Waughman, M. (1998) 'Excavations at Chigborough Farm', in Wallis, S. and Waughman, M. (eds.) 'Archaeology and the landscape in the lower Blackwater valley', *East Anglian Archaeology 82*: 59–108.

Weber, G. (2015) *Archäologische Grabungen am Zellhügel im Sommer 2015*, Geschichts- und Heimatverein Mainhausen.

Webster, J. (2001) 'Creolizing the Roman provinces', *American Journal of Archaeology* 105.2: 209–22.

Wedlake, W.J. (1982) *The excavation of the shrine of Apollo at Nettleton, Wiltshire, 1956–1971*, London: Society of Antiquaries of London.

Weeks, L. (2003) 'Worst foot forward: a guide to foreign insults', *Washington Post* April 11, 2003 online.

Weiß, M. (2019) Antike Tischkultur. Available at http://www.antike-tischkultur.de/beleuchtungmotivfuss.html [Date accessed 15/01/2019].

Weitzmann, K. (ed.) (1979) *Age of spirituality: late antique and early Christian art, third to seventh century*, New York: The Metropolitan Museum of Art.

Weninger, P. (1973) *Die Römer an der Donau*, Vienna: Amt der Niederosterreichischen Landesregierung.

Wessex Archaeology (2018) online *Remarkably preserved Roman remains from grave*.

West, S. (1989) *West Stow, Suffolk: the prehistoric and Romano-British occupations*, East Anglian Archaeology 48.

Weston, S. (1814) 'Description of a Roman altar found in the neighbourhood of Aldston Moor, in Cumberland' *Archaeologia* 17: 229–230.

Wheeler, R.E.M. (1923) *Segontium and the Roman occupation of Wales*, London: the Honourable Society of Cymmrodorion.

White, R.B. (1985) 'Excavations in Caernarfon 1976–1977', *Archaeologia Cambrensis* 134: 53–105.

Whitmore, A. (2018) 'Phallic magic: a cross-cultural approach to Roman phallic small finds', in Parker, A. and McKie, S. (eds.) *Material approaches to Roman magic: occult objects and supernatural substances*, Oxford: Oxbow Books: 17–32.

Wickenden, N.P. (1988) *Excavations at Great Dunmow*, Chelmsford: East Anglian Archaeology Report 41.

Wiedemer, H.R. (1962) 'Ausgrabung Königsfelden 1961', *Gesellschaft Pro Vindonissa Jahresbericht* 1961–1962: 19–47.

Wild, J.P. (1970) *Textile manufacture in the northern Roman provinces*, Cambridge: Cambridge Classical Studies.

Williams, R.J. and Zeepvat, R.J. (1994) *Bancroft: the late Bronze Age and Iron Age settlements and Roman temple-mausoleum*, Aylesbury: Buckinghamshire Archaeological Society.

Williate, M. and Corsiez, A. (2006) 'Une sandale en cuir gallo-romaine de Montigny-en-Ostrevent (Nord)', *Revue du Nord 5/2006* (no 368): 207–212.

Wilmott, T. (1982) 'Excavations at Queens Street, City of London, 1953 and 1960; and Roman timber-lined wells in London', *Transactions of the London and Middlesex Archaeological Society* 33: 55–61.

Wilmott, T. (2007) *The Roman amphitheatre in Britain*, Stroud: Tempus.

Willmott, T. (2018) Conversation with Elizabeth Shaw, 16 October.

Wilmouth, A. (2014) *Caractérisation du mobilier métallique des quartiers artisanaux est et ouest du vicus gallo-romain de Bliesbruck (Moselle)* v.4, Doctoral thesis, Université de Bourgogne.

Witcher, R.E. (2000) 'Globalisation and Roman imperialism: perspectives on identities in Roman Italy', in Heriing, E. and Loma, K. (eds.) *The emergence of state identities in Italy in the first millennium BC.*, London: Accordia Research Institute, University of London: 213–225.

Woodfield, P. (1978) 'Roman architectural masonry from Northamptonshire', *Northamptonshire Archaeology* 13: 67–86.

Woodward, A. (1992) *English Heritage book of shrines and sacrifice*, London: Batsford/English Heritage.

Woodward, A. and Leach, P. (1993) *The Uley shrines: excavation of a ritual complex on West Hill, Uley, Gloucestershire 1977–9*, English Heritage Archaeology Report 17.

Worrell, S. (2005) 'Finds reported under the Portable Antiquities Scheme', *Britannia* 36: 447–472.

Worsley, R. and Prowett, S. (1824) *Museum Worsleyanum*, London: Septimus Prowett.

Wrathmell, S., Nicholson, A. and West Yorkshire Archaeology Service (1990) *Dalton Parlours: Iron Age settlement and Roman villa*, Wakefield: West Yorkshire Archaeology Service.

Xanthopoulou, M. (2010) *Les lampes en bronze à l'époque paléochrétienne*, Turnhout: Brepols, Bibliothèque de l'Antiquité Tardive 16.

Yad Vashem (2021) online *The shoes on the Danube Promenade—commemoration of the tragedy*.

Zienkiewicz, J.D. (1986) *The legionary fortress baths at Caerleon, Volume 2: the finds*. Cardiff: National Museum of Wales.